C0-AZR-730

STP 1346

Alternative Bearing Surfaces in Total Joint Replacement

Joshua J. Jacobs and Thomas L. Craig, Editors

ASTM Stock #: STP1346

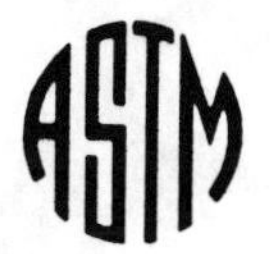

ASTM
100 Barr Harbor Drive
West Conshohocken, PA 19428-2959
Printed in the U.S.A.

ISBN: 0-8031-2494-5
ISSN: 1050-8104
Library of Congress Cataloging-in-Publication Data

Alternative bearing surfaces in total joint replacement / Joshua J.
Jacobs and Thomas L. Craig, editors.
p. cm. — (STP : 1346)
"ASTM stock number : STP 1346."
Proceedings of the Symposium on Alternative Bearing Surfaces in
Total Joint Replacement, held in San Diego, Calif., on Nov. 11-12, 1997.
Includes bibliographical references and index.
ISBN 0-8031-2490-2. — ISBN 0-8031-2490-2
1. Artificial joints—Bearings—Materials—Congresses.
2. Tribology—Congresses. I. Jacobs. Joshua J., 1956-
II. Craig, Thomas L., 1947- . III. Symposium on Alternative
Bearing Surfaces in Total Joint Replacement (1997 : San Diego,
Calif.) IV. Series: ASTM special technical publication ; 1346.
[DNLM: 1. Hip Prosthesis congresses. 2. Biocompatible Materials
congresses. 3. Friction congresses. 4. Materials Testing
congresses. WE 860 A466 1998]
RD686.A44 1998
617.4'720592—dc21
DNLM/DLC
for Library of Congress 98-47496
CIP

Peer Review Policy

Each paper published in this volume was evaluated by two peer reviewers and at least one editor. The authors addressed all of the reviewers' comments to the satisfaction of both the technical editor(s) and the ASTM Committee on Publications.

To make technical information available as quickly as possible, the peer-reviewed papers in this publication were prepared "camera-ready" as submitted by the authors.

The quality of the papers in this publication reflects not only the obvious efforts of the authors and the technical editor(s), but also the work of the peer reviewers. The ASTM Committee on Publications acknowledges with appreciation their dedication and contribution of time and effort on behalf of ASTM.

Printed in Fredericksburg, VA
December 1998

Foreword

This publication, *Alternative Bearing Surfaces in Total Joint Replacement,* contains 18 papers presented at the Symposium on Alternative Bearing Surfaces in Total Joint Replacement held in San Diego, California on November 11 and 12, 1997. The symposium was sponsored by the ASTM Committee F04 on Medical and Surgical Materials and Devices. Joshua J. Jacobs of Rush Medical College in Chicago, Illinois and Thomas L. Craig from Smith & Nephew Richards, Inc. of Memphis, Tennessee presided as symposium chairmen and are editors of the resulting publication. The editors would like to express their thanks to the ASTM staff members who assisted in the organization of the symposium and to those who assisted in the editorial process. The editors also wish to thank the many members of the F04 Committee who served as peer reviewers for the manuscripts contained herein.

Contents

Overview

Over the last decade, there has been a resurgence of interest in wear of the bearing surfaces in total joint replacement components. The most commonly used wear couple, cobalt-based alloy articulating with ultrahigh molecular-weight polyethylene, has had an excellent track record. However, there is an increasing recognition that long-term clinical failures of total joint replacement devices are attributable to the release of a relatively high volume of particulate wear debris generated from these bearings.

Numerous studies have documented that polyethylene is the most abundant wear particle within the tissues surrounding the implanted device. Thus, there has been an intense interest in the development and utilization of alternative bearing surfaces to mitigate the effects of particulate polyethylene debris. These effects include aseptic loosening and osteolysis, the most common long-term complications of total joint replacement. Although in widespread use in certain centers abroad, alternative bearing surfaces are currently in the developmental or early clinical trial stage in the United States. There are numerous manufacturing, regulatory, scientific, and clinical issues that need to be carefully examined prior to the widespread introduction of these devices. The goal of this symposium was to provide a forum for the discussion of these issues in the context of relevant standards development. There was broad participation in this symposium with speakers and attendees from Europe and North America representative of industry, academia, clinical practice, and the regulatory and standards communities.

This volume is presented in four sections. The first section has two papers on wear testing. The paper by Sauer, et al. is an exhaustive historical review of the clinical and laboratory wear performance of orthopedic bearing materials. This is a valuable contribution in that it provides a context with which to interpret many of the subsequent papers. The paper by Wimmer, et al. describes the development of a novel screening method for wear analysis that may prove helpful in the preclinical evaluation of alternative bearing surfaces.

The second section presents nine papers on metal-on-metal bearings. The first three papers concern general developmental issues. The paper by Poggie, et al. presents an overview of the effects of design, contact stress, and materials on the tribological performance of metal-on-metal bearings. Varano, et al. examine the metallurgy of the cobalt-base alloys used for modern generation metal-on-metal bearings, while Tesk, et al. discuss the potential applicability of glassy alloy surfaces for this application. The second three papers, by Cipera, et al.; Medley, et al.; and Chan, et al., discuss issues related to the characterization and tribological performance of these bearings based on in-vitro tests, including hip simulator studies. The latter paper also presents a numerical analysis, using elastrohydrodynamic lubrication theory, describing the lubrication regime in metal-on-metal bearings. The nature and thickness of the lubricant may be key factors that govern the clinical performance of these devices. The final three papers in this section, by Park, et al.; Reiker, et al.; and Scott, et al. present analyses of clinical retrievals of both first and second generation metal-on-metal components. Critical informatioin can be gleaned from such retrievals including the wear rate, wear mode, and patterns of surface damage and the relation of these parameters with design, metallurgy, geometry, and clinical performance. The paper by Scott, et al. deserves special mention as it was the recipient of the annual student award paper awarded by ASTM Committee F04.

The third section is comprised of four papers on ceramic bearings. Three of these papers originate from Europe, attesting to the longstanding clinical experience with these devices overseas. Papers by Richter, et al. and Cales, et al. address the tribological and mechanical behavior of ceramic-on-ceramic bearings. The paper by Armini, et al. examines the feasibility of using ceramic coatings on conventional metal balls to improve wear performance. Finally, Meunier, et al. present long-term clinical results of ceramic-on-ceramic bearings. This clinical information is quite valuable and provides key information to assess the applicability of these technologies to orthopedic practice.

The final section contains three papers on alternative polymeric bearings. The first two papers, by Megremis, et al. and Mosleh, examine the feasibility of using composite bearing materials where both the fiber and matrix are fabricated from ultrahigh molecular-weight polyethylene. Polineni, et al. examine the feasibility of using a composite polymeric material fabricated from carbon fibers and polyetheretherketone.

Following the symposium, concurrent breakout sessions, followed by a plenary session, were held to develop a consensus statement on the state-of-the-art of alternative bearings for total joint replacement vis-a-vis standards development. The following were felt to be the most urgent issues facing the standards community:

1) Development of meaningful screening tests which will accurately rank the wear performance of candidate bearings. The kinematics of such screen text should be carefully characterized;

2) The development of standard joint simulators which should be validated by the wear testing of known clinical failures. Such simulator testing will include a standard lubricant which produces wear rates and wear patterns consistent with clinical retrievals. In addition, simulation studies should be able to test ''worst case'' scenarios including the presence of third bodies;

3) The development of standardized tests to determine the effects of sterilization and aging on bearing surface performance, for both polymeric and ceramic bearing surfaces; and

4) Development of standard methods for i) characterization of the biocompatability and toxicity of wear debris, ii) the recovery of wear debris from hip simulator fluids and periprosthetic tissue, and iii) the characterization of the morphology of wear debris.

Wear of Orthopaedic Bearings

Willard L. Sauer[1] and Mary E. Anthony[1]

PREDICTING THE CLINICAL WEAR PERFORMANCE OF ORTHOPAEDIC BEARING SURFACES

REFERENCE: Sauer, W. L. and Anthony, M. E., **"Predicting the Clinical Wear Performance of Orthopaedic Bearing Surfaces,"** *Alternative Bearing Surfaces in Total Joint Replacement, ASTM STP 1346*, J. J. Jacobs and T. L. Craig, Eds., American Society for Testing and Materials, 1998.

ABSTRACT: A historical review of both laboratory and clinical wear performance of orthopaedic bearing materials and surfaces is presented. Over time, laboratory wear tests have been developed and used more frequently to support the introduction of new material couples. Historically, these methods have been unreliable, and, despite recent improvements, predicting clinical wear performance is still a challenging task. Orthopaedic wear is a highly multi-factorial process—successful simulation depends on the identification, modeling, and control of many critical factors. Clinical results themselves are highly variable, complicating efforts to establish clinical validation criteria for test methods. It is recommended that improvements be made in identifying the appropriate clinical targets for laboratory tests, and that increased effort be directed toward the optimization and standardization of wear test methods.

KEYWORDS: clinical wear, wear test, historical, biomaterials, surface, cobalt-chrome, UHMWPE, standards

---

The pioneering efforts of Sir John Charnley led to a breakthrough in the popularity and success of total hip arthroplasty in the early 1960's [*1,2*]. Similar developments occurred for total knee arthroplasty and other joint replacements in the following years. Although there have been significant improvements in device fixation and fatigue strength of materials and designs since then, relatively small improvements have been made in wear performance. Today, 35 years later, wear of the bearing surfaces remains a primary limitation of joint replacements.

Ideally, clinically predictive wear models would exist such that new materials and designs could be evaluated with confidence in comparative testing. In reality, even the best wear models still have significant uncertainty due to the multitude of clinical applications and parameters which influence the degree and mechanisms of wear.

---

[1] Manager, tribology research projects, and senior research engineer, respectively, Smith & Nephew, Inc., Orthopaedic Division, 1450 Brooks Road, Memphis, TN 38116.

Additionally, the multi-factorial nature of wear creates doubt in even the most carefully controlled clinical evaluation; thus, clinical validations of wear models, while necessary, still have various degrees of uncertainty.

Nevertheless, there are decades of clinical results which provide some indication of the relative wear performance of different materials and surfaces. Technologies for modeling wear have advanced rapidly in recent years and now have greater potential to predict clinical wear behavior.

The objective of this review is to examine the historical role and performance of laboratory wear testing in guiding the introduction of new bearing surfaces for total joint replacement and identify the approaches necessary to achieve more clinically predictive wear test methods. It should be noted that it is beyond the scope of this review to analyze the methods used in each study to explain contradictory or potentially flawed results. This issue will be addressed in a general sense. This review will focus on wear studies and limit the clinical application primarily to hip replacements. The rationale will, however, apply to other applications.

Orthopaedic Bearing Material Performance: Laboratory and Clinical

The historical performance of various orthopaedic bearing materials and surfaces is evaluated below. Results are summarized in brief to stay within a reasonable scope. The objective is to determine the degree of variability in results and to examine the role and success of wear testing in the introduction of new bearing surfaces.

Baseline Data: CoCr Head/UHMWPE Cup Wear

The cobalt-chromium (CoCr) head/UHMWPE (gamma-air-sterilized) cup wear couple will be considered the standard baseline condition. A collection of such results is summarized in Table 1 (hip simulator) and Table 2 (clinical).[2] The clinical data exhibit higher wear rates than the hip simulator data. This is due to at least five potential factors:

1. Clinical wear data rarely separate volume loss due to creep deformation from volume loss due to wear. Additionally, the conversion of clinical wear rates from linear to volumetric could overestimate wear.[2]

2. Laboratory tests are usually accelerated and may thus not account for time-dependent changes in the UHMWPE or the metal head which may accelerate clinical wear.

3. Clinical usage may average greater than one million cycles (steps) per year with large ranges in patient activity levels.

---

[2]It should be noted that volumetric wear values were converted from linear wear values for [15], [16], [19], [20], [23], [26], and [29]. The conversion was made assuming the head and cup radii were identical and a cylindrical tunnelling wear mechanism occurred. Linear wear rates were thus multiplied by the projected area of the head, πr^2, to determine the volumetric wear rates.

4. Potentially inappropriate test conditions such as water lubricant or linear motion have been used. In recent years, most hip simulator testing laboratories have incorporated the methods recommended by industry experts in the current ISO and ASTM draft standards. This is reflected in the relatively consistent data shown in Table 1, particularly for the post-1990 28 mm and 32 mm head data. This is not to suggest that these data are all clinically valid. It is the responsibility of each laboratory to substantiate its data with appropriate proof of clinical validity.

5. Clinical wear data are often expressed in terms of a *mean* wear or penetration rate. A given series, however, usually exhibits a broad range (see Figures 1 and 2) due to the distribution of low-demand to high-demand or problematic patients, the latter often involving third-body wear debris. The mean clinical wear rate might not be the proper target for laboratory testing if it is skewed by a disproportionate number of low-demand or problematic cases. Most contemporary laboratory test methods probably represent a high-demand, well-functioning patient.

TABLE 1--*CoCr/UHMWPE hip simulator wear comparison.*
(All wear rates are expressed in mm^3 per 1 million cycles.)

Study	22 mm head	28 mm head	32 mm head
Dowson et al. (1988)[*3*]	42		
Pappas et al. (1990) [*4*]			54
McKellop et al. (1992) [*5*]			28
Elloy (1993) [*6*]	30		
Greer et al. (1995) [*7*]		30	
Bragdon et al. (1996) [*8*]			26.4
Brummitt et al. (1996) [*9*]	6		
Bigsby et al. (1996) [*10*]			30.4
Hamilton et al. (1997) [*11*]		35	
Essner et al. (1997) [*12*]			37
McKellop et al. (1997) [*13*]		30	
Sanford et al. (1997) [*14*]		22.5	
Mean/S.D.	26 ± 18	29 ± 5	35 ± 11

Pre-Charnley Bearing Materials

In the early 1900's, orthopaedic wear test methods were practically non-existent. Candidate bearing materials for hip joint or surface replacement were simply introduced as clinical experiments. Glass, Viscaloid, Pyrex, and Bakelite were tried in the 1920's

TABLE 2--*CoCr/UHMWPE clinical hip wear comparison.*
(All wear rates are expressed in mm^3 per year.)

Study	22 mm head	28 mm head	32 mm head
Charnley et al. (1975) [*15*]	59		
Scheier et al. (1976) [*16*]	97		
Atkinson et al. (1985) [*17*]	152		
Livermore et al. (1990) [*18*]	48	48	84
Isaac et al. (1992) [*19*]	80		
Lazcano et al. (1993) [*20*]	45		
Kabo et al. (1993) [*21*]			88
Hernandez et al. (1994) [*22*]		139 (uncemented)	
		92 (cemented)	
Petersen et al. (1994) [*23*]	78 (loose)		
	31 (well-fixed)		
Berzins et al. (1995) [*24*]		59	
Callaghan et al. (1995) [*25*]	48		
Woolson et al. (1995) [*26*]		86	
Kesteris et al. (1996) [*27*]	57		148
Sychterz et al. (1996) [*28*]			39.8
Hailey et al. (1997) [*29*]	66		
Mean/S.D.	69 ± 33	85 ± 33	90 ± 44

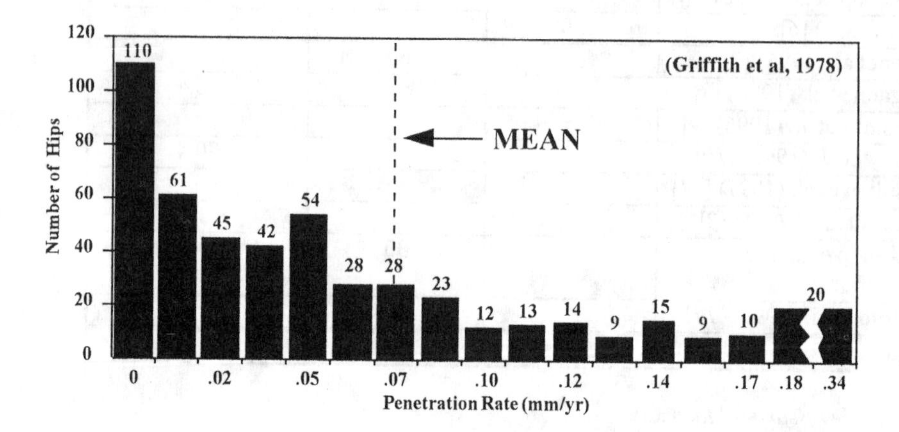

Figure 1: *Histogram of the distribution of UHMWPE cup linear wear (penetration) rates for 493 Charnley prostheses (22.25 mm head diameter), measured on radiographs, after an average of 8.3 years* in vivo. *Note the large distribution in wear rates relative to the mean of 0.07 mm per year. (Redrawn from Griffith et al. [30].)*

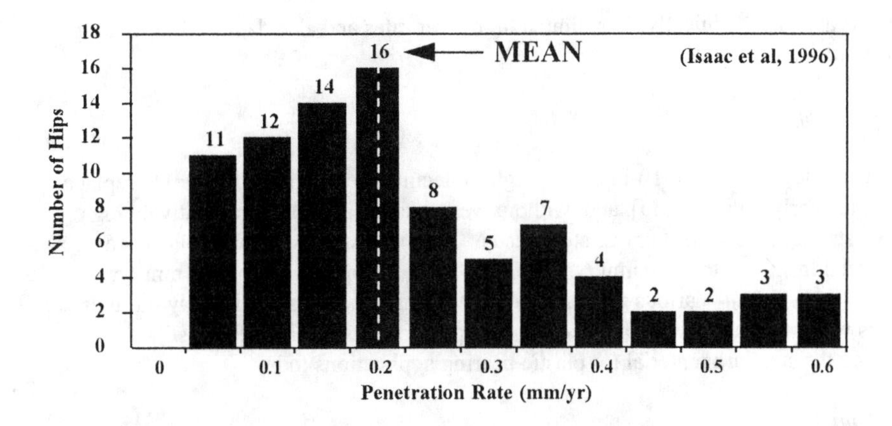

Figure 2: *Histogram of the distribution of UHMWPE cup linear wear (penetration) rates for 87* explanted *Charnley prostheses (22.25 mm head diameter), measured using the shadowgraph technique, after an average of 8.75 years* in vivo. *Note the higher mean wear rate of 0.204 mm per year, but a similarly large distribution in wear rates. (Redrawn from Isaac et al. [31].)*

and 1930's without success. Acrylic and nylon were tried in the 1940's and 1950's and were better, but still unsatisfactory. In 1943, AISI Type 302 stainless steel was proposed as an implant material. By 1952, the more corrosion-resistant Type 316 stainless steel was recommended, and soon, this and the low-carbon version (Type 316L) were being used successfully for femoral head bearing surfaces. CoCrMo alloys were adopted from the aerospace industry in the 1930's for dentistry; the first surgical grade alloy was called Vitallium. It soon found application in femoral head and acetabular cup applications and, along with 316L stainless steel, has exhibited successful clinical results through the present.

PTFE Cup

Charnley introduced PTFE (polytetrafluoroethylene) in 1957 [*32*], primarily to address the friction problems experienced with the Judet acrylic prosthesis. PTFE cups failed due to high wear rates [*33-35*], reported clinically from 835 to 2300 mm^3/yr [*33,34*] (8 to 20 times greater than UHMWPE clinical wear rates). When Charnley later developed wear test methods, he measured PTFE wear rates 500 to 1800 times greater than UHMWPE [*34,36*]. Others have since confirmed this finding [*37*]. Silica-filled

PTFE was also used clinically; it exhibited high wear rates and also damaged the mating stainless steel surface [*35*].

UHMWPE Cup

Charnley chose UHMWPE (ultra-high-molecular-weight polyethylene) to replace PTFE in the early 1960's [*1,35*], and, without wear data, achieved a comparatively high wear-resistant couple with stainless steel heads. The mean wear rate of the plastic cup was reduced from 835 to 2300 mm^3/yr (PTFE) [*33,34*] to approximately 103 mm^3/yr (UHMWPE; Table 3). Various grades of UHMWPE have been used clinically through the years with no conclusive differences in wear performance; UHMWPE is still considered the standard material for plastic bearing applications today.

HDPE Cup

It is not clear if HDPE (high density polyethylene) has been used clinically—the term HDPE often seems to be used interchangeably with UHMWPE even though it indicates a lower molecular weight range. In the U.S. (ASTM Specification for Ultra-High-Molecular-Weight Polyethylene Molding and Extrusion Materials (D 4020-92)), UHMWPE is defined as a polyethylene with a molecular weight average (M_w) of greater than approximately 3.1 million. The international specification (ISO 11542) defines UHMWPE with a much lower M_w: greater than approximately 1 million. Galante et al. [*38*] measured the wear rate of a HDPE to be approximately ten times higher than that of a UHMWPE. Using a sand slurry abrasion test, an ASTM Committee D20 task group demonstrated that polyethylene wear rate was constant for molecular weights above about 3 million, but increased by about 75% as molecular weights were decreased to 1 million [*39*].

CoCr Head/CoCr Cup

Metal-on-metal bearings were used for hip replacement before UHMWPE came into use [*40,41*]. In 1962, McKee began implanting the McKee-Farrar metal-on-metal hip prosthesis [*42*]. Other designs followed. In general, wear rates were low but early loosening rates were high. The latter was attributed to imprecise manufacturing. Interestingly, Charnley [*34*] later reported that with McKee's metal-on-metal hip, ". . . it is impossible to simulate satisfactory function in the laboratory," in contrast to successful clinical performance. CoCr-CoCr hips that did not fail early have generally exhibited excellent long-term performance. Due to recent concerns with UHMWPE wear, metal-on-metal has experienced renewed interest. A summary of laboratory and clinical results is given in Table 3.

Polyester Cup

Polyester (polyethylene terephthalate) was an alternative polymer bearing material introduced in the 1960's. Laboratory wear testing followed the clinical introduction of this material, with mixed results (Table 4). Semlitsch et al. [*53*] and Scales et al. [*54*] found polyester to perform better than UHMWPE. Semlitsch et al. [*53,55*] conducted hip simulator testing and found that irradiation of polyester improved its wear resistance 64 to 94%, to a level superior to UHMWPE. On the contrary, Dumbleton et al. [*56*], Walker et al. [*57*], and McKellop et al. [*37*] reported that the laboratory wear resistance of polyester was much worse than that of UHMWPE. Also, Capozzo et al. [*58*] conducted a hip simulator study and measured a wear rate of 180 $mm^3/10^6$ cycles for polyester vs. 21 $mm^3/10^6$ cycles for UHMWPE. Clinically, Scheier et al. [*16*] found that the wear performance of polyester was similar to that of UHMWPE. Dumbleton [*35*] and Willert et al. [*59*] reported that it was worse. Polyester cups were abandoned in the mid-1970's due to poor clinical wear performance. It should be noted that polyester performed better

TABLE 3--*Wear performance of CoCr-on-CoCr hips.*

	Study	Comparison of CoCr-CoCr to Metal-UHMWPE Wear	Comments
Hip Simulator *lab-to-lab: agreement (less wear)*	Streicher et al. (1990) [*43*]	0.02-0.03 mm linear wear at 1.8 million cycles	
	Farrar et al. (1997) [*44*]	0.46 $mm^3/10^6$ cycles vs. 20.76 $mm^3/10^6$ cycles	optimal diametral clearance: +.074 mm
	Scott et al. (1997) [*45*]	2.4 $mg/10^6$ cycles	most wear in first 500,000 cycles; minimize radial clearance
	Chan et al. (1997) [*46*]	20-100 times lower wear volume	optimal radial clearance: +.045 to +.090 mm
Clinical *clinical comparison: mostly in agreement (less wear)*	Dobbs (1981) [*47*]	survival at 20 years: metal-metal 33% metal-plastic 74%	
	Semlitsch et al. (1989) [*48*]	0.06 mm vs. 2.1 mm linear wear	
	Muller (1995) [*49*]	40 times less wear; much less tissue inflammation	
	Schmalzried et al. (1996) [*50*]	25 times lower linear wear	
	Doorn et al. (1997) [*51*]	25 times more particles than UHMWPE, but much smaller size; less adverse reactions	
	McKellop et al. (1997) [*52*]		metal/metal polishes out imperfections and 3-body abrasion

Lab vs. Clinical: Mostly in agreement (less wear)

as the cup component than as the head component. Early laboratory tests were typically not designed for specific applications.

Polyacetal Cup

Polyacetal (polyoxymethylene) was another alternative polymer bearing material introduced around 1970. Results were again mixed, but the Delrin grade appeared to perform much better than other grades such as Ertacetal, and better than polyester. Laboratory and clinical results are summarized in Table 5. Polyacetal has never been fully abandoned, but it is generally considered inferior to UHMWPE.

TABLE 4--*Wear performance of polyester for acetabular cups.*

	Study	Comparison to UHMWPE
Laboratory	Semlitsch et al. (1972) [*53,55*]	better
	Scales et al. (1972) [*54*]	better
lab-to-lab:	Dumbleton et al. (1974) [*56*]	much worse
conflicting, but	Walker et al. (1974) [*57*]	much worse
mostly increased	Capozzo et al. (1977) [*58*]	much worse
wear	McKellop et al. (1981) [*37*]	much worse
Clinical	Scheier et al. (1976) [*16*]	similar
	Willert et al. (1976) [*59*]	worse
clinical compar-ison: conflicting, but mostly increased wear	Dumbleton (1982) [*35*]	worse

Lab vs. Clinical: Similar (later results show increased wear)

PTFE, Polyester, Polyacetal, and UHMWPE Femoral Head/Metal Cup

These polymer head/metal cup combinations have all been tried clinically in the 1960's and 1970's but ultimately failed due to high wear of the polymer, performing worse as the convex component than the concave component [*35*]. Wear testing of these combinations has not been widely reported.

Alumina Head/UHMWPE Cup

Alumina ceramic bearing surfaces were introduced in the late 1960's. Significant laboratory wear testing has been conducted since around the time of clinical introduction through the present. Laboratory test results have indicated anywhere from no improvement over CoCr/UHMWPE to a large improvement. Clinical results have generally shown that the alumina head moderately reduces UHMWPE wear. These results are summarized in Table 6.

Zirconia Head/UHMWPE Cup

Zirconia was identified and introduced shortly after alumina as a means of further improving UHMWPE wear performance and improving resistance to ceramic fracture. Laboratory test results have indicated similar reductions in UHMWPE wear compared to alumina. Taylor et al. [*80*] reported hip simulator wear rates of 27 $mm^3/10^6$ cycles for CoCr and 11 $mm^3/10^6$ cycles for zirconia, a 59% reduction. McKellop et al. [*73*] reported 28.1 $mm^3/10^6$ cycles for CoCr and 21.9 $mm^3/10^6$ cycles for zirconia, a 22% reduction. Clinical results are still limited.

TABLE 5--*Wear performance of polyacetal for acetabular cups.*

	Study	Type of Polyacetal	Comparison to UHMWPE	Comments
Laboratory *lab-to-lab: conflicting*	Duff-Barclay et al. (1966) [*60*]	Delrin	much better	hip simulator: UHMWPE: 20 $mm^3/10^6$ cycles Delrin: 0.3 $mm^3/10^6$ cycles
	Amstutz (1968) [*61*]	Delrin	worse	
	Homsy et al. (1973) [*62*]	Delrin	worse	
	Galante et al. (1973) [*38*]	Delrin	worse	
	Shen et al. (1976) [*63*]	Delrin	better	
	Dumbleton (1979) [*64*]	Delrin	better	
	Clarke et al. (1980) [65]	Delrin	worse	
	Dumbleton (1981) [*66*]	Delrin	better	
	McKellop et al. (1981) [*37,67*]	Delrin	much worse	(28-200 times worse)
Clinical *clinical comparison: agreement for Delrin*	Clarke (1982) [*68*]	Delrin	similar	
	Dumbleton (1982) [*35*]	?	much worse	0.71 to 1.76 mm/yr wear (Stanmore prosthesis)
	Dumbleton (1979) [*64*] (1982) [*35*]	Delrin	similar	(Christiansen THP)

Lab vs. Clinical: Conflicting - more variability in laboratory testing

TABLE 6--*Wear performance of alumina heads.*

	Study	Comparison to Metal Head
	Semlitsch et al. (1977) [69]	95% reduced UHMWPE wear
	Wright et al. (1978) [70]	24% reduced UHMWPE wear
Hip Simulator	Niederer et al. (1978) [71]	93% reduced UHMWPE wear (9 $mm^3/10^6$ cycles vs. 134 $mm^3/10^6$ cycles)
lab-to-lab:	Wright et al. (1980) [72]	57% reduced UHMWPE wear (30 $mm^3/10^6$ cycles vs. 70 $mm^3/10^6$ cycles)
agreement (less wear)	McKellop et al. (1992) [73]	slightly increased UHMWPE wear, but alumina was rougher
	Weber (1981) [74]	50% reduced UHMWPE wear
	Semlitsch et al. (1989) [48]	38% reduced UHMWPE wear
	Oonishi et al. (1989) [75]	50% reduced UHMWPE wear
Clinical	Schuller et al. (1990) [76]	73% reduced UHMWPE penetration
	Zichner et al. (1992) [77]	cut penetration rate in half
clinical	Bragdon et al. (1995) [78]	no improvement
comparison: mostly in	Semlitsch et al. (1997) [41]	50% reduced UHMWPE wear
agreement (less wear)	Livingston et al. (1997) [79]	increased UHMWPE wear (Hylamer UHMWPE)

Lab vs. Clinical: Mostly in agreement (less wear)

TABLE 7--*Wear performance of alumina-on-alumina hips.*

	Study	Comparison to Metal/UHMWPE
Laboratory	Semlitsch et al. (1977) [69]	98% less wear in hip simulator
	Wallbridge et al. (1983) [81]	more potential for runaway wear
lab-to-lab: conflicting, but mostly favorable	Walter et al. (1985) [82] (1987) [83]	reduced wear
	Boutin et al. (1981) [84]	favorable
Clinical	Sawai et al (1981) [85]	runaway wear observed
	Boutin et al. (1987) [86]	favorable
clinical	Kummer et al. (1990)[87]	runaway wear observed
comparison:	Sedel et al. (1990) [88]	favorable
conflicting,	Borssen et al. (1991) [89]	osteolysis observed
but mostly	Mittlemeier et al.(1992) [90]	favorable
favorable	Sedel et al. (1994) [91]	favorable
	Boehlar et al. (1994) [92]	favorable

Lab vs. Clinical: Similarly conflicting, but mostly favorable

Alumina Head/Alumina Cup

Alumina ceramic-on-ceramic articulation has been used for total hip prostheses since 1970. No significant laboratory wear testing had been conducted at the time of clinical introduction. Since then, both laboratory testing and clinical results have been generally favorable with respect to wear behavior as shown in Table 7.

Carbon Fiber-Reinforced UHMWPE

Modifying UHMWPE by creating a carbon fiber-reinforced composite was proposed in the early 1970's, developed and tested for several years and then introduced for both hip and knee implants in the late 1970's. Additional laboratory studies and numerous clinical reports followed. These are summarized in Table 8. As shown, early laboratory tests were generally favorable, the clinical results were generally unfavorable, and the later laboratory results were also unfavorable.

Ti-6Al-4V Femoral Head

Titanium alloy (e.g., Ti-6Al-4V) was introduced as a potential bearing surface against UHMWPE in the late 1970's. By this time, laboratory wear testing had become much more established and there was an abundance of testing before and during the introduction of Ti-6Al-4V femoral heads and other articular applications. Both the laboratory and clinical results were mixed (as shown in Table 9). In general, Ti-6Al-4V was found to be an inferior bearing surface, compared to CoCr alloy, due to its susceptibility to abrasion. Wear testing in clean conditions did not predict this.

Ion-Implanted Ti-6Al-4V

Ion implantation of Ti-6Al-4V was developed in the mid 1980's to improve the abrasion resistance of Ti-6Al-4V. It was introduced for hip, knee, and shoulder bearing surfaces. Simulator test results ranged from no improvement (compared to untreated Ti-6Al-4V) to complete elimination of UHMWPE wear. These results are shown in Table 10. Clinical results have not been reported.

Ion-Implanted CoCr

Ion implantation of CoCr alloy was developed and introduced for hip and knee bearing surfaces in the early 1990's as a new means of reducing UHMWPE wear. Laboratory test results have varied significantly from increased UHMWPE wear to complete elimination of UHMWPE wear. These results are shown in Table 11. Clinical results have not been reported.

TABLE 8--Wear performance of carbon fiber-reinforced UHMWPE.

	Study	Comparison to Regular UHMWPE
Laboratory *lab-to-lab: conflicting*	Sclippa et al. (1973)[*93*]	no difference (carbon powder)
	Tetik (1973)[*94*]	short-term wear better, long-term wear worse
	Ainsworth et al. (1977)[*95*]	hip simulator: 88% reduction in wear (4.2 mg/10^6 cycles vs. 35.3 mg/10^6 cycles)
	Greer (1979)[*96*]	hip simulator: 74% reduction in wear (6.55 $mm^3/10^6$ cycles vs. 25.1 $mm^3/10^6$ cycles)
	Greer (1979)[*96*]	knee simulator: 77% reduction in wear (1.50 $mm^3/10^6$ cycles vs. 6.54 $mm^3/10^6$ cycles)
	Dumbleton (1981)[*66*]	similar
	McKellop et al. (1981)[*37,67,97*]	1.8 to 17 times more wear
	Peterson et al. (1988)[*98*]	worse (knee simulator)
Clinical *clinical comparison: mostly in agreement (increased wear)*	Wright et al. (1985)[*99*] 1988)[*100*]	no difference
	Wright et al. (1988)[*101*]	catastrophic failure in 2 cases caused by molding defects
	Kraay et al. (1994)[*102*]	slightly worse (MG knee)
	Chillag et al. (1995)[*103*]	worse

Lab vs. Clinical: Conflicting - clinical results showed generally more wear

TiN-Coated Ti-6Al-4V

TiN coating has been used as a bearing surface against UHMWPE since the late 1980's. Laboratory testing and clinical results have been limited. Pappas et al. [*4*] reported hip simulator wear rates of 56 $mm^3/10^6$ cycles for CoCr heads and 20 $mm^3/10^6$ cycles for TiN-coated Ti-6Al-4V heads, a reduction of 64%. Peterson et al. [*98*] reported that a TiN-coated Ti-6Al-4V femoral knee component remained undamaged after 500,000 knee simulator cycles, in contrast to an untreated Ti-6Al-4V component.

Heat-Pressed UHMWPE

A heat-pressing polishing technique for UHMWPE bearing surfaces was introduced during the 1980's. This technique was conducted for improved aesthetics [*128,129*]. There was little or no wear testing conducted to investigate the effects of this

TABLE 9--*Wear performance of Ti-6Al-4V for femoral head.*

	Study	Comparison to CoCr or 316LSS (total wear)
Laboratory *lab-to-lab: conflicting*	Galante et al. (1973) [*38*]	worse
	Miller et al. (1974) [*104*]	better
	Revell et al. (1978) [*105*]	worse under abrasive conditions
	McKellop et al. (1979) [*106*]	worse under abrasive conditions
	Greer (1980) [*107*]	same (hip simulator)
	McKellop et al. (1980) [*108*]	better under clean conditions, worse under abrasive conditions
	Rostoker et al. (1981) [*109*]	worse
	Dumbleton et al. (1981) [*66*]	same
	McKellop et al. (1982) [*110,111*]	worse (hip simulator)
	Starkebaum et al. (1983) [*112*]	better (hip simulator)
Clinical *clinical comparison: conflicting, but mostly increased wear*	Gruen et al. (1981) [*113*]	similar
	Clarke et al. (1982) [*68*]	similar
	Agins et al. (1988) [*114*]	worse
	Lombardi et al. (1989) [*115*]	worse
	Black et al. (1990) [*116*]	worse
	McKellop et al. (1990) [*117*] (1994) [*118*]	excellent under clean conditions, worse under abrasive conditions
	Cautilli et al. (1993) [*119*]	worse
	Kraay et al. (1994) [*102*]	susceptible to runaway wear under abrasive conditions

Lab vs. Clinical: Similar accelerated wear when abrasive conditions exist

surface modification on tribological behavior. A plethora of reports [*128-133*] of accelerated wear, however, indicated that heat-pressing adversely affected the clinical wear behavior of UHMWPE.

TABLE 10--*Wear performance of ion-implanted Ti-6Al-4V.*

	Study	Comparison to Untreated Ti-6Al-4V
Simulator *lab-to-lab: conflicting, but not increased wear*	McKellop et al. (1990) [*120*]	hip simulator: no difference in clean conditions, reduced Ti abrasion in PMMA particles
	Gilbertson et al. (1991) [*121*]	5 million cycle knee simulator: eliminated scratching and burnishing
	Rieu et al. (1991) [*122*]	hip simulator UHMWPE wear untreated: 11-53 $mm^3/10^6$ cycles ion-implanted: zero wear
	McKellop et al. (1994) [*123*]	hip simulator: no difference
Clinical	None reported	

TABLE 11--*Wear performance of ion-implanted CoCr.*

	Study	Comparison to Untreated CoCr
Laboratory *lab-to-lab: conflicting*	Sioshansi et al. (1991) [*124*]	elimination of UHMWPE wear (pin-on-disk)
	Poggie et al. (1992) [*125*]	2.8 times increase in wear (pin-on-disk)
	Taylor et al. (1992) [*80*]	56% reduced UHMWPE wear (hip simulator)
	McKellop et al. (1994) [*123*]	hip simulator: 0 - 2.5 million cycles: better 2.5 - 5.0 million cycles: worse overall: no significant effect
	Greer et al. (1994) [*126*]	10 N pin-on-disk: better 132 N pin-on-disk: worse
	Schmidt et al. (1995) [*127*]	hip simulator: no difference
Clinical	None reported	

HYLAMER™[3] and HYLAMER-M™[3]

In the late 1980's, "HYLAMER" and "HYLAMER-M" were developed and introduced. To create these materials, consolidated UHMWPE is subjected to a hot isostatic pressing (HIPing) procedure in a low-oxygen environment. This process results in a highly chain-extended UHMWPE (HYLAMER) or a moderately chain-extended UHMWPE (HYLAMER-M), the former designed for acetabular cup applications, the latter for tibial

[3]DePuy-DuPont Orthopaedics, Warsaw, IN.

component applications. The limited laboratory wear data is conflicting. Clinical reports have also been mixed. These results are summarized in Table 12.

TABLE 12--*Wear performance of HYLAMER.*

	Study	Comparison to Regular UHMWPE
Laboratory *lab-to-lab: conflicting*	Saum et al. (1992) [*134*]	30% less wear (pin-on-disk)
	Davidson et al. (1992) [*135*]	130% more wear (pin-on-disk)
	McKellop et al. (1992) [*5*]	no significant difference (hip simulator, 4 million cycle)
Clinical *clinical comparison: mostly in agreement (increased wear)*	Chmell et al. (1996) [*136*]	higher early failure rate due to eccentric wear
	Livingston et al. (1997) [*79*]	UHMWPE: 0.12 mm/yr, HYLAMER: 0.29 mm/yr (penetration rate)
	Sychterz et al. (1997) [*137*]	UHMPWE: 0.20 mm/yr, HYLAMER: 0.15 mm/yr (penetration rate)
	Schmalzried et al. (1997) [*138*]	HYLAMER: 0.43 mm/yr; high-demand patients
	Muratoglu et al. (1997) [*139*]	HYLAMER: 0.48 mm/yr

Lab vs. Clinical: Conflicting - clinical results tend to show more wear for Hylamer

Gamma Irradiation of UHMWPE

Gamma irradiation was first used to sterilize UHMPWE in the late-1960's. At the time, its effects on UHMWPE wear behavior had not been investigated. Numerous studies in the 1970's and 1980's, however, did investigate this and generally concluded that there was not a significant effect. In the last few years, the effects of radiation-induced crosslinking, chain scission, oxidation, and time-dependent degradation have been vigorously studied. Gamma irradiation does affect the wear behavior of UHMWPE. The nature of this effect, however, depends on many factors, such as radiation dosage, radiation and packaging atmosphere, UHMWPE characteristics, post-sterilization aging time and environment, and applied wear mechanisms. It is beyond the scope of this study to review all of the published results. Several laboratory studies have shown an adverse effect of gamma irradiation (Scales et al. [*140*], Dumbleton et al. [*56*], McKellop et al. [*37,141*], Fisher et al. [*142*], and Trieu et al. [*143*]) while several have shown a favorable effect (Wang et al. [*144*], Hamilton et al. [*145*], and McKellop et al. [*146*]). Adverse effects have been attributed to radiation-induced chain scission, oxidation, and aging while favorable effects have been attributed to radiation-induced crosslinking. Clinical observations have shown little effect of gamma sterilization (Streicher [*147*]) as well as significant adverse effects of gamma sterilization (White et al. [*148*], Sutula et al. [*149*], and Collier [*150*]); however, effects of recent packaging changes, free-radical scavenging methods, and shelf-aging limits have not yet been reported clinically.

Other Alternative Bearing Materials and Surfaces

Many other bearing materials and surfaces have been proposed and/or clinically introduced or are being evaluated. High-dose (100 to 200 Mrad) gamma irradiation of UHMWPE cups has been tested and implemented on a limited basis with favorable reports [*151,152*]. Cushion-form polyurethane bearings have been proposed as an alternative approach to achieve low wear in knees [*153*]. Polyacetal bearing against UHMWPE has exhibited favorable results [*154*]. Ion-implanted UHMWPE has exhibited favorable pin-on-disk [*155*] and hip simulator [*156*] results, but has not been tried clinically. On the metal side, diamond-like carbon (DLC) coatings have been proposed as a means of reducing UHMWPE wear [*157*]; however, some test results have shown an increase in UHMWPE articulating wear [*158*]. Oxygen diffusion hardening has been used to improve the wear performance of titanium alloy articulating surfaces [*159*]. Clinical results are still preliminary. Another proposed bearing surface is oxidized zirconium. Laboratory tests have been favorable [*160,161*], but clinical results are not yet known.

Currently, there is significant interest and investigation of crosslinked UHMWPE. This includes both radiation-crosslinked and chemically-crosslinked UHMWPE. A key reason for this recent activity is the discovery that crosslinking of UHMWPE chains, while not exhibiting an advantage under linear wear paths, does result in significant resistance to nonlinear (cross-shear) wear paths such as those believed to occur in hip wear. Improvements in test methods have been necessary to highlight the benefits of crosslinked UHMPWE. Although clinical validation is still incomplete, this example illustrates why it is critical that test methods are designed to account for the key factors for a given wear application. This will minimize misleading results such as those which have been generated in the past for alternative bearing materials and surfaces and have led to significant disagreement in their predicted performance.

Contradictory Results

As indicated in this review of clinical bearing material wear performance, contradictory results abound. It is beyond the scope of this review to analyze the causes of these contradictory results for each individual case. To provide a general explanation, a partial list of orthopaedic wear-related parameters (both laboratory and clinical) is given in Table 13. The overwhelming number of potential variables adds to the unpredictability of an already complex and inadequately understood UHMWPE wear behavior. The potential interactions between these parameters increase the complexity. Thus, it is easy to see why not only laboratory-to-clinical comparisons are difficult, but even apparently well-controlled laboratory-to-laboratory and clinical-to-clinical comparisons may contain many hidden variables. This explains the frequent contradictory results.

Even single-laboratory comparisons of materials and designs are potentially subject to many of the variables listed in Table 13. Meticulous attention to these potential sources of variability improves the confidence of the results. Clinical validation of the results, however, remains a key factor in establishing meaningfulness.

The Key to Predicting Clinical Wear Behavior - Clinically Validated, Standardized Wear Tests

Laboratory wear testing has historically played an inconsistent, but increasing, role in guiding the introduction of new bearing surfaces for total joint replacement. In the 1950's and 1960's, wear test methods were crude; components such as PTFE cups and metal-on-metal hips were introduced with little or no testing. In the 1970's and 1980's, wear test methods became more sophisticated and more frequently utilized. Test results for such devices as polyacetal cups and titanium alloy heads were mixed; these devices were introduced nevertheless. In many cases, the clinical results were also mixed. In recent years, wear test equipment and methods have improved dramatically due to significant research efforts at multiple laboratories. At the same time, sensitivity of the orthopaedic community to the wear performance of new bearing surfaces has significantly increased; thus, laboratory wear testing is now playing a much larger role than it ever has before.

Clarke [*68*] noted in 1982 that "much of the wear literature is either confusing or contradictory." While the improvements in hip simulator wear test and measurement procedures have apparently improved the results (Table 1), there is still a degree of uncertainty due to lack of standardization and incomplete validation of methods.

The majority of laboratory wear results reported in this review vary significantly and are not based on standardized methods. One exception is the pin-on-disk testing based on the ASTM Practice for Reciprocating Pin-on-Flat Evaluation of Friction and Wear Properties of Polymeric Materials for Use in Total Joint Prostheses (F 732-82). This method, however, has recently been invalidated, at least for hip wear conditions. Linear wear motion has been shown to generate inappropriate or misleading results for non-linear motion applications [*8,144,162,163,164*]. Another exception is the hip simulator testing based on the ASTM Guide for Gravimetic Wear Assessment of Prosthetic Hip Designs in Simulator Devices (F 1714-97). This standard, however, is only a guide. It is not specific with respect to some parameters such as load and motion inputs and it is not enforceable. These standards, as well as the ASTM knee simulator test method, are in the early stages of being revised into highly specified standard methods, reflecting the results of recent research, and distinguishing test parameters which appear to provide valid results from those which may generate misleading results. This is one important step towards the development of clinically predictive wear test methods.

Until, and possibly even after, the creation of universally-accepted wear test methods, clinical validation of these methods will remain an important requirement. Historically, clinical validation of methods has been lacking. Clarke [*68*] suggested, and McKellop [*165*] later reiterated, that laboratory studies should calibrate their methods by

TABLE 13--*Orthopaedic wear-related parameters for counterface/UHMWPE articulation.*

	Laboratory Parameters	Clinical Parameters
1. Contact Conditions	a. contact geometry	(same)
	b. specimen alignment	(same: surgical technique)
	c. motion path	(same)
	d. stroke length	(same)
	e. sliding velocity	(same)
	f. load/contact stress	(same: patient weight, activity)
	g. cyclic frequency	(same)
	h. periods of inactivity	(same)
	i. load-control vs. displacement-control	(same)
	j. component mismatch/tolerance issues	(same)
2. Lubricant Conditions	a. lubricant chemistry	(same)
	b. temperature	(same)
	c. replacement protocol	N/A
	d. particles/contaminants from other sources	(same)
	e. evaporation	N/A
	f. lubricant chemistry changes	biological equilibrium/changes
3. Counterface Conditions	a. surface finish	(same)
	b. specimen-to-specimen variations	(same)
	c. cleaning/chemical treatment of surface	(same)
	d. material grades	(same)
4. UHMWPE Conditions	a. surface finish	(same)
	b. specimen-to-specimen variations	(same)
	c. cleaning/chemical treatment of surface	(same)
	d. sterilization method/dose	(same)
	e. age of specimen at beginning of wear	(same)
	f. size/thickness of specimen	(same)
	g. molecular orientation/ fabrication effects	(same)
	h. material grades	(same)
5. Machine Variables	a. machine-to-machine variability	patient-to-patient variability
	b. fixturing/support variability	patient and surgical technique variability
	c. containment and fixture materials	N/A
6. Wear Mechanism Variables	a. break-in variability	(same)
	b. transfer film behavior	(same)
	c. wear mechanism transitions	(same)
7. Duration of Wear	a. cycles	(same: patient activity level)
	b. absolute time	(same)
8. Wear Measurement	a. gravimetric/volumetric/etc.	volumetric/radiographic/etc.

reproducing clinical wear rates and wear mechanisms of different materials. For example, mean clinical linear wear rates of the following polymer cup materials bearing against CoCr or stainless heads are roughly:

UHMWPE:	0.07 mm/yr
Delrin:	0.2 mm/yr
Polyester:	0.5 mm/yr
PTFE:	3.3 mm/yr

There is, however, significant uncertainty regarding the appropriate mean clinical values, as well as material grades and conditions, device characteristics, and surgeon and patient characteristics associated with these results. To identify the clinical target(s), factors such as these need to be identified and normalized. Should the mean clinical result be the target for laboratory testing? It is probably more appropriate to analyze the distributions in clinical results within each clinical series (such as those shown in Figures 1 and 2) and then determine where the proposed test conditions fit into these distributions. Other factors to consider include measurement criteria. Wear measurements for laboratory-tested specimens are often different from those for clinical specimens. To supplement wear rate data, it may be appropriate for laboratory studies to include wear debris characterizations and/or wear surface morphology analyses to compare with clinical results. Several recent studies have made progress towards such clinical validation criteria [*8,144,166,167*].

The standardization process should take these numerous factors into consideration to determine the targeted clinical results, determine criteria for clinical validation, and then develop methods which reproduce the targeted clinical results. Round-robin testing at multiple laboratories is recommended for determining reproducibility, particularly if there are significant differences in wear testing equipment [*168*]. Standardization not only eliminates the multitude of test methods (and corresponding variability in results), but the challenge in achieving this encourages the many experts in the field to combine forces and increase the probability of a successful outcome.

Though significant advances have been made, development and enforcement of laboratory tests which reliably predict results for alternative orthopaedic bearing materials and surfaces have still not occurred. We recommend that current efforts to establish and validate highly specified standard test methods for this purpose be expanded and accelerated.

References

[1] Mayor, M.B. and Collier, J.P., "The Technology of Hip Replacement," Scientific American, Science & Medicine, May/June 1994: 58-67.

[2] Davidson, J.A. and Georgette, F.S., "State of the Art Materials for Orthopaedic Prosthetic Devices," SME Technical Paper EM87-122, 1987.

[3] Dowson, D. and Jobbins, B., "Design and Development of a Versatile Hip Joint Simulator and a Preliminary Assessment of Wear and Creep in Charnley Total Hip Replacement Hip Joints," Engineering in Medicine, **17** (1988): 111-117.

[4] Pappas, M.J., Makris, G., and Buechel, F.F., "Comparison of Wear of UHMWPE Cups Articulating with Co-Cr and Ti-Ni Coated, Titanium Femoral Heads," Trans. 16th SFB (1990): 36.

[5] McKellop, H., Lu, B., and Li, S., "Wear of Acetabular Cups of Conventional and Modified UHMW Polyethylenes Compared on a Hip Joint Simulator," Trans. 38th ORS (1992): 356.

[6] Elloy, M., "Simulator Testing of Joint Prostheses: The Need for Realistic Simulator Testing," SERC/IMechE Annual Expert Meeting on Failure of Joint Prostheses, Bournemouth (Mechanical Engineering Publications, London) (1993): 79-82.

[7] Greer, K.W., Schmidt, M.B., and Tariah, I.B., "A Comparison of the Wear Properties of UHMWPE Produced from Two Powder Grades," Trans. 21st SFB (1995): 227.

[8] Bragdon, C.R., O'Connor, D.O., Lowenstein, J.D., Jasty, M., and Syniuta, W.D., "The Importance of Multidirectional Motion on the Wear of Polyethylene," Proc. Instn. Mech. Engrs./IMechE, **210** (1996): 157-165.

[9] Brummitt, K. and Hardaker, C.S., "Estimation of Wear in Total Hip Replacement Using a Ten Station Hip Simulator," Proc. Instn. Mech. Engrs./IMechE, **210** (1996): 187-190.

[10] Bigsby, R.J.A., Hardaker, C.S., and Fisher, J., "Wear of UHMWPE Acetabular Cups in a Physiological Hip Joint Simulator in the Anatomical Position," Trans. 5th World Biomaterials Congress (1996): 970.

[11] Hamilton, J.V., Schmidt, M.B., and Shah, C., "The Effects of Sterilization Dose on UHMWPE Wear Rates," Trans. 43rd ORS (1997): 782.

[12] Essner, A., Polineni, V.K., Schmidig, G., Wang, A., Stark, C., and Dumbleton, J.H., "Long Term Wear Simulation of Stabilized UHMWPE Acetabular Cups," Trans. 43rd ORS (1997): 784.

[13] McKellop, H.A., Shen, F.W., Yu, Y.J., Lu, B., and Salavey, R. "Effect of Sterilization Method on the Wear Rate of UHMW Polyethylene Acetabular Cups in a Hip Simulator," Trans. 43rd ORS (1997): 94.

[14] Sanford, W.M., Moore, W.C., McNulty, D., Frisinger, C., and Schmalzried, T.P., "Hip Simulator Study of the Effect of Study of the Effect of Sterilization and Oxidation on UHMWPE Wear," Trans. 43rd ORS (1997): 95.

[15] Charnley, J. and Halley, D., "Rate of Wear in Total Hip Replacement," Clin. Orthop., **112** (1975): 170.

[16] Scheier, H. and Sandel, J., "Wear Affecting the Plastic Cup in Metal-Plastic Endoprostheses," Total Hip Prostheses, N. Gschwend and H.U. Debrunner, Eds., Williams & Wilkins, Baltimore, MD, 1976: 186.

[17] Atkinson, J.R., Dowson, D., Isaac, G.H., and Wroblewski, B.M., "Laboratory Wear Tests and Clinical Observations of the Penetration of Femoral Heads into Acetabular Cups in Total Replacement Hip Joints. III: The Measurement of Internal Volume Changes in Explanted Charnley after 2-16 Years In Vivo and the Determination of Wear Factors," Wear, **104** (1985): 225-244.

[18] Livermore, J., Ilstrup, D., and Morrey, B., "Effect of Femoral Head Size on Wear of the Polyethylene Acetabular Component," J. Bone and Joint Surg., **72-A** (4) 1990: 518-528.

[19] Isaac, G.H., Wroblewski, B.M., Atkinson, J.R., and Dowson, D., "A Tribological Study of Retrieved Hip Prostheses," Clin. Orthop., **276** (1992): 115-125.

[20] Lazcano, M.A., Marin, J.M., Parroquin, J., and Sauri, J.C., "Wear of the Charnley Low Friction Arthroplasty Cup 18 to 22 Years," Scientific Exhibit SE52, 60th AAOS, 1993.

[21] Kabo, et al., J. Bone and Joint Surg., **75B** (1993): 254-257.

[22] Hernandez, J.R., Keating, E.M., Faris, P.M., Meding, J.B., and Ritter, M.A., "Polyethylene Wear in Uncemented Acetabular Components," JBJS, **76-B** (2) (1994): 263-266.

[23] Peterson et al., "Rate of In-Vivo Polyethylene Wear for Five Different Acetabular Components Used Over a Five to Twenty-Two Year Period," UHMWPE Workshop, ASTM F04 Spring Meeting, Montreal, 1994.

[24] Berzins, A., Sumner, R., Igloria, R., and Galante, J., "Wear Analysis of Autopsy-Retrieved Liners Based on Ultrasonic Measurements," Trans. 18th Society for Biomaterials Meeting, 1995: 92.

[25] Callaghan, J.J., Pedersen, D.R., Olejniczak, J.P., Goetz, D.D., and Johnston, R.C., "Radiographic Measurement of Wear in 5 Cohorts of Patients Observed for 5 to 22 Years," Clin. Ortho. Rel. Res., **317** (1995): 14-18.

[26] Woolson, S.T. and Murphy, M.G., "Wear of the Polyethylene of Harris-Galante Acetabular Components Inserted without Cement," J. Bone and Joint Surg., **77-A** (9) (1995): 1311-1314.

[27] Kesteris, U., Ilchmann, T., Wingstrand, H., and Onnerfalt, R. "Polyethylene Wear in Scanhip Arthroplasty with a 22 or 32 mm Head," Acta. Orthop. Scand., **67** (2) 1996: 125-127.

[28] Sychterz, C.J., Moon, K.H., Hashimoto, Y., Terefenko, K.M., Engh, C.A., and Bauer, T.W., "Wear of Polyethylene Cups in Total Hip Arthroplasty," J. Bone and Joint Surg., **78-A** (8) (1996): 1193-1200.

[29] Hailey, J.L., Ingham, E., Stone, M., Wroblewski, B.M., and Fisher, J., "Quantitative Comparison of Acetabular Cup Wear Rates and Femoral Head Damage in Explanted Charnley Hip Prostheses," Trans. 43rd ORS (1997): 853.

[30] Griffith, M., Sedienstein, M., Williams, D., and Charnley, J., "Socket Wear in Charnley Low Friction Arthroplasty of the Hip," Clin. Orthop., **137** (1978): 37-47.

[31] Isaac, G.H., Dowson, D., and Wroblewski, B.M., "An Investigation Into the Origins of Time-dependent Variation in Penetration Rates With Charnley Acetabular Cups - Wear, Creep, or Degradation?" Proc. Instn. Mech. Engrs./IMechE, **210** (1996): 209-216.

[32] Charnley, J., "Factors in the Design of an Artificial Hip Joint", in "Lubrication and Wear in Living and Artificial Human Joints," Proc. Inst. Mech. Eng., London, **181** (3J) (1966): 104.

[33] Charnley, J., Kamanger, A., and Longfield, M.D., "The Optimum Size of Prosthetic Heads in Relation to the Wear of Plastic Sockets in Total Replacement of the Hip," Med. Biol. Eng., **7** (1969): 31-39.

[34] Charnley, J., "Total Hip Replacement by Low-Friction Arthroplasty," Clin. Orthop., **72** (1970): 7-21.

[35] Dumbleton, J.H., "Prosthesis Materials and Devices - A Review," In Vitro and In Vivo Wear Measurements on Joint Prosthesis Materials and Devices, Chapter 20, 1982: 427-460.

[36] Charnley, J., "Plastics in Medicine and Surgery," Plastics and Rubber Institute, London, 1975.

[37] McKellop, H., Clarke, I., Markolf, K., and Amstutz, H., "Friction and Wear Properties of Polymer, Metal and Ceramic Prosthetic Joint Materials Evaluated on a Multichannel Screening Device," J. Biomedical Materials Research, **15** (1981): 619-653.

[38] Galante, J.O. and Rostoker, W., "Wear in Total Hip Prostheses. An Experimental Evaluation of Candidate Materials," Acta. Orthop. Scand., Suppl. 145, 1973.

[39] Wong, A.T., Meeting minutes from 11/14/94 ASTM D4020 Task Group.

[40] Amstutz, H.C. and Grigoris, P., "Metal on Metal Bearings in Hip Arthroplasty," Clin. Orthop., **329S** (1996): S11-S34.

[41] Semlitsch, M. and Willert, H.B., "Clinical Wear Behavior of Ultra-High Molecular Weight Polyethylene Cups Paired with Metal and Ceramic Ball Heads in Comparison to Metal-on-Metal Pairings of Hip Joint Replacements," Proc. Instn. Mech. Engrs./IMechE, **211**, Part H (1997): 73-88.

[42] McKee, G.K., "Total Hip Replacement - Past, Present, and Future," Biomaterials, **3** (1982): 130-135.

[43] Streicher, R.M., Schon, R., and Semlitsch, M., "Investigation of the Tribological Behavior of Metal-on-Metal Combinations for Artificial Hip Joints," Biomedizinische Technik, **35** (1990): 107-111.

[44] Farrar, R. and Schmidt, M.B., "The Effect of Diametral Clearance on Wear Between Head and Cup for Metal on Metal Articulations," Trans. 43rd ORS, February 1997: 71.

[45] Scott, R.A. and Schroeder, D.W., "The Effect of Radial Mismatch on the Wear of Metal on Metal Hip Prosthesis: A Hip Simulator Study," Trans. 43rd ORS, February 1997: 764.

[46] Chan F.W., Medley, J.B., Bobyn, J.D., Krygier, J.J., Podgorsak, G.F., and Tanzer, M., "Investigation of Parameters Controlling Wear of Metal-Metal Bearings in Total Hip Arthroplasty," Trans. 43rd ORS, Feb. 1997, p. 763.

[47] Dobbs, H.S., "Analysis and Prediction of Total Hip Replacement Performance," J. Mater. Sci., **16** (1981): 1204-1208.

[48] Semlitsch, M., Streicher, R.M., and Weber, H., Orthopaede, **18** (1989): 337-381.

[49] Muller, M.E., "The Benefits of Metal-on-Metal Total Hip Replacements," Clin. Orthop., **311** (1995): 54-59.

[50] Schmalzreid, T.P., Peters, P.C., Maurer, B.T., Bragdon, C.R., and Harris, W.H., "Long Duration Metal-on-Metal Total Hip Replacements with Low Wear of the Articulating Surfaces," 63rd Annual AAOS, February 1996: 385.

[51] Doorn, P., Campbell, P., Benya, P., Worrall, J., Salib, D., Kirchen, M., McKellop, H., and Amstutz, H., "The Application of Transmission Electron Microscopy to the Characterization of Metal Wear Particles from Metal-on-Metal Total Hip Replacements," Trans. 43rd ORS, February 1997: 70.

[52] McKellop, H., Campbell, P., Lu, B., Park, S.H., Doorn, P., and Dorr, L., "Clinical Wear Performance of Modern Metal-on-Metal Hip Arthroplasties," Trans. 43rd ORS, February 1997: 766.

[53] Semlitsch, M., "Increased Wear Resistance of Radiochemically Treated Polyester for Bioengineering Applications in Joint Surgery," Tech. Rep. 118, Sulzer Bros., Winterhur, Switzerland, 1972.

[54] Scales, J. and Lowe, S., "Choosing Materials for Bone and Joint Replacement," Engineering In Medicine, **1** (2) (1972): 52.

[55] Weber, B. and Semlitsch, M., "Total Hip Replacement with Rotation Endoprostheses: Problem of Wear," Arthroplasty of the Hip, G. Chapchal, Ed., Georg Thieme, Stuttgart, 1972: 71.

[56] Dumbleton, J., Shen, P., and Miller, E., "A Study of the Wear of Some Materials in Connection with Total Hip Replacement," Wear, **29** (1974): 163.

[57] Walker, P. and Erkman, M., "Variables Affecting Polymer Wear in Artificial Human Joints," Advances in Polymer Friction and Wear, Vol. 5B, Lieng-Huang Lee, Ed., Plenum Press, New York, 1974: 553.

[58] Capozzo, A., Cini, L., Pizzoferrato, A., Trentani, C., and Cortes, S., "Evaluation of Hip Arthroprostheses by Means of Body Environment Simulators," J. Biomedical Materials Research, **11** (1977): 657.

[59] Willert, H.G., and Semlitsch, M., "Tissue Reactions to Plastic and Metallic Wear Products of Joint Endoprostheses," Total Hip Prostheses, William & Wilkins, Baltimore, 1976: 205.

[60] Duff-Barclay, I. and Spillman, D., "Total Human Hip Joint Prostheses—A Laboratory Study of Friction and Wear," Proc. Inst. Mech. Eng., London, Part 3, **181** (1966): 90.

[61] Amstutz, H., "Polymers as Bearing Materials for Total Hip Replacement: A Friction and Wear Analysis," J. Biomedical Materials Research, **3** (1968): 547.

[62] Homsy, C. and King, J., "Friction and Wear Behavior of Prosthetic Cartilage Materials Under Simulated In-Vivo Conditions," Trans. 18th ORS, Washington D.C., 1973.

[63] Shen, C. and Dumbleton, J.H. "The Friction and Wear Behavior of Polyoxymethylene in Connection with Joint Replacement," Wear, **38** (1976): 291.

[64] Dumbleton, J., "Delrin as a Material for Joint Prostheses—A Review," in Corrosion and Degradation of Implant Materials, ASTM STP 684 B.C. Syrett and A. Acharya, Eds., American Society for Testing and Materials, 1979: 41.

[65] Clarke, I. and McKellop, H., "The Wear of Delrin 150 Compared to Polyethylene, Polyester, and PTFE," Mechanical Properties of Biomaterials, G.W. Hastings and D.F. Williams, Eds., John Wiley & Sons, New York, 1980: 27.

[66] Dumbleton, J.H., "The Tribology of Natural and Artificial Joints," Elsevier, Amsterdam (1981), Chap. 7-8.

[67] McKellop, H., "Wear of Artificial Joint Materials II: Twelve-Channel Wear-Screening Device: Correlation of Experimental and Clinical Results," Engineering In Medicine, **10** (1981): 123-136.

[68] Clarke, I., "Wear-Screening and Joint Simulation Studies Versus Materials Selection and Prosthesis Design," CRC Critical Reviews in Biomedical Engineering, Vol. 8, Issue 1, 1982: 29-91.

[69] Semlitsch, M., Lehmann, M., Weber, H., Doerre, E., and Willert, H., "New Prospects for a Prolonged Functional Life-Span of Artificial Hip Joints by Using the Material Combination Polyethylene/Aluminum Oxide Ceramic/Metal," J. Biomedical Materials Research, **11** (1977): 537.

[70] Wright, K.W.J. and Scales, J.T., Proceedings of the Third Conference on Mechanical Properties of Biomaterials and Bioceramics Symposium, Biological Engineering Society, Keele (1978).

[71] Niederer, P., Semlitsch, M., Doerre, E., and Dietschi, C., "Total Hip Arthroplasty with Ceramic-Polyethylene Articulation," Scientific Exhibit Presented at SICOT '78 XIV World Congress, Kyoto, Japan, Oct. 1978.

[72] Wright, K. and Scales, J., "The Use of Hip Joint Simulators for the Evaluation of Wear of Total Hip Prostheses," Evaluation of Biomaterials, G. Writer, J. Lerey, and K. de Grosst, Eds., John Wiley & Sons, New York, 1980: 135.

[73] McKellop, H., Lu, B., and Benya, P., "Friction, Lubrication and Wear of Cobalt-Chromium, Alumina, and Zirconia Hip Prostheses Compared on a Joint Simulator," Trans. 38th ORS, February 1992: 402.

[74] Weber, B.G., "Total Hip Replacement: Rotating Versus Fixed and Metal Versus Ceramic Heads," The Hip, 1981: 264-275.

[75] Oonishi, H., Igaki, H., and Takayama, Y., "Comparisons of Wear of UHMWPE Sliding Against Metal and Alumina in Total Hip Prosthesis," Bioceramics, **1** (1989): 272.

[76] Schuller, H. and Marti, R., "Ten-year Socket Wear in 66 Hip Arthroplasties—Ceramic Versus Metal Heads," Acta. Orthop. Scand., **61** (1990): 240.

[77] Zichner, L.P. and Willert, H-G., "Comparison of Alumina-Polyethylene and Metal-Polyethylene in Clinical Trials," Clin. Orthop., **282** (1992): 86-94.

[78] Bragdon, C.R., Jasty, M., Kawate, K., Elder, J., Lowenstein, J.D., and Harris, W.H., "Wear at the Ceramic on Polyethylene Articulation," Trans. 21st Society for Biomaterials Meeting, March 1995: 50.

[79] Livingston, B.J., Chmell, M.J., Reilly, D.T., Spector, M., and Poss, R., "The Wear Rate of Hylamer Cups is Higher Than Conventional PE and Differs with Heads from Different Manufacturers," Trans. 43rd ORS, February 1997: 141.

[80] Taylor et al., presented at 6th International Conference on Surface Modifications, Chicago, November 1992.

[81] Wallbridge, N., Dowson, D., and Roberts, E.W., "A Study of the Wear Characteristics of Sliding Pairs of High Density Polycrystalline Aluminum Oxide with Particular Reference to Their Use in Total Replacement Human Joints," Engineering In Medicine, **12** (1983): 23-28.

[82] Walter, A. and Plitz, W., "The Ring-on-Disc Method—Clinical Significance of a Wear-Screening Test of Biomaterials for Hip Joint Alloplasty," Bioceramics: Current Interdisciplinary Research, S.M. Perren and E. Schneider, Eds., Dordrect/Boston/Lancaster, Martinus Nijhoff, (1985): 129-134.

[83] Walter, A., "Wear-Screening of Ceramic-to-Ceramic Components for Total Hip Replacements by Ring-on-Disc and Joint Simulator Test," Ceramics in Clinical Applications, P. Vicenzini, Ed., Amsterdam, Elsevier, (1987): 159-168.

[84] Boutin, P., "THR Using Alumina-Alumina Sliding and Metallic Stem: 1330 cases and an 11 Years Follow-up," Orthopaedic Ceramic Implants, Proc. Jap. Soc. Orthop. Ceram. Implants, **1**, H. Oonishi and Y. Ooi, Eds., (1981): 11-19.

[85] Sawai, K., Niwa, S., Yamazaki, S., Honjo, H., Miki, S., Hori, M., and Hattori, T., "Unusual Excessive Wearing of the Ceramic Total Hip Implants Caused by Shaky Movement Between These Components," Orthopaedic Ceramic Implants, Proc. Jap. Soc. Orthop. Ceram. Implants , **1**, H. Oonishi and Y. Ooi, Eds., (1981): 51-57.

[86] Boutin, P., Christel, P., Dorlot, J.M., Meunier, A., Sedel, L., and Witvoet, J., "A View of 15 Years Results Obtained Using the Alumina-Alumina Hip Joint Prostheses," Ceramics in Clinical Applications, P. Vincenzini, Ed., Amsterdam, Elsevier, (1987): 297-303.

[87] Kummer, F.J., Stuchin, S.A., and Frankel, V.H., "Analysis of Removed Autophor Ceramic-on-Ceramic Components," J. Arthroplasty, **5** (1) (1990): 29-33.

[88] Sedel, L., Kerboull, L., Cristel, P., Meunier, A., and Witvoet, J., "Alumina-on-Alumina Hip Replacement—Results and Survivorship in Young Patients," J. Bone and Joint Surgery, **72B** (4) (1990): 658-663.

[89] Borssen, B., Karrholm, J., and Snorrason, F., "Osteolysis after Ceramic-on-Ceramic Hip Arthroplasty," Acta. Orthop. Scand., **62** (1) (1991): 73-75.

[90] Mittelmeier, H. and Heisel, J., "Sixteen-Years' Experience with Ceramic Hip Prostheses," Clin. Orthop., **282** (1992): 64-72.

[91] Sedel, L., Nizard, R.S., Kerboull, L., and Witvoet, J., "Alumina-Alumina Hip Replacement in Patients Younger Than 50 Years Old," Clin. Orthop., **298** (1994): 175-183.

[92] Boehlar, M., Knahr, K., Plenk, H. Jr., Walter, A., Salzer, M., and Schreiber, V., "Long-Term Results of Uncemented Alumina Acetabular Implants," JBJS, **76B** (1) (1994): 53-59.

[93] Sclippa, E. and Piekarski, J., "Carbon Fiber Reinforced Polyethylene for Possible Orthopaedic Uses," J. Biomedical Materials Research , **7** (1973): 59-70.

[94] Tetik, R., "Preliminary Evaluation of Polyethylene Graphite as a Material for Use in Total Hip Replacement," Proc. Inst. Med. Chic. (1973): 29.

[95] Ainsworth, R.D., Farling, G.M., and Bardos, D.I., "Human Surgical Implant Structural Devices of Carbon Fiber Reinforced Ultra-High Molecular Weight Polyethylene," Zimmer Technical Brief, 1977: 167-169.

[96] Greer, K.W., "Four Years of Wear Testing Experience on Three Joint Simulators," 11th Int. Biomaterials Sym., Clemson, April-May 1979.

[97] McKellop, H., Markolf, K.L., and Amstutz, H.C., "Comparative Wear of Conventional and Carbon Fiber-Reinforced UHMW Polyethylenes," Trans. 27th ORS, 1981: 168.

[98] Peterson, C.D., Hillberry, B.M., and Heck, D.A., "Component Wear of Total Knee Prostheses Using Ti-6Al-4V, Titanium Nitride Coated Ti-6Al-4V, and Cobalt-Chromium-Molybdenum Femoral Components," J. Biomedical Materials Research, **22** (1988): 887-903.

[99] Wright, T.M., Bartel, D.L., and Rimnac, C.M., "Carbon Fiber-Reinforced UHMWPE for Total Joint Replacement Components," Composites in Biomedical Engineering, **21** (1985): 1-3.

[100] Wright, T.M., Rimnac, C.M., Faris, P.M., and Bansal, M., "Analysis of Surface Damage in Retrieved Carbon Fiber-Reinforced and Plain Polyethylene Tibial Components from Posterior Stabilized Total Knee Replacements," J. Bone and Joint Surgery, **70-A** (9) (1988): 1312-1319.

[101] Wright, T.M., Astion, D.J., Bansal, M., Rimnac, C.M., Green, T., Insall, J.N., and Robinson, R.P., "Failure of Carbon Fiber-Reinforced Polyethylene Total Knee-Replacement Components," J. Bone and Joint Surgery, **70-A** (6) (1988): 926-932.

[102] Kraay, M.J., Goldberg, V.M., Brown, S.A., and Merritt, K., "Clinical Experience with Ti-6Al-4V Miller Galante Total Knee Replacements," Symposium on Medical Applications of Titanium, ASTM F04 Fall Meeting, Phoenix, AZ, November 1994.

[103] Chillag et al., "Symposium: The Relationship Between Polyethylene Quality and Wear," Contemporary Orthopaedics, **30** (1) (1995): 75-76.

[104] Miller, D., Ainsworth, R., Dumbleton, J., Page, D., Miller, E.H., and Shen, G., "A Comparative Evaluation of the Wear of Ultrahigh Molecular Weight Polyethylene Abraded by Ti-6Al-4V," Wear, **28** (1974): 207.

[105] Revell, P.A., Weightman, B., Freeman, M.A.R., and Roberts, B.V., "The Production and Biology of Polyethylene Wear Debris," Arch. Orthop. Traum. Surg., **91** (1978): 167.

[106] McKellop, H., Clarke, I., Markolf, K., and Amstutz, H., "Wear Properties of New High Strength Alloys for Prosthetic Joints," Trans. 25th ORS, February 1979.

[107] Greer, K., "Hip Simulator Wear Testing Summary for Ti-6Al-4V," Tech. Memo #319, Zimmer, Warsaw, IN, January 1980.

[108] McKellop, H., Kirkpatrick, J., Markolf, K., and Amstutz, H., "Abrasive Wear of Ti-6Al-4V Prostheses by Acrylic Cement Particles," Trans. 26th ORS, February 1980.

[109] Rostoker, W. and Galante, J.O., "The Influence of Titanium Surface Treatments on the Wear of Medical Grade Polyethylene," Biomaterials, **2** (1981): 221-224.

[110] McKellop, H.A. and Clarke, I.C., "Evolution and Evaluation of Materials-Screening Machines and Joint Simulators in Predicting In Vivo Wear Phenomena," Functional Behavior of Orthopaedic Biomaterials, Vol. II: Applications, Chap. 3, P. Ducheyne and G.W. Hastings, Eds., CRC Press, Boca Raton, FL, 1983: 51-85.

[111] McKellop, H., Redfern, F., Okuda, R., and Clarke, I., "Correlation of Hip Joint Simulator Wear Tests with Clinical Experience," Trans. 8th Society for Biomaterials Meeting, April 1982.

[112] Starkebaum, W. and Woodman, J.L., "Metallic Wear of Total Hip Components: A Joint Simulator Study," Trans. 9th Society for Biomaterials Meeting, April 1983: 9.

[113] Gruen, T.A., Espiritu, E.T., McGuire, P., Hull, D., and Sarmiento, A., "In-Vivo Performance of Titanium Alloy Total Hip Replacement Femoral Components," ASTM Symposium On Use of Titanium, Phoenix, AZ, May 1981.

[114] Agins, H.J., Alcock, N.W., Bansal, M., Salvati, E., Wilson, P.D., Pellici, P.M., and Bullough, P.G., "Metallic Wear in Failed Titanium Alloy Total Hip Replacement," J. Bone and Joint Surgery, **70-A** (1988): 347-356.

[115] Lombardi, A.V., Mallory, T.H., Vaughn, B.K., and Drouillard, P., "Aseptic Loosening in Total Hip Arthroplasty Secondary to Osteolysis Induced by Wear Debris from Titanium-Alloy Modular Femoral Heads," J. Bone and Joint Surgery, **71-A** (9) (1989): 1337-1342.

[116] Black, J., Sherk, H., Bonini, J., Rostoker, W.R., Schajowicz, F., and Galante, J.O., "Metallosis Associated with a Stable Titanium-Alloy Femoral Component in Total Hip Replacement. A Case Report." J. Bone and Joint Surgery, **72-A** (1990): 126-130.

[117] McKellop, H.A., Sarmiento, A., Schwinn, C.P., and Erbamzadeh, E., "In Vivo Wear of Titanium-Alloy Hip Prostheses," J. Bone and Joint Surgery, **72-A** (1990): 512-517.

[118] McKellop, H., Rostlund, T., Ebramzadeh, E., and Sarmiento, A., "Wear Properties of Titanium Alloy Bearing Surfaces of Total Hip Prostheses in Laboratory Tests and In-Vivo," Symposium on Medical Applications of Titanium, ASTM F04 Fall Meeting, Phoenix, AZ, November 1994.

[119] Cautilli, G.P., Beight, J.L., Yao, B., Hozack, W.J., and Rothman, R.H., "A Prospective Review of 303 Cementless Universal Cups with Emphasis on Wear as Cause of Failure," Scientific Exhibit SE51, 60th Annual AAOS Meeting, February 1993.

[120] McKellop, H.A. and Rostlund, T.V., "The Wear Behavior of Ion-Implanted Ti-6Al-4V against UHMW Polyethylene," J. Biomedical Materials Research, **24** (1990): 1413-1425.

[121] Gilbertson, L., "Effects of Nitrogen Ion Implantation on the Medical Properties of Ti-6Al-4V," presented at Workshop on Ion Implantation of Medical Devices, ASTM F04 Spring Meeting, Atlantic City, NJ, May 1991.

[122] Rieu, J., Pichat, A., Rabbe L-M., Rambert, A., Chabrol, C., and Robelet, M., "Structural Modifications Induced by Ion Implantation in Metals and Polymers Used for Orthopaedic Prostheses," Surface Modification Technologies V, T.S. Sudarshan and J.F. Braza, Eds., The Institute of Materials, 1992: 155-165.

[123] McKellop, H., "Alternate Femoral Heads," presented at the 22nd Annual Hip Society Meeting, New Orleans, February 27, 1994.

[124] Sioshansi, P., "Ion Implantation of Cobalt-Chromium Prosthetic Components to Reduce Polyethylene Wear," Orthopedics Today, August 1991: 24-25.

[125] Poggie et al., presented at 6th International Conference on Surface Modifications, Chicago, November 1992.

[126] Greer, K.W. and Jones, D.E., "The Importance of Standardization of Wear Test Parameters in the Simulation of Knee Wear Mechanisms," Trans. 20th Society for Biomaterials Meeting, April 1994: 408.

[127] Schmidt, M.B., Lin. M., and Greer, K.W., "Wear Performance of UHMWPE Articulated Against Ion Implanted CoCr," Trans. 21st Society for Biomaterials Meeting, March 1995: 230.

[128] Bleobaum, R.D., Nelson, K., Dorr, L.D., Hofmann, A.A., and Lyman, D.J., "Investigation of Early Surface Delamination Observed in Retrieved Heat-Pressed Tibial Inserts," Clin. Orthop., **269** (1991): 120-127.

[129] Kobayashi, S. and Terayama, K., "Rapid Tibial Polyethylene Failure in Porous-coated Anatomic Total Knees as a Cause of Clinical Failure," Contemporary Orthopaedics, **26** (6) (1993): 567-576.

[130] Knight, J.L., Gorai, P.A., Atwater, R.D., and Grothans, L., "Tibial Polyethylene Failure After Primary Porous-Coated Anatomic Total Knee Arthroplasty," J. Arthroplasty, **10** (6) (1995): 748-757.

[131] Mintz, L., Tsao, A.K., McCrae, C.R., Stulberg, S.D., and Wright, T.M., "The Arthroscopic Evaluation and Characteristics of Severe Polyethylene Wear in Total Knee Arthroplasty," Clin. Orthop., **273** (1991): 215-222.

[132] Wright, T.M., Rimnac, C.M., Stulberg, S.D., Mintz, L., Tsao, A.K., Klein, R.W., and McCrae, C., "Wear of Polyethylene in Total Joint Replacements," Clin. Orthop., **276** (1992): 126-134.

[133] Blunn, G.W., Joshi, A.B., Lilley, P.A., Engelbrecht, E., Ryd, L., Lidgren, L., Hardinge, K., Neider, E., and Walker, P. "Polyethylene Wear in Unicondylar Knee Prostheses," Acta. Orthop. Scand., **63** (3) (1992): 247-255.

[134] Saum, K., "Past, Present, and Future of Polyethylene," presented at Harvard Combined Orthopedic Grand Rounds, December 1992.

[135] Davidson, J.A., Poggie, R.A., Mishra, A.K., Salehi, A., and Harbaugh, M.E., "Increased Wear and Contact Stress From Increased Polyethylene Stiffness in Prosthetic Knee and Hip Articulation," Proc. 7th International Conf. On Biomed. Eng., Singapore, December 1992.

[136] Chmell, M.J., Poss, R., Thomas, W.H., and Sledge, C.B., "Early Failure of Hylamer Acetabular Inserts Due to Eccentric Wear," J. Arthroplasty, **11** (3) 1996: 351-353.

[137] Sychterz, C.J., Shah, N., and Engh, C.A., "Radiographic Evaluation of Femoral Head Penetration Into Polyethylene Liners: Hylamer vs. Enduron," Trans. 43rd ORS, February 1997: 140.

[138] Schmalzried, T.P., Szuszczewicz, E.S., Campbell, P.C., and McKellop, H.A., "Femoral Head Surface Roughness and Patient Activity in the Wear of Hylamer," Trans. 43rd ORS, February 1997: 787.

[139] Muratoglu, O.K., Imlach, H., Estok, D., Ramamurti, B., Sedlacek, R., Jasty, M., and Harris, W.H., "Analysis of Eight Retrieved Hylamer Acetabular Components," Trans. 43rd ORS, February 1997: 852.

[140] Scales, J.T. and Wright, J.W.J., "Experimental Methods for the Assessment of Wear of Materials Potentially Useful for Endoprostheses," Acta. Orthop. Belg., **41** (Suppl. 1) (1975): 160.

[141] McKellop, H., Griffin, G., and Clarke, I., and Markolf, K., "Increased Wear of UHMW Polyethylene After Gamma Radiation Sterilization," Trans. 26th ORS, February, 1980: 99.

[142] Fisher, J., Reeves, E.A., Isaac, G.H., Saum, K.A., and Sanford, W.M., "Comparison of the Wear of Aged and Non-aged Ultrahigh Molecular Weight Polyethylene Sterilized by Gamma Irradiation and by Gas Plasma," J. Mater. Sci.: Materials in Medicine, **8** (1997): 375-378.

[143] Trieu, H.H., Jahan, M.D., Buchanan, D.J., Thomas, D.E., Morris, L.H., Needham, D.A., Rouleau, J.P., Haggard, W.O., Conta, R.L., and Parr, J.E., "Relationships Between Free Radicals, Oxidative Degradation and Wear Resistance of UHMWPE Tibial Components," Scientific Exhibit, 64th AAOS Meeting, February 1997.

[144] Wang, A., Stark, C., and Dumbleton, J.H., "Mechanistic and Morphological Origins of Ultra-High Molecular Weight Polyethylene Wear Debris in Total Joint Replacement Prostheses," Proc. Instn. Mech. Engrs./IMechE, **210** (1996): 141-155.

[145] Hamilton, J.V., Schmidt, M.B., and Greer, K.W., "Improved Wear of UHMWPE Using Gamma Sterilization and a Vacuum-Foil Package," Scientific Exhibit, 64th AAOS Meeting, February 1997.

[146] McKellop, H.A., Shen, F.W., Yu, Y. J., Lu, B., and Salovey, R., "Effect of Sterilization Method on the Wear Rate of UHMW Polyethylene Acetabular Cups in a Hip Simulator," Trans. 43rd ORS, February 1997: 94.

[147] Streicher, R.M., "Influence of Ionizing Irradiation on Properties and In Vivo and In-Vivo Long-Term Behavior of UHMWPE," Trans. 20th Society for Biomaterials Meeting, April 1994: 119.

[148] White, S.E., Paxson, R., Whiteside, L., and Tanner, M., "The Effects of Sterilization on Wear in Total Knee Arthroplasty," Trans. 1996 Knee Society Meeting, Paper #22, February 1996.

[149] Sutula, L.C., Collier, J.P., Saum, K.A., Currier, B.H., Currier, J.H., Sanford, W.M., Mayor, M.B., Wooding, R.E., Sperling, D.K., Williams, I.R., Kasprzak, D.J., and Surprenant, V.A., "Impact of Gamma Sterilization on Clinical Performance of Polyethylene in the Hip," Clin. Orthop., **319** (1995): 28-40.

[150] Collier, J.P., "The Effects of Sterilization Polyethylene," Orthopaedic Special Edition, **2** (2) (1996): 33-35.

[151] Oonishi, H., Ishimaru, H., and Kato, A., "Effect of Cross-Linkage by Gamma Radiation in Heavy Doses to Low Wear Polyethylene in Total Hip Prostheses," J. Mater. Sci.: Materials in Medicine, **7** (1996): 753-763.

[152] Oonishi, H., Kuno, M., Tsuji, E., and Fujisawa, A., "The Optimum Dose of Gamma Radiation—Heavy Doses to Low Wear Polyethylene in Total Hip Prostheses," J. Mater. Sci.: Materials in Medicine, **8** (1997): 11-18.

[153] Caravia, L., Jin, Z.M., Dowson, D., and Fisher, J., "Friction and Wear of Polyurethane Materials in Cushion Form Bearing for Artificial Joints," Trans. 4th World Biomaterials Congress, Berlin, April 1992: 606.

[154] McKellop, H.A., Rostlund, T., and Bradley, G., "Evaluation of Wear in an All-Polymer Total Knee Replacement. Part I: Laboratory Testing of Polyethylene on Polyacetal Bearing Surfaces," Clinical Materials, **14** (1993): 117-126.

[155] Sioshansi, P., "Wear Reduction of UHMWPE Through Ion Implantation," Spire Corporation Technical Report, March 23, 1993.

[156] Rieu, J., Pichat, A., Rabbe, L-M., Rambert, A., Chabral, C., and Robelet, M., "Ion Implantation Effects on Friction and Wear of Joint Prosthesis Materials," Biomaterials, **12** (1991): 139-143.

[157] Dearnaley, G., presented at 4th World Biomaterials Congress, Berlin, April 1992.

[158] Lilley, P.A., Walker, P.S., and Blunn, G.W., "Potential Reduction of UHMWPE Wear in TKR by Ion-Implantation and DLC Coatings," Trans. 41st ORS, February 1995: 117.

[159] Streicher, R.M., Weber, H., Schon, R., and Semlitsch, M., "New Surface Modification for Ti-6Al-7Nb Alloy: Oxygen Diffusion Hardening (ODH)," Biomaterials, **12** (1991): 125-129.

[160] White, S.E., Whiteside, L.A., McCarthy, D.S., Anthony, M., and Poggie, R.A., "Simulated Knee Wear with Cobalt Chromium and Oxidized Zirconium Knee Femoral Components," Clin. Orthop., **309** (1994): 176-184.

[161] Poggie, R.A., Wert, J.J., Mishra, AK., and Davidson, J.A., "Friction and Wear Characterization of UHMWPE in Reciprocating Sliding Contact with Co-Cr, Ti-6Al-4V and Zirconia Implant Bearing Surfaces," Wear and Friction of Elastomers, ASTM STP 1145, Robert Denton and M.K. Keshaven, Eds., American Society for Testing and Materials, Philadelphia, 1992.

[162] Wang, A., Polineni, V.K., Essner, A., Sokol, M., Sun, D.C., Stark, C., and Dumbleton, J.H., "The Significance of Nonlinear Motion in the Wear Screening of Orthopaedic Implant Materials," Journal of Testing and Evaluation, **25** (2) (1997): 239-245.

[163] McKellop, H.A., "Comparison Between Laboratory Wear Tests and Clinical Performance of Past Bearing Materials," ASTM F04 Workshop on Characterization and Performance of Articular Surfaces, American Society for Testing and Materials, Denver, CO, May 17, 1995.

[164] Walker, P.S., Blunn, G.W., and Lilley, P.A., "Wear Testing of Materials and Surfaces for Total Knee Replacement," J. Biomedical Materials Research, **33** (1996): 159-175.

[165] McKellop, H., Letter to ASTM, Nov. 17, 1994.

[166] Clarke, I.C., Gustafson, A., Jung, H., and Fujisawa, A., "Hip-Simulator Ranking of Polyethylene Wear," Acta. Orthop. Scand., **67** (2) (1996): 128-132.

[167] McKellop, H.A., Campbell, P., Park, S.-H., Schmalzried, T.P., Grigoris, P., Amstutz, H.C., and Sarmiento, A., "The Origin of Submicron Polyethyene in Total Hip Arthroplasty," Clin. Orthop., **311** (1995): 3-20.

[168] Wright, T.M. and Goodman, S.B., Eds., Implant Wear: The Future of Total Joint Replacement, American Academy of Orthopaedic Surgeons, 1996: 96-97.

Markus A. Wimmer[1], Roman Nassutt[1], Frank Lampe[2], Erich Schneider[1], and Michael M. Morlock[1]

A NEW SCREENING METHOD DESIGNED FOR WEAR ANALYSIS OF BEARING SURFACES USED IN TOTAL HIP ARTHROPLASTY

REFERENCE: Wimmer, M. A., Nassutt, R., Lampe, F., Schneider, E., and Morlock, M. M., **"A New Screening Method Designed for Wear Analysis of Bearing Surfaces Used in Total Hip Arthroplasty,"** *Alternative Bearing Surfaces in Total Joint Replacement, ASTM STP 1346*, J. J. Jacobs and T. L. Craig, Eds., American Society for Testing and Materials, 1998.

ABSTRACT: New technologies of surface treatment are speculated to reduce or prevent the generation of polyethylene particles. These new (spherical) bearing surfaces need to be evaluated with an appropriate testing method. Results from testing of flat surfaces are - in general- difficult to interpret.
A bi-axial *"pin-on-ball"* device utilising commercially available components of artificial joints has been developed. The contact zone kinematics in hip joints according to in-vivo conditions are approximated. First results are promising: a phase shift between the pin and ball oscillations produced quasi-elliptical displacement trajectories, similar to the ones which are reported to take place during gait. The "pin-on-ball" set-up allowed to identify subtle characteristics of friction and generated a wear pattern which matched the features known from retrieval studies. Therefore, this new testing device might be an interesting alternative to common screening devices.

KEYWORDS: wear, friction, hip prostheses, contact kinematics, material testing

Nomenclature

t	time
x_o	initial x-coordinate of a point on the pin surface

[1] Ph.D. Student, Ph.D. Student, Dr.sc.tech., Head, and Ph.D. Assistant Professor, respectively, Biomechanics Section, Technical University Hamburg-Harburg, 21071 Hamburg, Germany.
[2] MD, Orthopedic Surgeon, Department of Orthopedics, General Hospital Barmbek, 22337 Hamburg, Germany.

y_o	initial y-coordinate of a point on the pin surface
F_n	normal load
M_t	frictional moment (torque)
R	radius of the femoral head
μ	coefficient of friction
φ_p	phase difference of pin and ball oscillation
$\phi(t)$	oscillation of the ball
$\psi(t)$	oscillation of the pin
ω_b	frequency of oscillation of the ball
ω_p	frequency of oscillation of the pin
Φ	amplitude of oscillation of the ball
Ψ	amplitude of oscillation of the pin
ø	diameter

Introduction

There has been growing concern about ultra-high-molecular-weight polyethylene (UHMWPE) debris generated during normal function in total hip replacement (THR). The generated particles originate from the acetabular bearing surface of the hip joint and have been associated with foreign body mediated bone resorption (osteolysis). Subsequent problems such as component loosening were described in numerous studies [1, 2, 3] and new technologies of surface treatment have been examined with respect to their potential to reduce or prevent UHMWPE wear. The wear properties of polymers against various counterbodies are typically assessed with relatively simple wear screening machines [4].

Common screening machines are the pin-on-disc or pin-on-flat designs. The pin usually represents the polymer, which is slid over a uni-directional rotating disk or reciprocating plate, respectively. The surface finish of a flat disk or plate, however, might cause problems when new technologies of surface treatment for alternative bearing surfaces in THR are evaluated: the artificial hip joint consists of a spherical metal or ceramic femoral head running in a UHMWPE socket. The polishing and coating procedures applied to the head might not be reproducable for a disk or plate, since the technology differs between spherical and flat [5].

Screening tests are intended to approximate the sliding conditions encountered in-vivo as close as possible. Care is taken to simulate similar surface pressures, sliding speeds and lubrication conditions in the pin-on-disc configuration. However, recently it has become evident that especially the contact zone kinematics influences the wear of certain polymers, including UHMWPE. Under otherwise the same conditions, higher wear rates have been observed, when an additional pin rotation was imposed on the rotating disk. Thereby the contact zone displacement trajectories changed from linear to curvilinear and, thus, influenced the creation and loss of polymer transfer films on the counterface [6].

An analysis of displacement trajectories during human locomotion on the acetabular bearing surface revealed, that the wear tracks form quasi-elliptical to rectangular paths [7]. Those paths vary widely in shape as well as in length over the contact area, but all cross each other during the cyclic motion pattern of gait. It has been suggested that the surface would experience multi-directional shear forces, which disturbes the structural alignment of UHMWPE and, thus, affects wear [7]. Further studies were able to demonstrate that the crossing of the wear tracks accelerates the formation of particulate debris [8]. Consequently this has been incorporated in hip simulators [9] which, however, are rather costly for the initial stage of material evaluation. Devices for early screening which simulate those important aspects of wear, are not yet available.

The objective of the study was to develop a bi-axial screening device for the determination of friction and wear of THR bearing surfaces. The testing configuration should account for the appropriate contact zone kinematics as well as the specific bearing geometry to reflect realistic wear properties.

Theoretical Considerations

The pin-on-ball concept

Based on the requirements mentioned above, a bi-axial *"pin-on-ball"* concept has been developed for friction and wear analyses of joints (Figure 1). The interface is comprised by a concave pin which is pressed onto a conforming ball. The pin is intended to represent the same geometrical and morphological features (e.g. machining marks) as original hip cups. The ball consists of a commercially available femoral head.

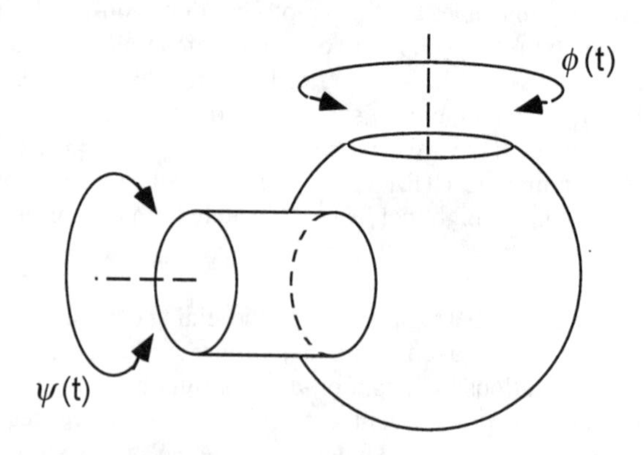

FIG. 1: *The functional principle of the pin-on-ball arrangement. A cylindrical pin with a conforming frontal plane is pressed radially onto a ball. The rotationary motion of the ball and the pin are orthogonal to each other.*

The center of the contact area between pin and ball is positioned on the equatorial circumference of the ball. A two-dimensional interface motion is generated by axial, independent oscillation of pin and ball. Thereby the instantaneous angle of oscillation of the ball is given by

$$\phi(t) = \Phi \cdot \sin(\omega_b t) \tag{1}$$

with Φ as the angular amplitude and ω_b as the frequency of oscillation of the ball. In a similar manner, the oscillation of the pin with respect to an axis perpendicular to $\phi\,(t)$ can be described:

$$\psi(t) = \Psi \cdot \sin(\omega_p t + \varphi_p); \tag{2}$$

whereby Ψ is the angular amplitude and ω_p the frequency of oscillation of the pin, while φ_p describes the phase shift of the oscillation of the pin in comparison to the ball.

Displacement trajectories within the contact area

The combination of oscillating pin and oscillating ball produces a complex interface motion. In order to visualize this motion, the displacement trajectories of specific locations of the contact area are calculated and plotted for a complete cycle of oscillation. In other words, the paths of several representative points of the ball on the pin surface are determined.

The spherical contact area of the pin on the ball is developed into a plane and described in cartesian coordinates x and y (Figure 2). While the ball rotates about an axis parallel to the y-axis and, thus, produces an interface motion in x-direction only, the pin rotates about the z-axis (coming out of the plane) and produces a motion in x- and y-direction. The amplitude of this motion rises with growing distance from the origin. Using equations (1) and (2), the location of point A at time t is given by

$$\bar{s}_A(t) = \begin{pmatrix} x_A(t) \\ y_A(t) \end{pmatrix} = \begin{pmatrix} \Phi \cdot \sqrt{R^2 - y^2}\,\sin(\omega_b t) + \sqrt{x_0^{\,2} + y_0^{\,2}}\,\cos\left[\Psi \cdot \sin(\omega_p t + \varphi_p) + \arctan\left(x_0/y_0\right)\right] \\ \sqrt{x_0^{\,2} + y_0^{\,2}}\,\sin\left[\Psi \cdot \sin(\omega_p t + \varphi_p) + \arctan\left(x_0/y_0\right)\right] \end{pmatrix} \tag{3}$$

with the initial conditions for the location $(x_o;\, y_o)$ of A at the time $t = 0$: $-\pi/2 < x_o/y_o < \pi/2$ and $y_o \neq 0$. The displacement trajectory of any single point is, therefore, governed by the parameters Φ, Ψ, ω_b, ω_p and φ_p.

The results for certain values of these parameters are illustrated in Figure 2. While shape and length of a trajectory change dependent on the position of the selected point, it becomes obvious that only a difference in phase of $\phi(t)$ and $\psi(t)$ generates a quasi-elliptical path (Figure 2b, c, d), otherwise a curvilinear path is achieved (Figure 2a). The ratio of the main axes of the ellipse is dependent on the ratio Ψ/Φ, while its circumference (i.e. the length of the path) is governed by the absolute values of Ψ and Φ. The trajectories of adjacent points cross each other during a cycle. A difference in frequency of ball (ω_b) and pin (ω_p) oscillation produces such crossings already for the path of a single point, since the shape of the path changes from elliptical to more complex forms, e.g. an eight (Figure 2d).

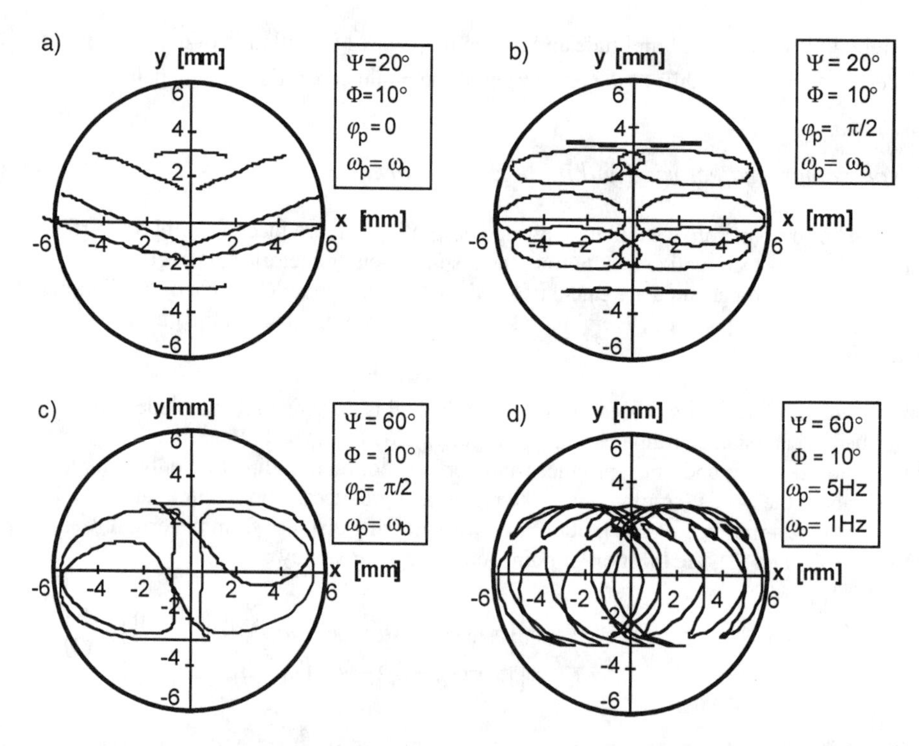

FIG. 2: *Motion trajectories of examplary points (8 points in a.) and b.), 4 points in c.) and d.) plotted on the surface of a pin of 12mm diameter: a) Biaxial oscillatory motion with no phase and frequency difference leads to nearly linear paths, b) introducing a phase shift causes elliptical trajectories, c) changing the ratio of pin and ball oscillation amplitude causes a widening of the trajectories, d) a difference in oscillation frequency causes a permanently changing phase shift and self-crossing path on the articulating surface.*

Experimental Design

Methods

The design of the pin-on-ball device is based in principal on the concept outlined in section 2. However, not one but two opposing pins were pressed onto an interposed femoral head and three of the devices are placed in series (Figures 3). This arrangement has two distinct advantages: a self-balancing of each device is achieved (i.e. no extra bearings are needed to compensate the applied contact force), and 3 times two wear specimens are evaluated at a time.

The two UHMWPE pins (cylindrical, ø 12 mm) are pressed against the ball (ø 22 ... 32 mm) using a pneumatic short-stroke cylinder driven by a central pressure control device. The pins and the contact load actuator are arranged in a closed load frame, establishing a closed compression mechanism (Figure 4). This mechanism generates an equivalent normal load on both pins. High precision bearings guarantee proper alignment of the pins. The loading magnitude is adjustable (constant or dynamic) and is recorded using a force sensor (range 0 ... 1kN, sensitivity ±1%). In order to generate the oscillatory motion of the pins, each complete load frame is pivoted around a horizontal axis and driven by an own electric engine with a crank shaft (Figure 3b). The oscillatory motion of

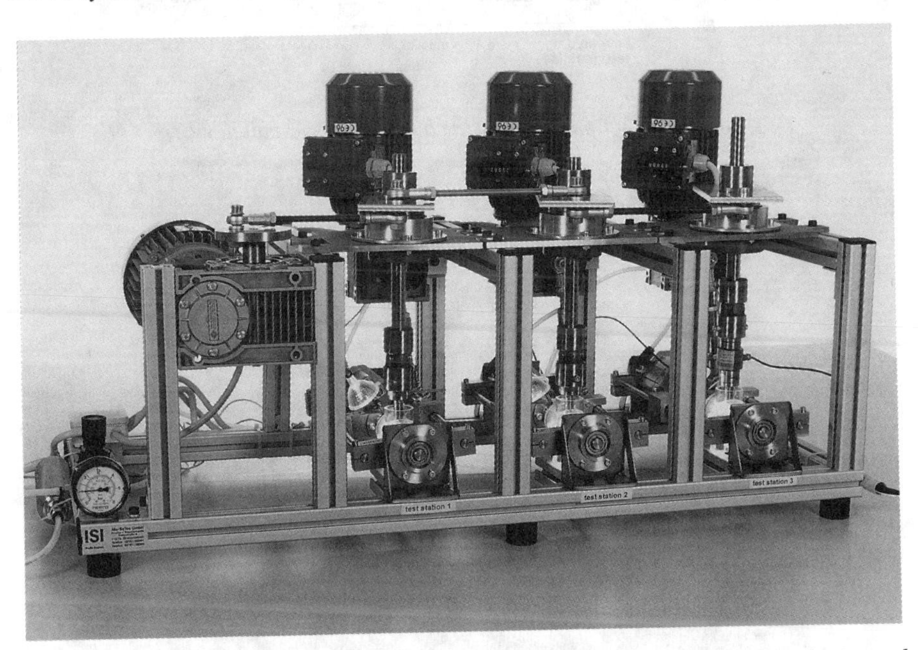

FIG. 3a: *The complete three-station pin-on-ball-testing device. Each of the three horizontal axes are powered by a separate electric motor. The vertical motion axes are connected by a central crank gear mechanism,*

each ball is also electromotively driven by a central engine, whereby the vertical motion axes of the balls are connected by a crank gear (Figure 3a,3b). Each vertical shaft carries an adapter for taper conjunction with the prosthesis' head. The shaft was transversally displacable in z-direction and an unilever joint allows the ball to adjust for any constraints in x- and y- direction during oscillatory motion. One of the three vertical driving shafts is equipped with a torque sensor (10 Nm, ±1%) as illustrated in Figure 4.

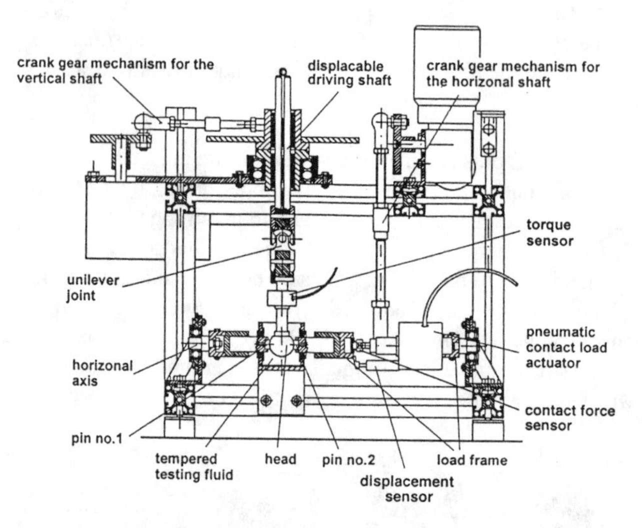

FIG. 3b: *Cross-sectional view of the bi-axial pin-on-ball device*

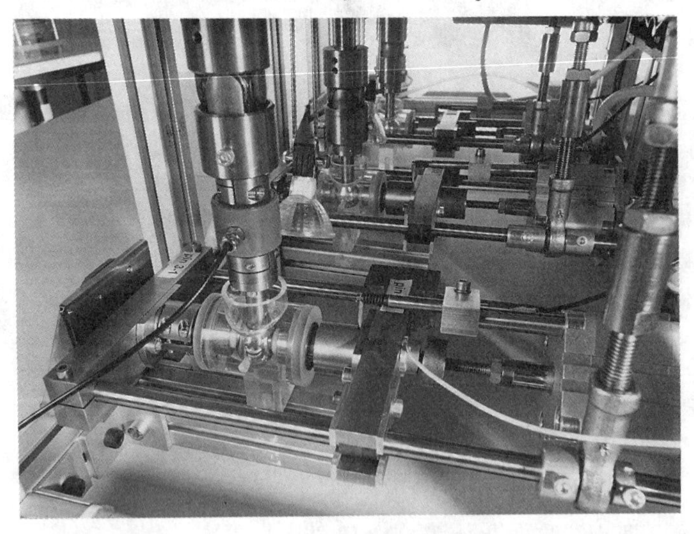

FIG. 4: *The closed load frame with the pneumatic actuator for contact load application. The vertical shaft of the front station carries the torque sensor for frictional measurements.*

Both, the self-adjusting pin holder of the load frame and the cardanic suspension of the ball guarantees self-alignment and -adjustment of the conforming joint during the process of wear. The equatorial contact situation of the pin-on-ball arrangement uses the maximum lever-arm for the determination of the friction moment. Furthermore, the orthogonal arrangement of force application and moment acquisition prevents signal cross talk during measurements. For lubrication, the pin-on-ball interfaces are placed in a plexiglass container with tempered fluid (37°C). The lateral openings for the pins are sealed using radial Simmer® rings (Figure 4).

Pilot Study: Friction Measurements

The first friction tests were conducted applying a sinusoidal ±20° motion of 1Hz frequency to the vertical shaft. The horizontal axis was kept fixed throughout the experiment. Thus the pins did not rotate. Frictional moments were measured during continuous oscillating motion of 250,000 cycles at a constant contact load of 500 N and distilled water (37°C) as lubricant. Data acquisition frequency was set to 1.5 kHz and measurements were taken every 10 minutes for a interval of 5 seconds. The friction coefficient μ was calculated from the measured frictional moment M_t, the contact force F_n and the radius R of the femoral head:

$$\mu = \frac{M_{t.}}{2 \cdot R \cdot F_n}; \tag{4}$$

Five commercially available cobalt-chromium alloy (CoCr) heads and five CoCr heads coated with amorphous hydrogenated carbon (a-CH) were tested against UHMWPE pins. The conforming surface of the pin (clearance of 0.2 mm) was machined using the same tools and production processes as for original hip cups. The cylindrical diameter of the pins was 12 mm, and their length 7 mm. Creep of the UHMWPE pins was reduced by metal-backing 5 of these 7 mm.

Pilot Study: Wear Measurements

In order to evaluate the difference on wear between uni- and multi-directional sliding, two CoCr heads (ø 32 mm) were tested. The first CoCr head was examined according to the above (uni-directional) protocol, while a second CoCr head was analysed applying an additional sinusoidal motion of 1Hz frequency to the pin. The range of motion of the pin was set to ±10°. The phase difference between ball and pin oscillation was set to π/2. Both wear trials were executed simultaneously: in the first station of the pin-on-ball device, motion around the horizontal axis was prevented by turning off the respective motor; in the second station, the motor for the horizontal axis was adjusted according to the specifications above, and the third station was left empty.

Linear wear was measured using LVDT displacement sensors with a sensitivity of ±0.1 μm. Each displacement sensor was mounted on the self-adjusting pin holder, recording the total of wear (and deformation) of two opposing pins. To reduce measurement artefacts due to creep and swelling, both wear systems were preloaded and presoaked for 20 hours with the same contact load, as used for testing. The CoCr heads (R_a=0.04 μm) and the UHMWPE pins were fabricated and mounted as stated above. Distilled water of 37°C served as lubricant. After 650,000 cycles, the UHMWPE pins were removed from the pin holders and morphologically characterised using polarised light microscopy (LM) and scanning electron microscopy (SEM). The samples were coated with gold prior to SEM analysis.

Results

Friction Measurements

At each reversal point of the sinusoidal motion, a peak in frictional moment was found, commonly referred to as the static friction (Figure 5a). Once sliding motion was initiated, friction decreased continuously until it changed its sign after the reversal of motion. The mean value of friction during the sliding phase is referred to as the dynamic coefficient of friction (Figure 5a). It is about three times higher for the a-CH coated heads than the CoCr heads throughout the measurement: 0.12 ± 0.01 respectively 0.04 ± 0.02 (Figure 5b). The latter finding corresponds to published data of earlier studies [10].

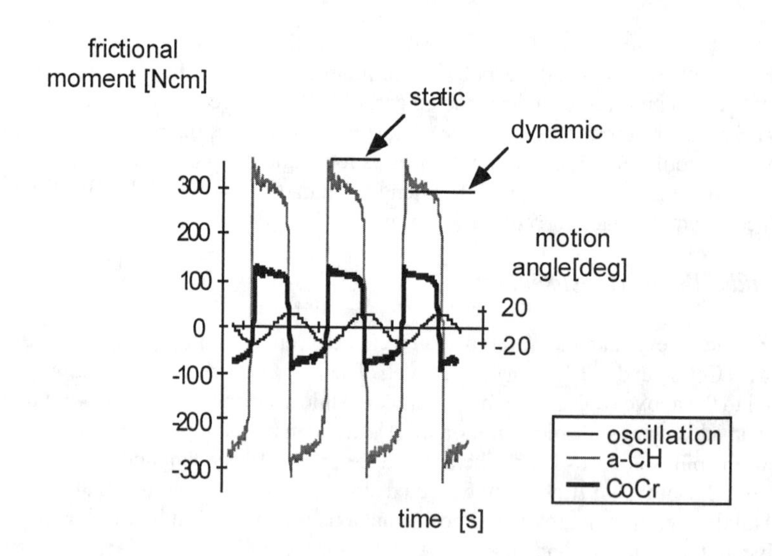

FIG. 5: a) *The equatorial frictional moment at CoCr and a-cH coated CoCr heads paired with UHMWPE-pins.*

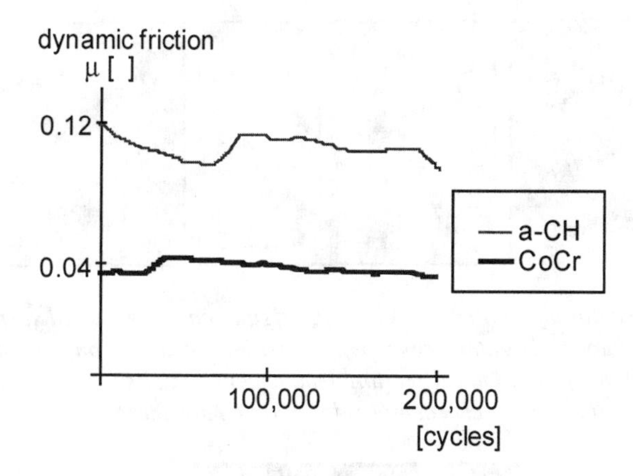

FIG. 5: b) *The frictional coefficien t vs. test duration.*

Linear wear as a function of time is dependent on the operating conditions (Figure 6). For both, the uni- and multi-directional testing mode, a steady-state wear rate was reached after about 100,000 cycles (running-in). During the steady-state period, the linear increase of wear was about 40% higher for the multi-directional mode as compared to uni-axial mode which reached 12.9 μm / 10^6cycles respectively 18.2 μm / 10^6cycles. The degressive wear loss during the period of running-in was also higher for the multi-directional mode.

The morphological differences between the worn surfaces for both testing modes are striking. While the sliding direction was clearly visible at the pins from the uni-directional testing, no preferred wear tracks could be detected on the multi-directionally tested pins (Figures 7). The latter rather appeared burnished (polished) in the region of contact, as it is described for the high wear region of retrieved acetabular liners [11, 12]. Furthermore, closer examination revealed a finely textured surface in this polished area (Figure 8). Those microfeatures are also described from retrieved hip cups [12].

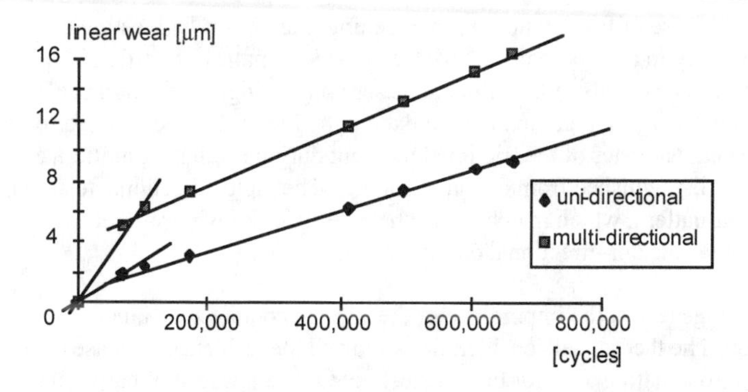

FIG. 6: *Linear wear for the multi- and uni-directional testing. Running-in was achieved after about 100,000 cycles followed by a steady state (linear) period of wear.*

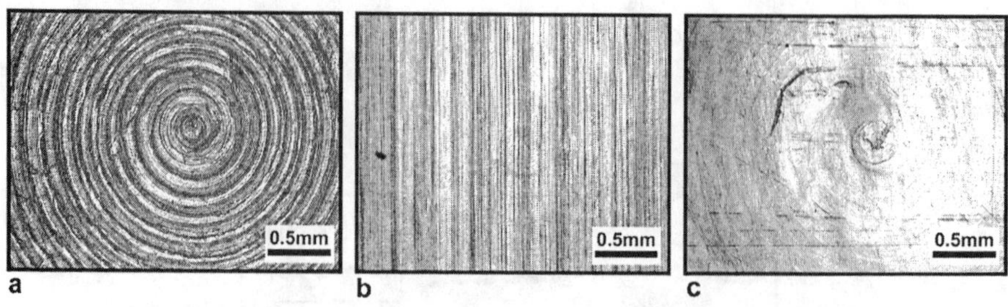

FIG. 7: *a) The circular machining marks of the original concave frontal surface of the UHMWPE pins (polarized light microscopy), b) straight scratches on the polyethylene surface after 650,000 cycles of uni-directional movement, c) polished wear pattern after 650,000 cycles of multi-directional movement.*

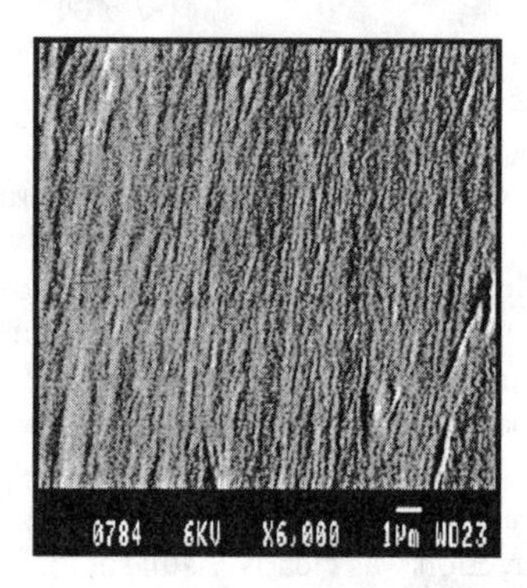

FIG. 8: *Micron sized elongated ripples are visible on the polished area of the muli-directional tested pins using SEM (5kV).*

Discussion

For the purpose of friction and wear screening, the pin-on-ball testing concept offers the possibility to approximate the contact zone kinematics of artificial hip joints as occurring in vivo. The results of the pilot studies are promising: the friction coefficients were highly reproducible and comparable to data in the literature. The set-up allowed to identify subtle characteristcs of the frictional moment during oscillating motion, e.g. static friction could be distinguished from dynamic friction. The multi-directional testing mode generated a wear pattern, which matched the characteristics known from retrieved cups quite well, whereas the uni-directional did not.

The findings reflect the importance of the applied contact zone kinematics during wear evaluation. The theoretical considerations showed the influence of phase difference between the two oscillating axes for bi-axial testing. Only a phase shift between pin and ball oscillation produces quasi-elliptical trajectories which are reported to take place during human locomotion [7]. This illustrates that it is not appropriate to think in purely physiological frames (e.g. the ball oscillation represents the flexion / extension motion pattern, the pin characterises the abduction / adduction during gait), but to think in terms of contact kinematics and to adjust the motion of the testing device in order to get trajectories of the the shape desired.

The different magnitudes of wear during running-in between the two testing modes might be due to a faster removal of machining marks by multi-directional shear forces at the surface. However, it is also possible that left-over constraints (e.g. an angular mismatch of the pins) are responsible for the differences. This needs closer investigation as do the wear rates during the steady-state period: assuming that a normal patient walks about one million cycles per year, both testing modes produced wear rates (about 0.01 mm) which are smaller as known from in-vivo [13] and joint simulator [14] studies: Livermore et al. [13] reported 0.1 ± 0.06 mm linear wear per year for 32 mm heads during time in service, while Saikko et al. [14] published a wear rate corresponding to 0.005 to 0.24 mm/year for metallic heads against polyethylene. Whereby it should be kept in mind that a screening test does not seek to duplicate service wear rates, the generation of smaller wear rates with the pin-on-ball screening device might have two reasons: firstly, the UHMWPE samples were preloaded. Thus, the results reflect mostly wear since creep had nearly stopped (Figure 9); secondly, the applied 500 N contact force is at the lower end of physiological loading. Further studies are required to support the interpretations of these pilot studies, since the experimental variability of the testing configuration needs to be addressed.

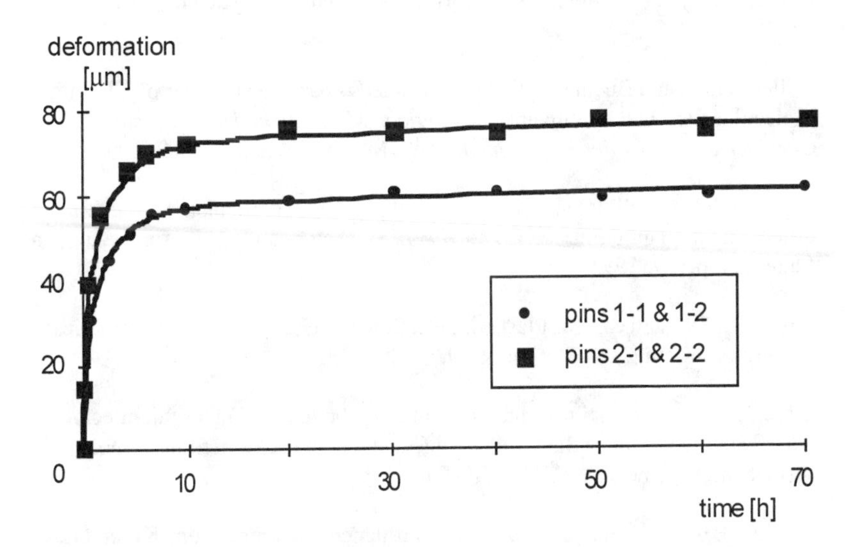

FIG. 9: *Results of a creep experiment with four UHMWPE pins (ø32mm) loaded with a contact force of 500N. After about 15 hours, a plateau in deformation was reached. Therefore, the pins were preloaded for 20 hours. Then, displacement data evaluation was set to zero before starting the oscillating wear tests.*

In summary, probe geometries identical to THR are utilised for friction and wear analyses. This design feature permits to use commercially available heads and does not require any custom made testing samples. This seems to be particularly important when evaluating surface coatings. Frictional moments and linear wear of the probes can be relatively easy monitored due to the self-balancing principle of the testing specimens. While this design configuration allows to evaluate two opposing contact areas at a time, the ball itself can be turned into a new starting position after the end of test and used for two or more additional trials dependent on the oscillation amplitude chosen. Those attributes might make the pin-on-ball apparatus an interesting alternative for common screeningdevices.

Acknowledgements

The a-CH coating of the heads was applied at the Frauenhofer Institute (Braunschweig, Germany), while all other tested specimens, including the polyethylene pins, were manufactured and supplied by the following implant manufacturing companies: gb-implantattechnik GmbH, Essen and MTM Mauk Medizintechnik GmbH, Hamburg, Germany.

References

[1] Harris, W.H., "The Problem is Osteolysis", *Clinical Orthopaedics*, Vol. 311, pp. 48-53, 1995.

[2] Willert, H.G., and Buchhorn, G. H., "Particle Disease due to Wear of Ultrahigh Molecular Weight Polyethylene", *Biological, Material, and Mechanical Considerations of Joint Replacement*, B.F. Morrey,Ed., pp. 87-102, 1993.

[3] Clarke, I., Campbell, P., and Kossovsky, N., "Role of Particulate Biomaterials in Osteolysis Implant Failure", *ASTM STP 1144*, American Society for Testing and Materials, p.199, 1993.

[4] Bayer, R., "Wear Tests for Plastics: Selection and Use", *ASTM 701* , American Society for Testing and Materials, 1980.

[5] Mäschig, K., "Allgemeine Grundlagen und Methoden der Dünnschichttechnik zur Oberflächenvergütung (Basic knowledge and methods of thin film technology for surface improvement)", *SYNTEXT* , Frankfurt , 1988.

[6] Briscoe, B.J., and Stolarski, T.A., "The Influence of Contact Zone Kinematics on Wear Process of Polymers", *Wear*, Vol. 149, pp. 233-240, 1991.

[7] Ramamurti, B.S., Bragdon, C.R., O´Connor, D.O., Lowenstein, J.D., Jasty, M., Estok, D.M., and Harris, W.H., "Loci of Movement of Selected Points on the

Femoral Head during Normal Gait", *Journal of Arthroplasty*, Vol. 11, pp. 845-852, 1996.

[8] Bragdon, C.R., O'Connor, D.O., Lowenstein, J.D., Jasty, M., and Harris, W.H., "Development of a New Pin on Disc Testing Machine for Evaluating Polyethylene Wear", *Trans. 10th Conf. ESB*, p. 114, 1996.

[9] Bragdon, C.R., O'Connor, D.O., Lowenstein, J.D., Jasty, M., and Harris, W.H., "Comparison of Polyethylene Wear and Polyethylene Debris Generated on New Hip Simulator Versus Direct Measurements of In Vivo Wear", *Trans. 43rd ORS*, Vol. 22 , p.120, 1997.

[10] O'Kelly, J., Unsworth, A., Dowson, D., and Wright, V., "An Experimental Study of Friction and Lubrication in Hip Prostheses", *Engineering in Medicine*, Vol. 8, pp.153-159, 1979.

[11] Cooper, J.R., Dowson, D., Fisher, J., Isaac, G.H., and Wroblewski, B.M., "Observations of Residual Sub-Surface Shear Strain in the Ultrahigh-Molecular-Weight-Polyethylene Acetabular Cups of Hip Prostheses", *Journal of Material Science and Materials for Medicine*, Vol. 5, pp. 52-57, 1994.

[12] McKellop, H.A., Campbell, P., Park, S-H., Schmalzried, T.P., Grigoris, P., Amstutz, H.C., and Sarmiento, A., "The Origin of Submicron Polyethylene Wear Debris in Total Hip Arthroplasty", *Clinical Orthopaedics*, Vol. 311, pp. 3-20, 1995.

[13] Livermore, J., Ilstrup, D., and Morrey, B., "Effect of Femoral Head Size on Wear of the Polyethylene Acetabular Component", *Journal of Bone and Joint Surgery*, Vol. 72-A, pp. 518-528, 1990.

[14] Saikko, V.O., Paavolainen, P.O., and Slätis, P., "Wear of the polyethylene acetabular cup. Metallic and ceramic heads compared in a hip simulator", *Acta Orthopaedica Scandinavica*, Vol. 64, pp. 391-402, 1993.

Metal–on–Metal Bearings

Robert A. Poggie[1]

A Review Of The Effects Of Design, Contact Stress, And Materials On The Wear Of Metal-On-Metal Hip Prostheses

REFERENCE: Poggie, R. A., "**A Review of the Effects of Design, Contact Stress, and Materials on the Wear of Metal-On-Metal Hip Prostheses,**" *Alternative Bearing Surfaces in Total Joint Replacement, ASTM STP 1346*, J. J. Jacobs and T. L. Craig, Eds., American Society for Testing and Materials, 1998.

Abstract: The clinical and tribological history of metal-on-metal (MOM) hip bearings indicates mixed clinical performance. Low wear and excellent twenty-year clinical performance is reported, as is early loosening and high wear. Contemporary tribological studies of MOM hip implants combined with improved Co-Cr-Mo materials has led to more predicable wear performance, and provided an understanding of the dichotomy in historical clinical performance. Historical failures of MOM bearings can be attributed to one or more of the following: poor control of sphericity and radial clearances greater than 200 μm (high wear), poor implant design and/or cementing technique, inadequate radial clearance via matched head-cup pairs (seizing and high friction), and unpredictable Co-Cr-Mo microstructure and large carbides (two and three body wear). And conversely to these failure modes, the success of contemporary MOM bearings can be attributed to the following: modern machine tools are capable of reliably manufacturing MOM bearings with sphericity of +/- 3 to 5 μm, linear head penetration wear rates of about 5 to 20 μm per year (million cycles) are reliably achieved, and contemporary high carbon (0.25% C) wrought Co-Cr-Mo alloys possess homogenous microstructures with carbides less than 5 μm in size. Furthermore, contemporary radial clearances of 35 to 50 μm result in maximum Hertzian contact stresses of about 25 to 50 MPa, which is 50 times less than the compressive yield strength of Co-Cr-Mo (2700 MPa) or about 20 times less than the tensile yield strength. Therefore, mechanical damage due to excessive contact stress probably does not contribute to bearing failure. Rather, the optimum radial clearance is related to an optimized balance between maintenance of fluid film lubrication and avoidance of bearing seizure due to interference of opposing asperities and/or entrapment of third-body particles. The literature suggests 25 to 45 μm as the optimum radial clearance for 28 and 32 mm diameter head-cup components.

Keywords: wear, metal-on-metal, contact stress, Co-Cr-Mo, hip implants, tribology, orthopaedics

[1]Director of Applied Research, Implex Corp., 80 Commerce Drive, Allendale, NJ 07401.

Introduction

Interest in MOM bearings has been increasing over the past few years due to concerns regarding polyethylene wear and osteolysis. Several recent studies of MOM wear by researchers such as Medley, McKellop, Farrar, Chan, St. John, and Bobyn indicate that MOM can produce between 1/25 and 1/100 times less volumetric wear than polyethylene-metal components. However, the clinical performance of MOM bearings has been mixed. Excellent, twenty year survivorship has been widely reported, as has high friction, wear, and pre-mature implant failure. For example, Dobbs [*1*] reported 53% survivorship at 11 years for several types of MOM hips implanted from 1963 to 1972. Wilson and Scales [*2*] encountered high friction and premature loosening of MOM hips, and determined that sphericity was non-uniform, and that surface finish was irregular. In 1970, Amstutz [*3*] reported unacceptable wear and premature loosening of the McKee-Farrar prosthesis.

Converse to this unflattering picture of MOM performance, excellent clinical performance has been reported. For example, Muller stated in 1990 [*4*] "with the present metal-on-metal articulations it is now possible to stop using polyethylene." Muller's statement was based on the claim that no revisions (3 years in-vivo) had been performed on contemporary bearings implanted from 1987 to 1990. In hip simulation wear testing and frictional torque measurements, Streicher et.al. [*5*] determined that linear MOM wear was about 2 to 4 μm per year after run-in, and that friction was extremely low. Recently, McKellop et.al. [*6*] reported low linear wear (a few microns per year) for three contemporary MOM bearings, and that hip simulation wear was similar to low in-vivo wear rates measured on retrieved McKee-Farrar, Ring, and Mueller prostheses. In hip wear simulation testing, Chan et.al. [*7*] clearly showed decreasing wear with decreasing diametrical clearance and surface roughness, and attributed the results to enhanced fluid film lubrication. Numerous other papers written since the mid-1960's provide a mixed review of MOM performance; but the majority of papers published recently show favorable results.

The dichotomy in the MOM literature is primarily attributed to highly variable bearing design and materials factors in the 1960s and 1970s, and the fact that contemporary bearings possess more refined materials and precise dimensional tolerances. For example, many of the early MOM bearings (1960s to 1970s) possessed variable sphericity values (>25 μm) due to machine tool limitations, and such variability is no longer the case. Modern machining techniques are capable of sphericity deviations of less than 5 μm, and dimensional tolerances which reliably permit radial clearances of 25 to 40 μm. A second issue is that some 1st generation designs were fabricated by lapping matched head and cup bearing pairs. The result was very low diametrical clearance, which in turn often resulted in high friction and premature implant loosening. Another important issue associated with early MOM designs was excessive radial clearance, which in turn caused poor fluid film lubrication and high wear. And regarding changes in cobalt base materials from the 60s to the present, the early MOM bearings were cast Co-Cr-Mo while today's bearings are fabricated from wrought Co-Cr-Mo. In summary, advancements in materials and machining technology over the past 15 years, and identification of optimal radial clearances, are probably responsible for the low wear of contemporary MOM bearings.

Materials and Methods

Co-Cr-Mo Alloys

Since the 1960s, MOM hip bearings have historically been manufactured from Co-28Cr-6Mo with about 0.2 to 0.3% carbon. A minority of MOM implants have been manufactured from low carbon (0.05% C) Co-Cr-Mo alloy. Co-Cr-Mo alloys are well known for their excellent resistance to galling-type wear. Most researchers have attributed this behavior to the high mechanical stability of the passive oxide which forms on chromium containing alloys, combined with the high hardness and toughness of cobalt based super alloys. In the 1960s, Co-Cr-Mo alloy used in orthopaedics was typically cast and heat-treated, and contained relatively large, irregular grains and carbides.

Contemporary wrought Co-Cr-Mo alloys contain about 0.25%C and 0.15% N, which both contribute to solid solution interstitial strengthening and carbide formation. Solid solution strengthening increases hardness of the matrix phase (meta-stable FCC) as well as work hardening potential, both of which increase wear resistance. C and N also promote carbide formation, which increases hardness and resistance to wear. However, carbides are capable of increasing wear via two and three body abrasion, and by perturbation of fluid film lubrication. Figure 1a shows the typical microstructure of a high carbon Co-Cr-Mo alloy (CCM+, CarTech Inc., Reading, PA). The average carbide size of the alloy shown in 1a is 2.4 by 4 μm, with a carbide volume fraction of about 5%. Figure 1b shows the typical microstructure of a low carbon alloy (CCM alloy, CarTech Inc.). The average carbide size shown in 1b is about 1.4 μm, with a volume fraction of carbide of 0.3%.

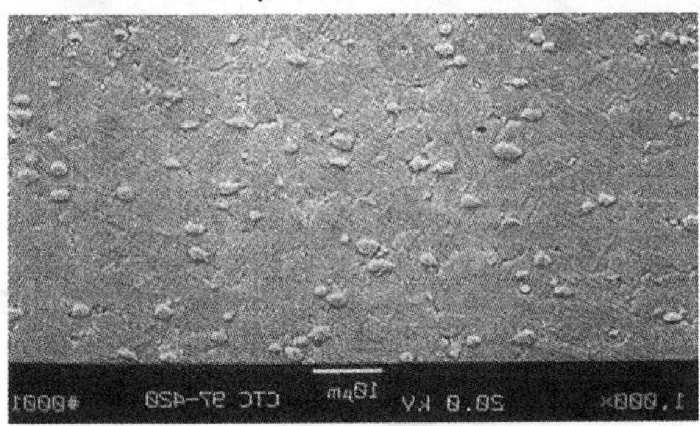

FIG. 1a – *Scanning electron micrograph of CarTech CCM+ alloy. Note the uniform, refined grain structure and uniform dispersion of carbides.*

Wrought Co-Cr-Mo alloys typically possess high strength, hardness, and ductility. The mechanical properties of the high carbon alloy shown in Figure 1a are typically: Yield strength (Y.S.) of 935 MPa (135 ksi), ultimate tensile strength (UTS) of 1365 MPa (198 ksi), elongation of 26%, Young's modulus of elasticity of 210 GPa (30 Msi), Rockwell hardness of 43 "C", and a compressive YS of about 2700 MPa using Archard's approximation of 3 x Y.S. The low carbon alloy possesses very similar mechanical properties, with the measurable difference being a 4% lower UTS and 18% higher ductility. It should be noted that contemporary MOM bearings fabricated from high and low carbon alloys typically conform to the requirements of ASTM F-1537-94.

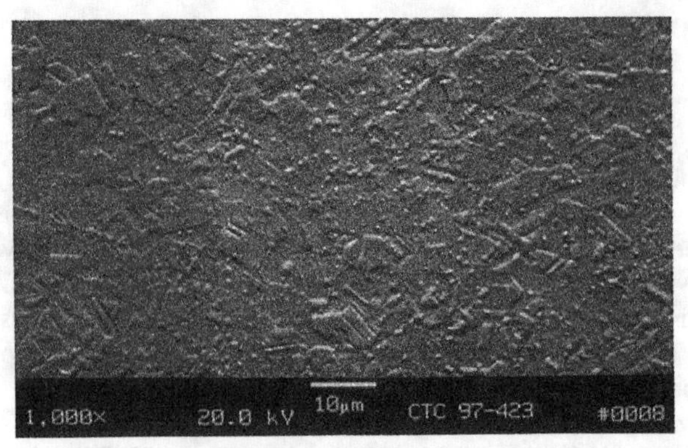

FIG. 1b – *Scanning electron micrograph of CarTech CCM alloy. Note uniform, refined grain structure and lesser size and volume fraction of carbides as compared to 1a.*

Hertzian Elastic Contact Stress

Application of Hertzian Elastic Stress Theory to circular contacts for MOM bearings indicates that contact stress is very low in relation to alloy strength. The Hertz stress formulae are shown below in Figure 2, and Figures 3a and 3b show contact stress as a function of radial clearance for MOM, ceramic-on-ceramic (COC), and polyethylene-on-metal (Poly & Co-Cr) bearings for a 3300 N (742 pounds) load and a 28 mm head.

Tribology - Hertzian Elastic Contact

$$\text{Max elastic stress} = \left[\frac{(6 \times \text{load} \times E^{*2})}{(\pi^3 R^2)}\right]^{1/3}$$

$R = [1/R_1 + 1/R_2]^{-1}$ $E^* = [(1-v_1^2)/E_1 + (1-v_2^2)/E_2]^{-1}$

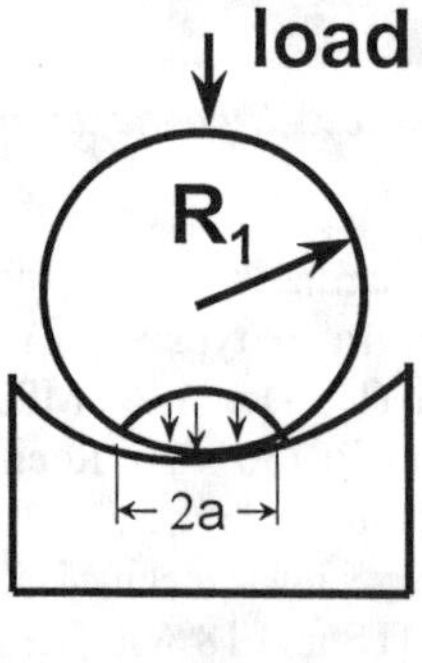

load

R_1

← 2a →

a = 1/2 contact width

Max stress in subsurface at about 0.7 x a

E* - normalized modulus

v - Poissons ratio

FIG. 2 – *Hertzian contact conditions and theory applied to MOM bearings.*

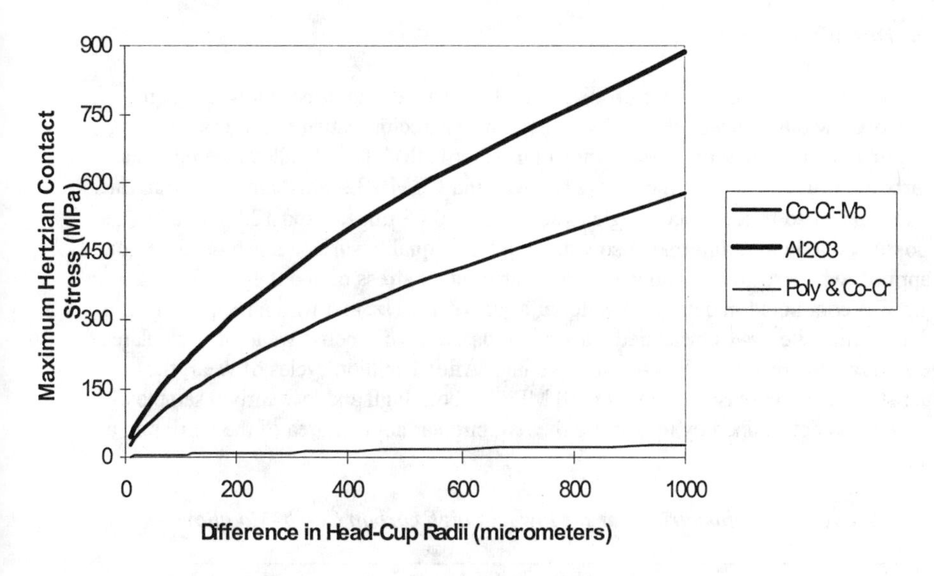

FIG. 3a – *Maximum Hertzian contact stress as a function of radial clearance; 0 to 1.0 mm, for MOM, COC, and Poly & Co-Cr bearings.*

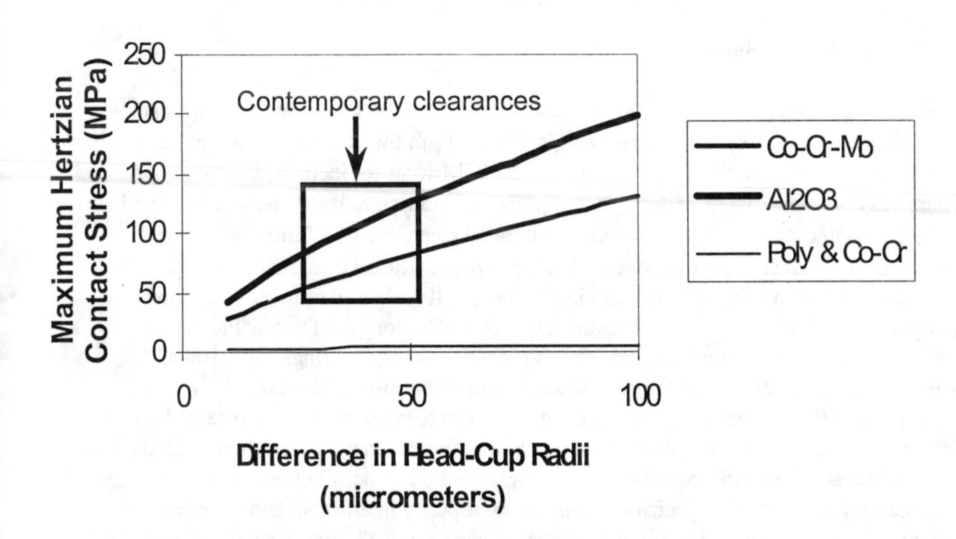

FIG. 3b – *Maximum Hertzian contact stress as a function of radial clearance; 0 to 100 μm, for MOM, COC, and Poly & Co-Cr bearings.*

Pin-On-Disc Wear

Comparative reciprocating pin-on-disc (RPOD) wear testing of both low and high carbon Co-Cr-Mo alloys was performed using a linear, reciprocating motion (stationary, loaded pin and a reciprocating disc within a DI water bath). The Co alloys were high and low carbon wrought CarTech Inc. alloys (CCM+ and CCM). 32 mm diameter, 7 mm thick discs were polished to a surface roughness of 0.03 to 0.05 μm Ra, and 12.7 mm diameter pins possessed a 5 cm radius end, also with an implant quality surface finish. A 3.3N load was applied, which resulted in an initial Hertzian contact stress of about 147 MPa. Testing was conducted in deionized water at a rate of 1.5 Hz, and with a reciprocating length of 2 cm. Wear was measured via weight loss, and volumetric wear was calculated. Table 1 shows the results of RPOD wear testing. After 1 million cycles of wear, the contact stress had decreased to about 0.18 MPa for both high and low carbon samples. This value was determined by measuring the flat, circular contact area of the worn pin, and dividing by the normal load.

TABLE 1 - *Volumetric wear for low and high carbon Co-Cr-Mo alloys*

	High Carbon Co-Cr-Mo Volumetric Wear (mm^3), n=4, std. dev. 10%	Low Carbon Co-Cr-Mo Volumetric Wear (mm^3), n=4, std. dev. 10%
0 – 1 million cycles	**0.94**	**1.00**
1 – 2 million cycles	**0.97**	**1.09**
2 – 3 million cycles	**0.69**	**0.91**

Discussion and Conclusions

Radial Clearance – The literature published since the 1980s indicates the optimal radial clearance with respect to least wear is 25 to 40 μm for 28 and 32 mm diameter components. For example, Chan et.al. showed MOM wear to decrease for radial clearances decreasing from 55 to 15 μm [*7*]. Farrar and Schmidt [*8*] showed head and cup wear (2 million cycles) to be 0.384 mm^3 for a radial clearance of 37 μm, with wear increasing at radial clearances above and below 37 μm. Radial clearance strongly influences contact stress, as shown in Figures 3a and 3b. However, given a compressive strength of 2700 MPa for Co-Cr-Mo and a tensile yield strength of 935 MPa, and in comparison to the maximum contact stress for contemporary bearings (50 - 100 MPa); gross plastic deformation and fatigue does not contribute to MOM wear. Rather, as Medley et.al. [*9*] have demonstrated previously, an increasing radial clearance and contact stress rapidly decreases the effectiveness of the thin film lubricant layer, thereby leading to increased wear. A significant draw back to low radial clearances in the 5 to 25 μm range is the increased potential for seizing promoted by asperity interaction and third body entrapment. During the wear of Co-Cr alloys, it has been well documented that carbides contained in Co-Cr-Mo alloys are liberated from the base matrix material. Once liberated, a carbide may become entrapped and re-lodged within the soft matrix material of both the head and cup, which in turn retards relative motion between the opposing surfaces. In summary, the optimal radial clearance is a balance between high clearance/high stress and associated breakdown of lubricant, and low clearance and bearing seizure. Based on current industry manufacturing practices and published research, the optimum radial clearance is in the range of 25 to 45 μm.

Co-Cr-Mo Alloys – Co-Cr-Mo alloys are characterized by a high resistance to abrasive and galling type wear, both necessary for low wear for MOM hip bearings. The mechanical properties of high and low carbon alloys are similar, and significantly above that required for resisting gross mechanical damage during hip articulation. Both alloys possess refined, homogeneous grain structures and carbide dispersions. This is a substantial improvement over MOM bearings fabricated from cast Co-Cr-Mo in the 1960s and 1970s, which were often characterized by poor surface finishes, irregular surface geometry, and unacceptably high clinical wear. The primary distinguishing feature in microstructure for contemporary high and low carbon Co-Cr-Mo alloys is the difference in volume fraction of carbides, with high carbon possessing about 5% carbide and low carbon possessing 0.3% carbide. High carbon alloys have dominated MOM bearings since the 1960s, while a minority of low carbon MOM bearings have been employed in Austria. A review of the literature (hip simulation wear testing) suggests that high carbon Co-Cr-Mo wears slightly less than low carbon Co-Cr-Mo [*10*]. The RPOD results shown in Table 1 support these findings.

Acknowledgments

The author would like to thank Greg Del Corso of CarTech Inc., who provided the scanning electron micrographs and materials properties of the high carbon and low carbon Co-Cr-Mo alloys discussed herein, and also John Medley of the University of Waterloo for his input regarding MOM wear and fluid film lubrication.

References

[1] Dobbs, H. S., "Survivorship of Total Hip Replacements," *Journal of Bone and Joint Surgery*, Vol. 62-B, No. 2, May, 1980, pp. 168-173.

[2] Wilson, J. N. and Scales, J. T., "Loosening of Total Hip Replacements with Cement Fixation, Clinical Findings and Laboratory Studies," *Clinical Orthopaedics and Related Research*, No. 72, 1970, pp. 145-160.

[3] Amstutz, H. C., "Complications of Total Hip Replacement," *Clinical Orthopaedics and Related Research*, No. 72, 1970, pp. 123-137.

[4] Muller, M. E., "The Benefits of Metal-on-Metal Total Hip Replacements," *Clinical Orthopaedics and Related Research*, No. 311, pp. 54-59.

[5] Streicher, R. M., Schon, R., and Semlitsch, M. F., "Investigation of the Tribological Behavior of Metal-On-Metal Combinations for Artificial Hip Joints," *Biomedizinische Technik*, Vol. 35, No. 5, 1990, pp. 107-111.

[6] McKellop, H., Campbell, P., Lu, B., Park, S-H, Doorn, P., and Dorr, L., "Clinical Wear Performance of Modern Metal-On-Metal Hip Arthroplasties," 23rd Soc. for Biomaterials, New Orleans, 1997, 190 pp.

[7] Chan, F. W., Bobyn, J. D., Medley, J. B., Krygier, J. J., Podgorsak, G. F., and Tanzer, M., "Design Factors That Control Wear of Metal-Metal Total Hip Implants," 23rd Soc. for Biomaterials, New Orleans, 1997, 77 pp.

[8] Farrar, R., and Schmidt, M. B., "The Effect of Diametrical Clearance on Wear Between Head and Cup for Metal On Metal Articulations," 43rd Annual Orthopaedic Research Society, San Francisco, CA, 1997, 71 pp.

[9] Medley, J. B., Chan, F. W., Krygier, J. J., and Bobyn, J. D.,"Comparison of Alloys and Designs in a Hip Simulator Study of Metal On Metal Implants," *Clinical Orthopaedics and Related Research*, August, 1996 Supplement, Volume 239, pp. S148-S159.

[10] Medley, J. B., Dowling, J. M., Poggie, R. A., Krygier, J. J., and Bobyn, J. D., "Simulator Wear of Some Commercially Available Metal On Metal Hip Implants," *presented at the 1997 ASTM Symposium on Alternative Bearing Surfaces in Total Joint Replacement*, San Diego, CA, ASTM STP publication pending.

Rocco Varano,[1] Steve Yue,[1] J. Dennis Bobyn,[2] and John B. Medley[3]

Co-Cr-Mo ALLOYS USED IN METAL-METAL BEARING SURFACES

REFERENCE: Varano, R., Yue, S., Bobyn, J. D., and Medley, J. B., **"Co-Cr-Mo Alloys Used in Metal-Metal Bearing Surfaces,"** *Alternative Bearing Surfaces in Total Joint Replacement, ASTM STP 1346*, J. J. Jacobs and T. L. Craig, Eds., American Society for Testing and Materials, 1998.

ABSTRACT: The microstructure, crystallography, mechanical properties and tribological properties of an ASTM Standard Specification for Thermomechanically Processed Cobalt-Chromium-Molybdenum Alloy for Surgical Implants (F1537-94) were studied in this work. The effects of room temperature compression and carbon content on the above characteristics were also analyzed. Increasing amounts of deformation resulted in a decrease in the number of annealing twins in the microstructure. Also observed was an increase in the volume fraction of the hexagonal-closed-packed phase from the metastable face-centered cubic phase due to a strain-induced transformation. The higher carbon alloy had a lower volume fraction of this strain-induced phase. When subjected to mechanical testing, the low carbon and high carbon alloys exhibited an increase in both the yield strength and ultimate tensile strength with increasing amounts of deformation. In addition, the low carbon alloy experienced higher amounts of work hardening in comparison to the high carbon alloy. Friction studies conducted on these alloys revealed a higher coefficient of friction for the higher carbon alloy and no significant effect of strain-induced transformation on the friction characteristics.

---

[1] M. Eng. Student and Ass. Prof., Department of Metallurgical Engineering, McGill University, Montreal, Quebec, Canada H3A 2B2.

[2] Ass. Prof., Jo Miller Orthopaedic Research Laboratory, Montreal General Hospital, Montreal, Quebec, Canada H3G 1A4.

[3] Ass. Prof., Department of Mechanical Engineering, University of Waterloo, Waterloo, Ontario, Canada N2L 3G1.

KEYWORDS: carbides, face-centered-cubic, friction coefficient, hexagonal-closed-packed, neutron diffraction, strain-induced transformation, strength, twins, wear

---

Concerns about wear debris related to peri-implant inflammation and osteolysis have led to a renewed interest in alternate bearing technologies for total hip replacements. The reintroduction of metal-metal bearings made of cobalt-chromium-molybdenum (Co-Cr-Mo) alloys has made use of improved design and manufacturing to avoid the problems of equatorial seizing and implant loosening that plagued first generation metal-metal bearings a quarter of a century ago.

The purpose of this work was to manipulate the microstructure and crystallography of Co-Cr-Mo alloys and investigate their influence on the friction and mechanical properties. This fundamental metallurgical approach may lead to optimization of the tribological properties of metal-metal hip bearings [*1*]. The family of Co-Cr-Mo alloys that are suitable for self-bearing applications include both cast and wrought materials with either low or high carbon (C) contents. In the past, particular attention has been paid to the effect of carbides on the mechanical and wear-resistant properties of the material. Clearly, lower carbon levels will result in fewer carbides. However, of equal interest is the presence of "twins" in the alloy. The presence of "twins" is often considered to be a precursor to strain-induced transformation (SIT). This is expected in the lower C alloy because C is a face-centered cubic (FCC) stabilizer [*2*]. The lower C alloy will be more prone to undergo a SIT to the stable hexagonal close packed (HCP) structure. Such a transformation will influence the mechanical properties and the tribological properties of these alloys, depending on the characteristics of the transformation, including the susceptibility of the FCC to SIT. Therefore, changes in C levels could affect tribological properties through changes in both the carbide and SIT characteristics of the Co-Cr-Mo microstructure.

Materials and Methods

Materials

In order to assess the effects of carbon content on the microstructural properties of the material, two ASTM F1537-94 alloys were used (Table 1). The bulk material was machined into cylindrical specimens with dimensions of 8.25 mm in height and 5.50 mm in diameter, prior to deformation processing.

TABLE 1--*ASTM F1537-94 alloy composition (in wt%).*

Alloy	Cr	Mo	C	Ni	Si	Mn	Fe	N	Co
Low C	27.82	5.77	0.054	0.50	0.68	0.64	0.12	0.162	Bal.
High C	26.99	5.55	0.197	0.49	0.09	0.73	0.12	0.096	Bal.

Deformation

To investigate the phenomenon of SIT, as-received specimens were subjected to room temperature uniaxial compression, since it is close to the final working temperature in hip implant applications. During compression, the surfaces were lubricated with molybdenum grease to reduce the friction between the anvils and the specimen during compression. The specimens were deformed at a strain rate of -0.0015 s^{-1} to a total permanent strain of -0.05, -0.15 and -0.25. Deformation of the cylindrical specimens also produced a slightly barreled shape, in preparation for friction testing (Fig. 1), but not significantly enough to have affected the strength data.

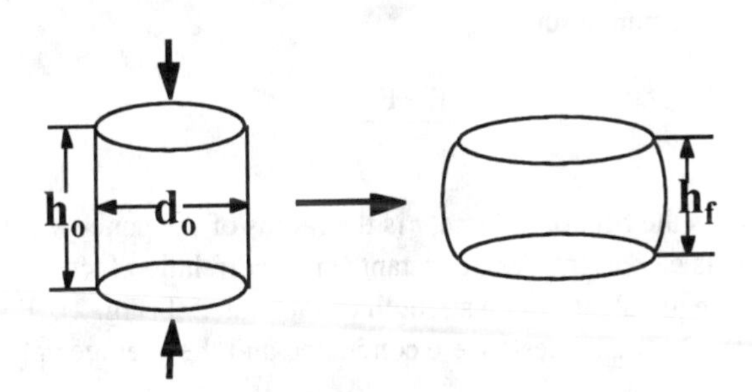

FIG. 1--*Plastic deformation of specimens under uniaxial compression (h_o=initial height, h_f=final height and d_o=initial diameter).*

Metallography

The specimens were cut and mounted in bakelite for microstructural analysis using the usual grinding and polishing techniques. After final polishing, the specimens were electroetched in an acid solution of 60% vol. nitric acid (HNO_3) - 40% vol. distilled water at 5V for 10 - 25 s. The specimens were then analyzed using a JEOL 840 Scanning Electron Microscope (SEM).

Neutron Diffraction

Characterization of SIT was performed on a DUALSPEC C2 neutron powder diffractometer at AECL, Chalk River, Ontario, Canada. The device utilizes an 800 multichannel detector with a 80 degree scanning capacity (i.e., it can pick up a signal every 0.1 degrees). Since neutrons penetrate the entire specimen, a crystallographic analysis of the bulk specimen was attained. The scan time for each sample was one hour.

Mechanical Testing

The mechanical properties of the material were acquired by shear punch testing [*3*]. Thin discs were sliced from the barreled specimens using a diamond cutting wheel and the discs were ground using 600 grit silicon carbide paper to a thickness of ~ 300 μm. The strain rate was 0.0015 s^{-1} and the stress was calculated by dividing the load by the circumferential area of the punch surface:

$$\sigma = \frac{P - F}{C \cdot 2\pi r t} \quad (1)$$

where, P is the load, F is the frictional force, r is the radius of the punch, t is the thickness of the specimen and C is a constant. The constant C is a correlation factor between the punch strength and the equivalent tensile strength of the material (Fig. 2). For each experimental condition, 3-5 punch tests were conducted and the average value was taken.

Friction Testing

The coefficient of friction of both alloys was determined using a reciprocating cylinder-on-flat friction apparatus. Details of this apparatus have been described elsewhere [*3*]. The specimens were mounted on a "sled" (shown in Fig. 3) which remained stationary against a reciprocating baseplate of the same material. Pure sliding friction of the barreled specimens in contact with a flat counterface was achieved, under dry conditions. The baseplate reciprocated at a frequency of 0.5 Hz and the normal load used for each specimen was 8.0 N. The friction force and corresponding coefficient of friction were measured using two strain-gauged hanging beams as force transducers,

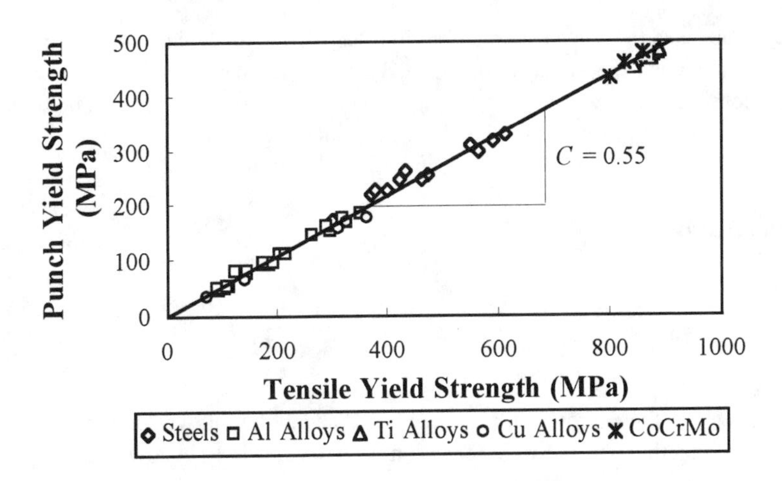

FIG. 2--*Correlation between the punch and the tensile yield strengths for various alloys* [3].

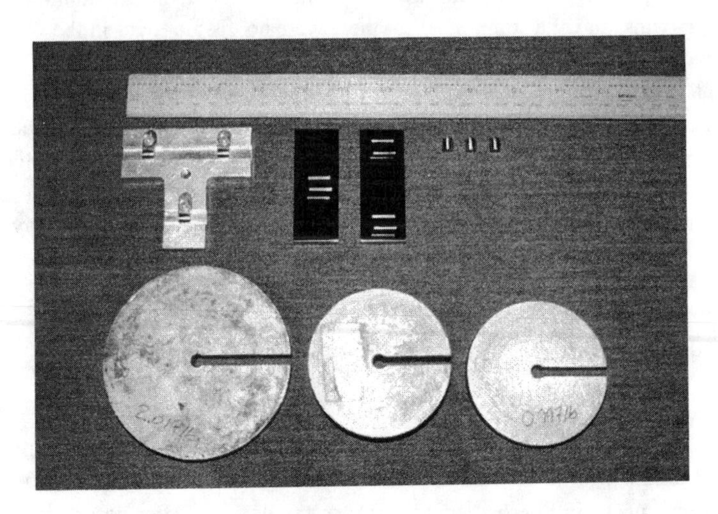

FIG. 3--*Test components used in friction study.*

which were connected to the sled via high-tension steel wires. Since this was a preliminary study, one experiment was conducted per each test condition. Each experiment consisted of 3 specimens tested simultaneously. Therefore, the friction force per specimen was determined by dividing the total friction force by 3.

Results and Discussion

Metallography

SEM photos of the microstructures of the low C and high C alloys, after room temperature deformation, are shown in Figs. 4 and 5, respectively. The low C alloy revealed a relatively fine microstructure (avg. grain size ~ 4.5 μm) with randomly distributed carbide precipitates and some grain boundary carbides. In addition, annealing twins were present in the microstructure and were found to traverse the grains. Annealing twins are very common in FCC metals, such as Co, that possess low stacking fault energies. As the material was deformed, there was a reduction in the number of these annealing twins, and at a strain of -0.25, there were no visible twins in the microstructure. This was an indication that SIT might have occurred.

The high C alloy revealed a slightly coarser microstructure (avg. grain size ~ 6.5 μm) with more carbide precipitates (which can be seen at the grain boundaries), due to the higher C content (Fig. 5). The annealing twins were more pronounced, possibly due to the coarser microstructure. As with the low C alloy, as the amount of deformation increased, the number of annealing twins was reduced, suggesting that SIT may have occurred.

Neutron Diffraction

Neutron diffraction studies of the low C and high C alloys revealed a predominately FCC crystal structure prior to deformation. An example of this is shown in Fig. 6 for the low C alloy (the γ peaks in Fig. 6a denote FCC crystal planes). After deformation (Fig. 6b), there were new peaks which emerged due to neutron scattering of HCP crystal planes (these planes are denoted by ε). It was found that peak broadening occurred (as shown in Fig. 6b), suggesting particle nucleation of this new HCP phase. The volume fraction of the HCP phase was determined from the neutron data, and is shown in Fig. 7. It was found that the higher C content lowered the volume fraction of the HCP phase ($p>0.01$) which was formed by SIT (probably due to the fact that C is an FCC stabilizer,

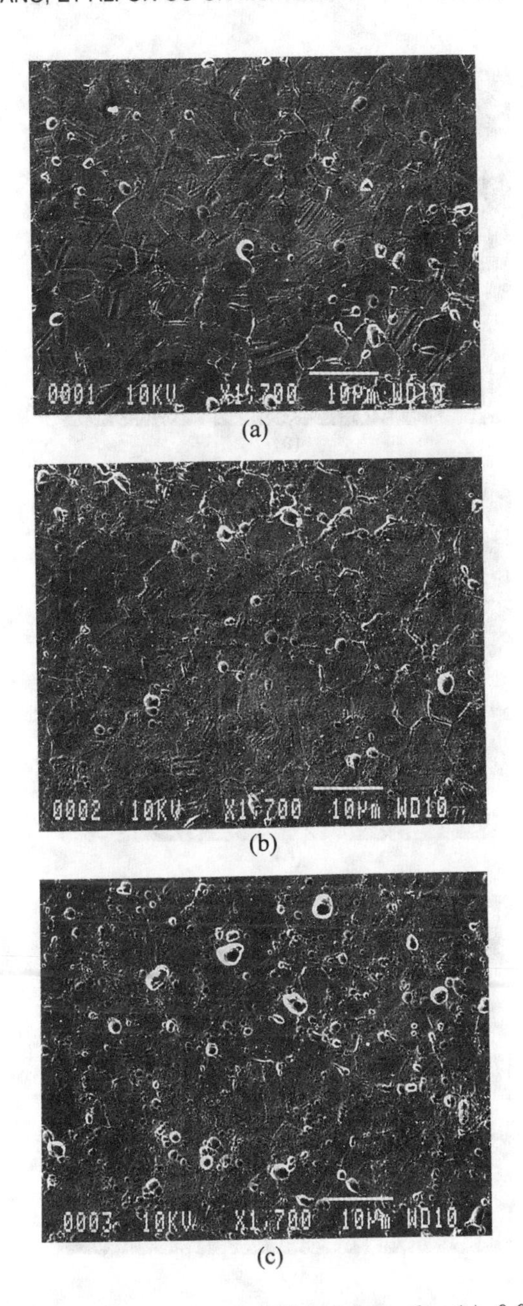

FIG. 4--*Microstructures of low C alloy deformed to (a) -0.05 strain, (b) -0.15 strain and (c) -0.25 strain (magnification 1700x).*

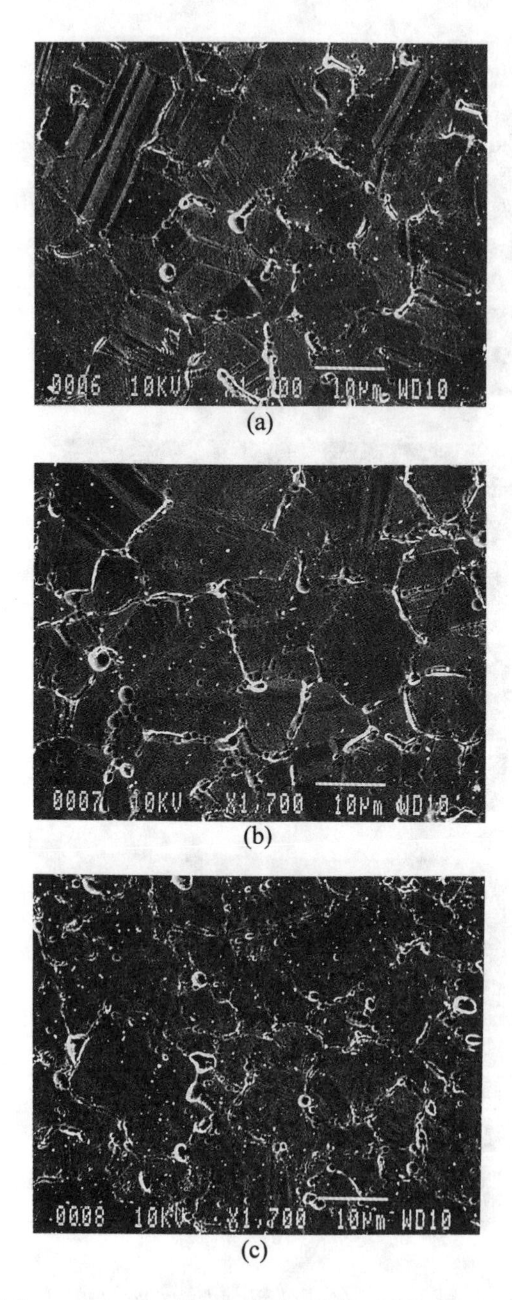

FIG. 5--*Microstructures of high C alloy deformed to (a) -0.05 strain, (b) -0.15 strain and (c) -0.25 strain (magnification 1700x).*

although grain size could be a factor as well). Increasing amounts of deformation increased the volume fraction of the HCP phase.

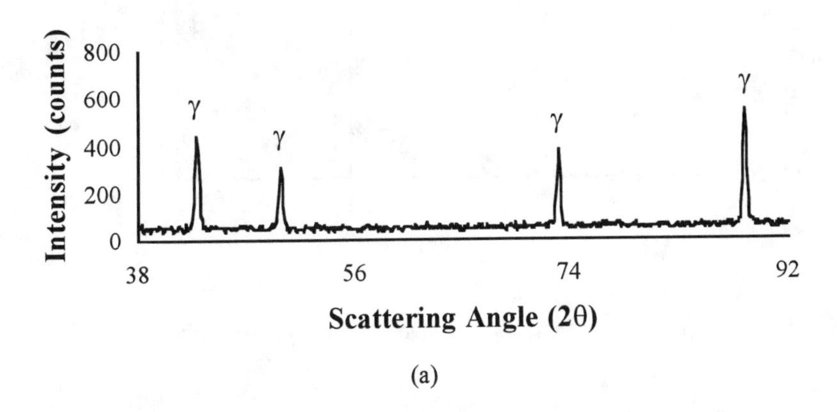

(a)

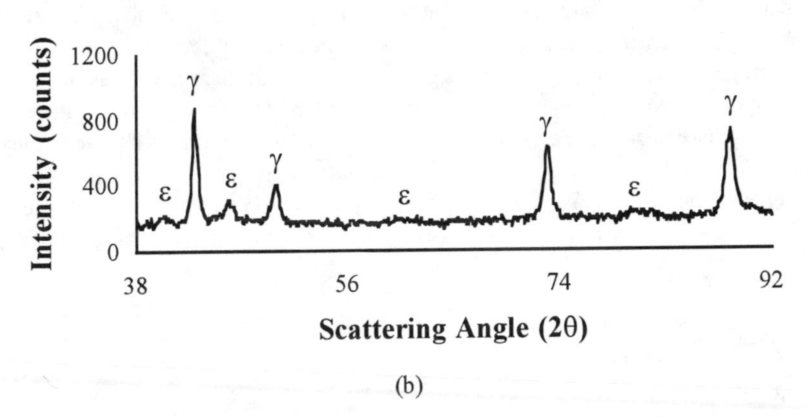

(b)

FIG. 6--*Typical neutron diffraction spectra for low C alloy: (a) before compression and (b) after compression.*

Mechanical Testing

The shear punch test indicated that both the low C and high C alloys showed an increase in the yield strength (YS) and ultimate tensile strength (UTS) after deformation (Figs. 8 and 9). The low C alloy experienced higher amounts of work hardening during mechanical testing ($p>0.01$), which may have been a result of the higher volume fraction of the HCP phase from SIT.

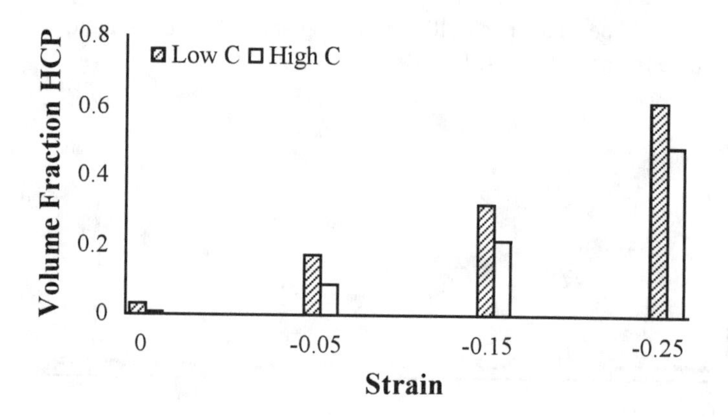

FIG. 7--*Volume fraction of HCP phase due to SIT for low C and high C alloys.*

In addition, the somewhat unexpected increase in the UTS can be explained by the occurrence of SIT (altering the materials properties), or the fact that the UTS was exceeded during uniaxial compression of the specimens, prior to shear punch testing.

Although the overall percent elongations of the Co-Cr-Mo alloy were lower than more ductile biomaterials (e.g., polyethylene and Titanium-6%Aluminum-4%Vanadium), little or no significant losses to the ductility of the material after compression were observed (Figs. 10 and 11). This may be explained by a transformation induced plasticity (TRIP) effect caused by SIT of the remaining FCC to HCP during punch testing [*5*].

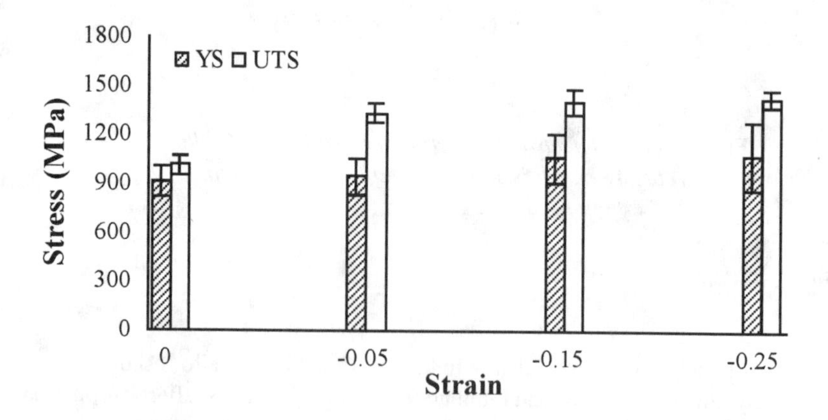

FIG. 8--*Yield and ultimate tensile properties for low C alloy.*

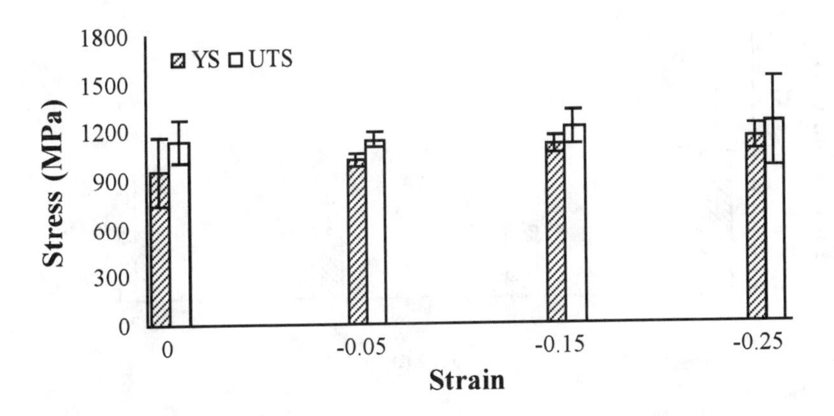

FIG. 9--*Yield and ultimate tensile properties for high C alloy.*

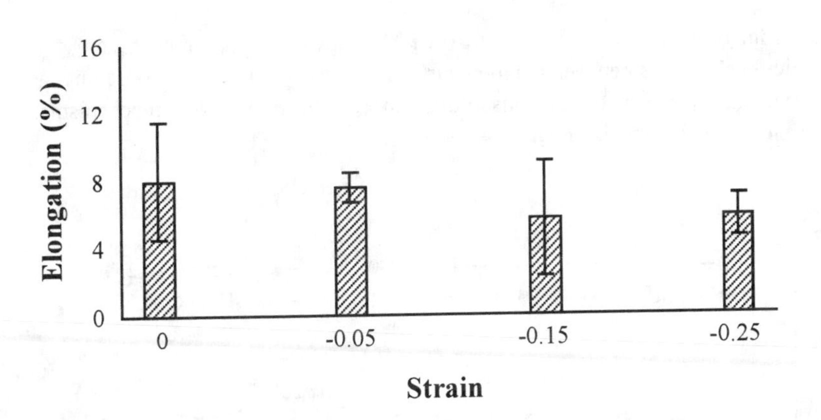

FIG. 10--*Percent elongation for low C alloy.*

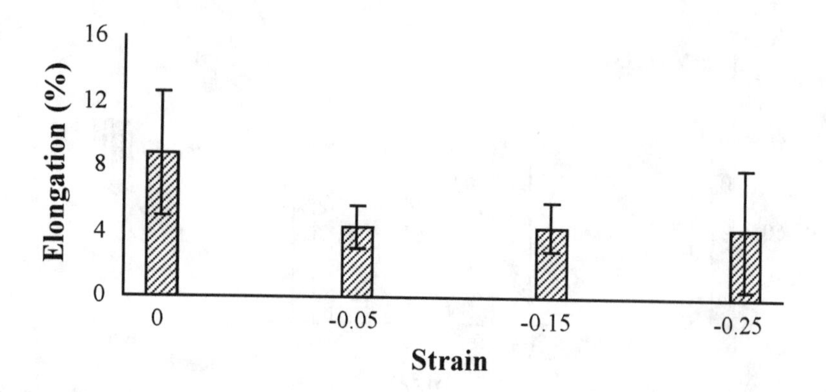

FIG. 11--*Percent elongation for high C alloy.*

Friction Testing

Knowledge of the friction behavior of Co-Cr-Mo alloys is important because excessive frictional torques between the joint surfaces can cause component loosening, as was the case in early metal-metal implants. Furthermore, with similar wear mechanisms, higher friction is usually associated with higher wear.

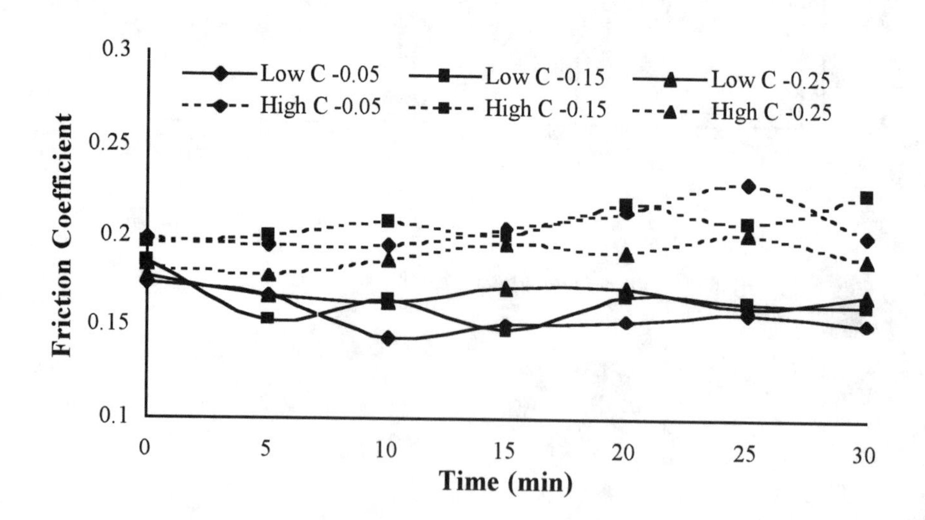

FIG. 12--*Friction coefficients for both low C and high C alloys.*

Overall, the friction coefficients for the high C specimens were higher than the low C specimens (Fig. 10), probably due to the increased number of carbide precipitates in the microstructure. The results also showed that there was a minor effect of SIT on the friction coefficient. This can be explained by the fact that the presence of these carbide precipitates in the microstructure may have had an overriding effect on the friction behavior. Also, asperity-asperity interactions may have transformed the surface structure in the case of specimens not subjected to compression prior to friction testing. Since a minimum number of tests were conducted in this area, an analysis could not be performed to determine the statistical significance of these results. Further tests (perhaps of longer duration) should be conducted in order to clarify this behavior.

Conclusions

This study revealed that alloy ASTM F1537-94 undergoes SIT when deformed at room temperature, and that the volume fraction of the HCP phase increases with increasing amounts of deformation. In addition, the neutron diffraction studies indicated that C is an FCC stabilizer. It was also found that the low C alloy experienced large amounts of work hardening during mechanical testing and there was no significant loss to the percent elongation for both the low C and high C alloys after prior compression deformation. Finally, the friction study revealed that varying amounts of SIT had no significant effect on the friction behavior. However, there was a definite effect of C content on the coefficient of friction (i.e., higher C content resulted in a higher friction coefficient for all strain values).

Based on this study, the low C alloy still remains a candidate for metal-metal joint replacement. However, further investigations of the effect of microstructure on the friction and wear performance of these alloys are required.

Acknowledgments

The authors would like to acknowledge John Root and his team for their invaluable assistance during the neutron diffraction studies, which were conducted at Atomic Energy of Canada Limited (AECL), in Chalk River, Ontario, Canada. The authors would also like to acknowledge Ernst Huber of the Mechanical Engineering Department at the University of Waterloo, whose technical assistance was essential in conducting the friction experiments.

Financial support was given by the Medical Research Council of Canada (MRC), the Fonds pour la Formation de Chercheurs et l'Aide à la Recherche (FCAR), and the Natural Sciences and Engineering Research Council (NSERC) of Canada.

References

[*1*] Chan, F. W., Bobyn, J. D., Medley, J. B., Krygier, J. J., Yue, S. and Tanzer, M. "Engineering Issues and Wear Performance of Metal on Metal Hip Implants," *Clinical Orthopaedics and Related Research*, No. 333, 1996, pp. 96-107.

[*2*] Sims, C. T. "A Contemporary View of Cobalt-Base Alloys," *Journal of Metals*, Vol. 21, 1969, pp. 27-42.

[*3*] Wanjara, P., Drew, R. A. L. and Yue, S. "Shear Punch Test for Strength and Ductility Measurements of Ti-6Al-4V/Tic Particulate Reinforced MMC's," *Titanium '96*, Vol. 3, 1996, pp. 2851-2858.

[*4*] Cipera, W. M. and Medley, J. B. "Reciprocating Cylinder-on-Flat Test for Co-Cr-Mo Metal-on-Metal Contacts," *Alternative Bearing Surfaces in Total Joint Replacement*, 1998.

[*5*] Banerjee, B. R., Capenos, J. M. and Hanser, J. J., *Application of Fracture Toughness Parameters to Structure Metals*, Gordon and Breach Science Publishers Inc., New York, 1966.

John A. Tesk, [1] and Christian E. Johnson [2]

GLASSY ALLOYS AS POTENTIAL BEARING SURFACES FOR ORTHOPAEDIC IMPLANTS

REFERENCE: Tesk, J. A. and Johnson, C. E., "**Glassy Alloys as Potential Bearing Surfaces for Orthopaedic Implants,**" *Alternative Bearing Surfaces in Total Joint Replacement, ASTM STP 1346*, J. J. Jacobs and T. L. Craig, Eds., American Society for Testing and Materials, 1998.

ABSTRACT: Glassy (amorphous) metals have some unique properties that may render them attractive candidates for the coating of metal-implant bearing surfaces. Metastable glasses of metal alloys, with uniform compositions and homogeneous structures that are not attainable under usual quasi-equilibrium processing conditions, can often be made to produce alloys with exceptional corrosion resistance and high hardness. The absence of secondary phases argues for resistance to abrasive and asperity- initiated wear. One method of producing glassy alloys is electrodeposition. Glassy coatings from nanometers to millimeters thick can be produced. Unique compositions, such as single-phase, amorphous, cobalt-phosphorus alloys [*3,9*] or glass-like coatings of cobalt-chromium-carbon [*6,7*] alloys (those referred to by this name throughout the text have layers of amorphous chromium and cobalt that are known to have carbon dispersed throughout the chromium), can be made.

KEYWORDS: amorphous metals, glassy alloys, orthopaedic joint surfaces, orthopaedic joint surface coatings, corrosion resistant coatings, wear resistant coatings, wear of ultrahigh molecular weight polyethylene, wear resistant implants

---

Because wear debris from orthopaedic implants has been implicated as a major cause for the end-of-effective-service of orthopaedic implants [*1,2*] there is a strong interest in exploring new bearing designs, including new material couples that may reduce wear debris effects and, hence, help to prolong effective implant service. While modifications of existing materials and mechanical designs must surely be investigated, the potential of new technologies should also be explored for what they may have to offer

---

[1] Coordinator, Biomaterials Programs, Polymers Division

[2] Physical Scientist, Metallurgy Division, National Institute of Standards and Technology, Gaithersburg MD. 20899

and for what may be learned toward solving the problem.

What is described in this paper are three examples of recent developments in alloy coating technology at the National Institute of Standards and Technology. The coating alloys are glassy and consist of cobalt-phosphorous, cobalt-chromium-carbon, and chromium-carbon. These serve to illustrate the potential applicability of metallic glasses for improving the wear resistance of orthopaedic joint bearing couples, including those involving Ultrahigh Molecular Weight Polyethylene (UHMWPE). Among the properties of metallic glasses that may make them interesting for coatings as bearing surfaces are their high hardness, which also translates into high yield strengths, and good corrosion resistance. The properties of several glassy alloys are given here to illustrate desirable properties that can be attained. These indicate the potential usefulness of glassy alloys for applications to orthopaedic implants. The following sections provide some indication of their potential suitability as coatings on orthopaedic implants.

Fabrication

One way to produce metallic glasses is by electrodeposition, which is a facile method for applying coatings. By this method metallic glasses can be produced that have a variety of structures and properties. They may be produced as alloys of single phase structures or as mixed- phase, layered, structures of which one or all of the layers may be glassy, each with differing, predominate, elemental compositions. By control of the electrodeposition times, voltages, voltage waveforms, solutions and other characteristics of processing, the compositions and thicknesses of the layers can be controlled.

The cobalt-phosphorous, cobalt-chromium-carbon, and chromium carbon systems are specifically discussed (carbon is an element that is carried into the system from organic components of the electrolyte). Layers in these systems may be homogenized by annealing treatments to produce either amorphous materials or materials with nanocrystalline structures and/or finely dispersed precipitates (at early stages the precipitates are too fine to be detected optically or analyzed by x-ray diffraction but hardness changes indicate their presence).

Composition and Properties

Cobalt-Phosphorous Alloys

In 1993 Ratzker[3] et. al. described a method for fabricating dental prosthetic frameworks of metallic glasses, composed of cobalt and phosphorous, for use in resin-retained, fixed-partial-dentures. The alloys described contained preferred mass fractions of ca 88 % cobalt and 12 % phosphorous. The alloy samples had high hardnesses, ranging from Knoop Hardness numbers (HKs) of ca 620 kg/mm^2 to 1100 kg/mm^2 (the latter was obtained following one hour at 350 °C). The HK tests were taken from film cross sections, supported around the edges by 100 um nickel deposits, at loads of 100 g. Based on the method of Tabor [*4*], yield strengths calculated from HKs (ca 3 MPa/HK) indicate that these alloys are exceptionally strong, having yield strengths ranging from ca 1,920 MPa to 3,300 MPa (270,000 psi to 478,000 psi). These estimates compare favorably with the minimum yield and tensile strength requirements for cobalt-chromium-molybdenum alloys as given in ASTM specifications F-75 and F-1537, i.e.; 517 MPa and 897 MPa respectively. Such high strength is what was sought for the purpose of fabricating very thin prostheses for conservative tooth preparations. In addition, the corrosion potentials were ca 150 mV vs. hydrogen electrode potentials for the as-deposited alloy. These are alloys may be considered noble but their corrosion potentials are lower than those for polished cobalt-chromium-molybdenum dental alloy, which were found to be ca + 700 mV (the dental alloy is close in composition to that required for orthopaedic implant alloys according to ASTM F-75 and ASTM F-1537). Conversely, the corrosion current of the cobalt-phosphorous alloy is comparable to or better than (less than) that for the dental alloy and there was no evidence of pitting in the deposit.

The brittle nature of the glassy alloys is a potential detriment for use in the dental application and is certainly not a desirable feature for use as the main structural component of orthopaedic prostheses. However, this may actually be a favorable property for coatings on orthopaedic bearing surfaces to produce wear resistant bearing couples for orthopaedic implants. For example, unscratched, amorphous, diamond-like carbon coatings (ADL) have been described as resistant to scratch development by third body wear, and scratched ADL surfaces produced seven times (7 x) less wear on UHMWPE than did scratched stainless steel surfaces that were used for wear comparisons [*5*]. The explanation given was that the lack of ductility in the ADL coatings prevented the build-up of hilled material along scratches, due to plastic flow as the scratches were produced. The glassy alloys may behave in a similar manner.

Chromium-Carbon Alloys

Two other, related, examples of developments in glassy alloys that appear more interesting, because of the closer proximity of possible alloy compositions to those cobalt-chromium-molybdenum alloys described in ASTM F-75 and ASTM 1537, are those of Johnson [*6,7*] et.al. and Soltani [*8*]. These authors describe glassy, layered-structured, chromium-carbon alloys and cobalt-chromium-carbon alloys (Figs. 1 & 2).

The HKs of as-deposited glassy chromium are ca 800 kg/mm^2 to 850 kg/mm^2. The HKs were taken on film cross sections, supported around the edges by 100 um nickel deposits, at 50 g loads. The maximum HK (Fig. 3), attainable after a one hour heat treatment at 650 °C, is 1850 kg/mm^2 (for comparison, the HKs of highly pure zirconia and highly pure alumina are ca 1160 kg/mm^2 and 2100 kg/mm^2, respectively; hence, it may be possible to attain ceramic-like bearing properties when glassy derived coatings are applied to modular implant components). The heat-treated version just begins to display, by x-ray diffraction, evidence of carbide precipitation and a crystalline state that is probably nanocrystalline (as of this writing this has not yet been determined). In this condition the material is still expected to be brittle, but extremely hard, homogeneous with very finely dispersed precipitates, corrosion resistant, and strong). While the technology for deposition of chromium has been available for years, glassy coatings >ca 10 um could not be made. The Johnson et.al. advancement allows deposition of glassy coatings with thicknesses of 500 um or more. An interesting wear test result is that from a dry sliding-wear test against sintered tungsten carbide; wear of as-deposited chromium-carbon metal glass was 1/8 (12 %) of the wear rate of the tungsten carbide.

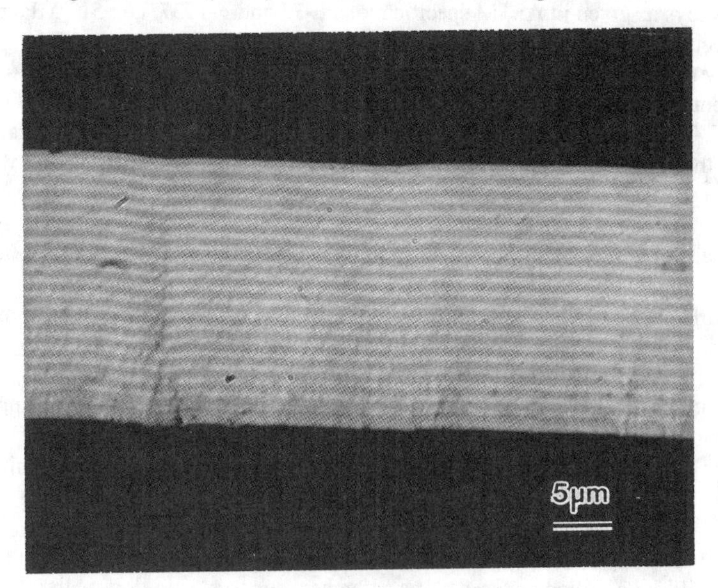

Fig. 1.Photograph of a layered structure from a cobalt-chromium-carbon alloy. A structure with ca 1.0 um thick layers was chosen for clear illustration. Layers as thin as 10 nm or less can be produced (Magnification. = 2000 X).

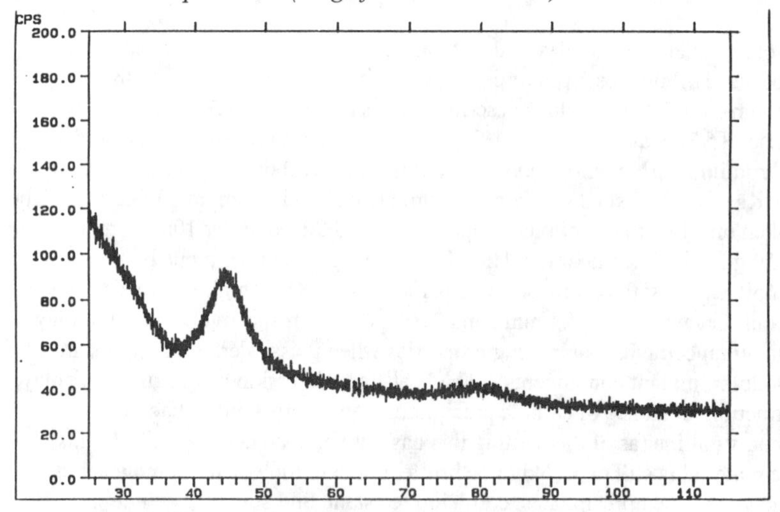

Fig. 2. X-ray diffraction showing the broad pattern from glassy cobalt-chromium multilayer deposit. The horizontal axis is the diffraction angle, 2θ., (resolution 0.01°). The vertical axis is the intensity in counts per second (CPS), for which the estimated standard uncertainty is ca 2 CPS.

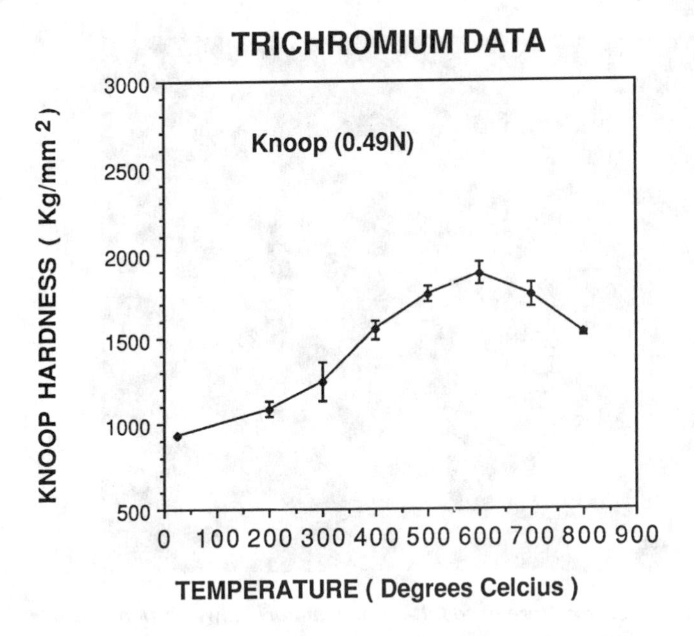

Fig.3. Knoop hardness number, HK, from glassy chromium deposit after heat treatments for one hour at the temperatures indicated.

Cobalt-Chromium-Carbon Alloys

The alloys of glassy cobalt-chromium-carbon are about as hard and strong as those of chromium-carbon and can be produced in thick coatings as well. HKs are: (693 ± 7.6) kg/mm^2, with a value of (692.4 ± 5.4) kg/mm^2 from measurements along the layer directions, and (694.8 ± 14.4) kg/mm^2 across the layers (± is the estimated standard uncertainty of the measurements). The HKs were taken from film cross sections, supported around the edges by 100 um nickel deposits, at loads of 25 g (Fig.4). Each layer is alternating glassy chromium and glassy cobalt; it is known that carbon exists in the chromium layer and it is expected that carbon also exists in the cobalt layer. By controlling the as-deposited layer thicknesses and selecting heat treatments, it is expected that the layered alloys may be homogenized to produce either glassy or nanocrystalline structures with a variety of compositions. If necessary, it should be possible to add molybdenum as a third element (if needed for resistance to pitting or crevice corrosion). The behavior of cobalt-chromium-carbon alloys is expected to be similar to that of the chromium-carbon alloys for which more data exists.

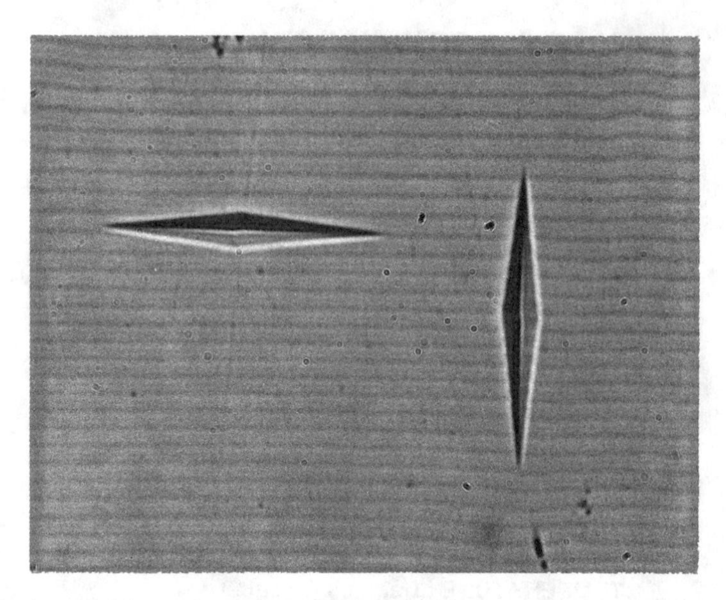

Fig.4. As-deposited layered structure of cobalt-chromium-carbon with Knoop hardness indentations (Magnification. = 2000 X).

Discussion and Conclusions

The resistance of the glassy cobalt-phosphorous alloys to pitting, the expected superior corrosion resistances of the glassy chromium-containing alloys, and the high hardnesses of these alloys render them interesting for further consideration for use as wear-resistant components of orthopaedic joint bearing couples. Because such alloys can be formed by electrodeposition, they can be readily deposited as shape-conforming coatings to bearing surfaces. The ability to heat treat these alloys to achieve a variety of properties and structures renders them attractive for attaining optimal performance characteristics. However, the adherence of any coating would need to be determined. If an as-deposited coating had poor adherence there is a possibility that it could be diffusion bonded to the underlying structure, producing an intermediate structural layer that adheres and also bonds well to the subsequently deposited coating. The results from the wear tests of Cr-C against tungsten carbide indicate that good bonding is possible with as-deposited coatings. In an as-deposited, glassy-state, a coating may have a lower elastic modulus than the underlying substrate alloy and, if so, this could conceivably be a benefit in stress transfer, depending on coating thickness. While mechanical properties may be changed by heat treatments, alloys composed of elements such as Co-P will form phosphides, which could completely change their corrosion properties [*9*], hence, structure and composition can very strongly interact to determine potential usefulness.

It is concluded that glassy alloys have unique properties that make them attractive for consideration as orthopaedic implant bearing surfaces. The Co-Cr-C system glassy alloy described appears to offer a good basis for further investigation and compositional modification because of its proximity to the composition of Co-Cr-Mo alloys currently used in orthopaedics. For all glassy alloys, factors such as adherence, apparent fracture toughness, corrosion resistance, structure and composition, and toxicity need to be considered.

Acknowledgment The authors gratefully acknowledge the assistance of Jasper P. Mullen in generation of x-ray diffraction and hardness data.

References

[1] Peters Jr., PC, Engh, GA, Dwyer, KA, and Vinh, TN, "Osteolysis After Total Knee Arthoplasty Without Cement," J. Bone Joint Surg, July, 1992, 74 (6): pp. 864-86.

[2] Schmalzreid, T P, Jasty, M, and Harris, WH, Preiprosthetic Bone Loss in Total Hip Arthroplasty: "The Role of Polyethylene Wear Debris and the Concept of the Effective Joint Space," J. Bone Joint Surg, July, 1992, 74A (6): 849- 863.

[3] Ratzker, M., Lashmore, D.S., and Tesk, J.A., U.S. Patent No. 5,316,650, Electroforming of Metallic Glasses for Dental Applications, 31 May 1994.

[4] D. Tabor, The Hardness and Strength of Metals, J. Inst Metals, 79: 1-18, 1951.

[5] Hailey, J.L., Furkins, P., Buttler, R., Lettington, A.H., and Fisher, J., "A Tribological Evaluation of Amorphous Diamond Like Carbon Coating for Use in Total Joint Replacement," Proceedings of 5th World Biomaterials Congress, Toronto, Canada, May 29 - June 2, 1996, 785.

[6] Johnson, C.E., Lashmore, D.S., and Soltani, E., U.S. Patent No. 5,415,763, Methods and Electrolyte Compositions for Electrodepositing Chromium Coatings, 16 May, 1995.

[7] Johnson, C.E., Lashmore, D.S., and Soltani, E., U.S. Patent 5,672,262, Methods and Electrolyte Compositions for Electrodepositing Metal-Carbon Alloys, 30 Sept., 1997.

[8] Soltani, E.C., Cobalt-Chromium Multilayer Alloys, Thesis submitted for degree of Master of Science, The University of Maryland, 1992.

[9] Helfand,MA, Clayton, CR, Ciegle, RB, and Sorenson, NR, "The Role of P in Anodic Inhibition of an Amorphous Co-20P Alloy in Acidic Electrolytes," J. Electrochem Soc, August 1992, 139 (8), pp. 2121-2127 .

Wendy M. Cipera[1] and John B. Medley[1]

TRIBOLOGICAL INVESTIGATIONS OF COBALT-BASED ALLOYS IN METAL-ON-METAL CONTACTS USING A RECIPROCATING CYLINDER-ON-FLAT APPARATUS WITH BOVINE SERUM LUBRICANTS

REFERENCE: Cipera, W. M. and Medley, J. B., **"Tribological Investigations of Cobalt-Based Alloys in Metal-on-Metal Contacts Using a Reciprocating Cylinder-on-Flat Apparatus with Bovine Serum Lubricants,"** *Alternative Bearing Surfaces in Total Joint Replacement, ASTM STP 1346*, J. J. Jacobs and T. L. Craig, Eds., American Society for Testing and Materials, 1998.

ABSTRACT: Retrieval studies have shown higher wear of metal-on-metal hip implants, on average, than found in simulator testing. The investigation of a simplified metal-on-metal contact under conditions of boundary lubrication might provide some insight into this behavior. Thus, the purpose of the present study was to perform exploratory tribological investigations using a linear reciprocating cylinder-on-flat apparatus under such conditions. Wrought cobalt-based alloys of high and low carbon content were tested in four lubricants, most containing bovine serum, for 3600 or 36000 cycles. The motion was sinusoidal with a stroke length of 13 mm. The load per cylinder was 50.5 N giving an average contact stress similar to metal-metal hip implants in simulators and *in vivo*. Some elementary analyses of lubrication conditions and the influence of mechanical vibrations caused by the tangential dynamics of the apparatus were presented. The main results consisted of friction and wear measurements. In the limited number of experiments performed, it was observed that alloy carbon content did not influence friction or wear for up to 36000 cycles, nor did additives in the bovine serum lubricant designed to discourage calcium-type deposits on the surfaces. Wear factors were calculated and provided an approximate prediction of some simulator wear in the initial period . Increasing the bovine serum content of the lubricant caused the friction to rise significantly thus suggesting a role of serum elements in metal-on-metal tribology. As a consequence of the work reported here, the application of cobalt-based alloys with low carbon content was encouraged and the use of the additives to suppress surface deposits was recommended in simulator testing.

KEYWORDS: friction, wear, cylinder-on-flat, metal-on-metal, cobalt-based alloys, hip implants, tribology, orthopaedics

---

[1]Graduate Student and Associate Professor, respectively, Department of Mechanical Engineering, University of Waterloo, Waterloo, ON N2L 3G1, Canada

A comparison between simulator and retrieval wear of metal-metal hip implants was made by Medley et al [*1*] in which linear least squares fits were performed on their simulator data and a selection of retrieval data from McKellop et al [*2*]. The agreement seemed quite good but if the simulator data values were examined more closely; a log least squares fit (of the form y = B log x + A), which reflected the rapid decline in initial wear rate, might have provided a better representation (Fig. 1). So, if the wear rate in the simulator remained low beyond 1.5 million cycles, as suggested by the log least squares curve fit, it was apparent that, in the long term, the simulator wear would seriously underestimate the average wear from retrievals. However, the retrieval data was very scattered and some of the retrieved implants showed very low wear, even after 24 years *in vivo*, which suggested that simulators might be able to represent some of these cases. A possible explanation for this rather confusing situation was the possibility that fluid film lubrication was less prevalent in individuals from which hips implants were retrieved than in the simulator used by Medley et al [*1*]. As fluid film lubrication became less prevalent, boundary lubrication with some direct surface contact and adhesive/abrasive wear would occur more extensively. Therefore, it would be useful to perform tribological investigations under controlled conditions of boundary lubrication.

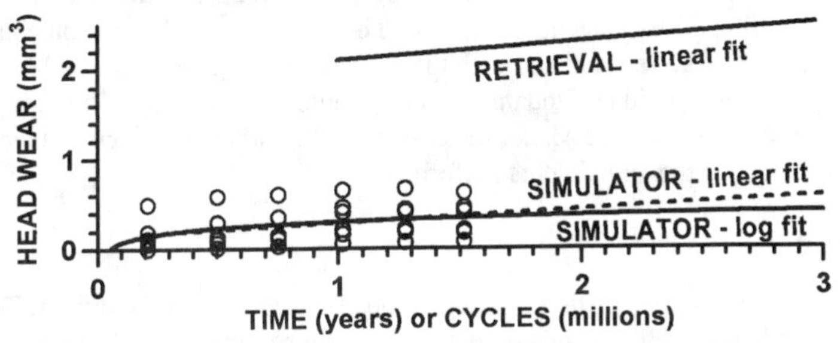

FIG. 1-- *Least squares linear fits for some retrieval and simulator data as presented by Medley et al [1] compared with a least squares log fit of the simulator data.*

One approach to creating conditions of boundary lubrication for metal-metal surfaces was to develop an apparatus with a pin-on-flat configuration, such that the specimen geometry precluded conventional fluid film lubrication. Only two such studies were found in the literature and neither one performed any assessment of the possibility of fluid film lubrication. A reciprocating sphere-on-flat apparatus was used by Walker and Erkman [*3*] with a 11 mm radius stationary sphere and a 58.9 N load. The speed of the flat surface was given as 1 mm/s (whether the motion was sinusoidal or of a square wave form was not clear). Various lubricants were used including synovial fluid, and a high molecular weight protein was shown to be important for lubrication. Using a Hertzian formula [*4*], the average contact stress was calculated as 764 MPa. Assuming that the given velocity was an average value, and using it in a steady state film thickness formula [*4*] along with a lubricant viscosity (corresponding to healthy synovial fluid [*5*]) of 0.01 Pa s, the central film thickness was calculated to be 0.2 nm. The given centerline-average (CLA) roughness of the flat surface was 0.1 μm which could be used to estimate a combined root mean square (RMS) roughness of 0.18 μm and then a lambda value of 0.0011 following the methods described in Medley et al [*4*]. Such a low lambda suggested that fluid film lubrication would not occur [*6*] and showed that conditions of boundary lubrication could be created using a pin-on-flat apparatus.

Streicher et al [*7*] used a sphere-on-disc apparatus with continuous motion of the flat disc surface at a speed of 10 mm/s. In this case, the sphere radius was 1.5 mm, the load was 2.46 N and most of the tests were run in a mixture of 30% bovine serum with Ringer's solution, which could be estimated to have a viscosity of about 0.0015 Pa s. A CLA surface roughness of 0.04 μm was given. Following the same calculation procedure as above, the average contact stress was 1000 MPa and the lambda value was 0.0013 which once again indicated conditions of boundary lubrication.

The above two studies [*3, 7*] provided some useful insights but were performed under quite high contact stresses compared to those likely to occur in vivo. Given the tribological complexity of these metal-metal contacts and the limited number of investigations performed, further study was warranted.

Thus, the purpose of the present study was to perform an exploratory investigation of friction and initial wear (up to 36000 cycles) under conditions of boundary lubrication with various lubricants using a linear reciprocating cylinder-on-flat apparatus with specimens of cobalt-based alloy. The cylinder-on-flat configuration and the linear (uni-axial) motion of the flat surface were chosen to simplify the contact and thus facilitate the tribological investigation of the remaining features. The influence of alloy carbon content and lubricant composition were examined with the intent of helping develop simulator wear protocols as well as providing fundamental insight into the metal-metal tribology. The present paper was based on the MASc thesis of the first author [*8*] which contained somewhat more details of the experiments performed.

Materials and Methods

The test specimens were made of wrought cobalt-based alloy (ASTM F 1537-94) of either about 0.05% or 0.20% carbon content. The surfaces were cleaned and passivated (ASTM F86) which included emersion in 20 - 40 % by volume of nitric acid for 30 minutes because this procedure was considered likely to be followed for hip implants. In the testing, contacting surfaces were always of the same carbon content.

The lubricants in the test program involved a variety of components (Table 1) combined to form bovine serum solutions (Table 2). Thus, the various lubricants (L1, L2, etc.) each had differing protein contents. Some solutions had ethylene diamine tetraacetic acid (EDTA) added to them to suppress the formation of calcium-type surface deposits.

Eleven experiments were performed with either lubricant L1 or L2; the first four for 36000 cycles and the remaining seven for 3600 cycles (Table 3). Additional tests of 300 cycles each for various lubricants were performed afterwards on the specimens of experiments numbers 5, 6, 7 and 8 in which lubricants L1, L3 and L4 were used in the sequences shown in Table 4.

The cylinder-on-flat apparatus (Fig. 2 and 3) had a uni-axial sinusoidal motion of the lower plate in which the flat test specimens were mounted. The motion of the lower plate was measured by a linear variable displacement transducer (LVDT).

A constant load was applied through an upper "sled" and cylindrical test specimens, all of which was held stationary by steel wires attached to "friction transducers" consisting of two strain-gauged cantilever beams of vertical orientation.

TABLE 1--*Components used in creating the lubricants.*

No.	Description	Purpose
C1	filter sterilized bovine calf serum*	analogue for synovial fluid
C2	ethylene diamine tetraacetic acid (EDTA), 20 mM in distilled water	suppress calcium-type surface deposits
C3	Fungizone** in distilled water	anti-fungal agent
C4	streptomycin** (type of penicillin)	anti-bacterial agent
C5	distilled water	produce different protein contents

*supplied by HyClone Laboratories, Inc., Logan UT
**supplied by Life Technologies, Inc., Grand Island, NY

TABLE 2--*Volumetric composition of the lubricants.*

Lubricant	Volumes, ml					Descriptive
	C1	C2	C3	C4	C5	Identification
L1	500	20	5	3	0	serum+EDTA
L2	500	0	5	3	0	serum
L3	150	6	1.5	0.9	369.6	28%serum+EDTA
L4	0	0	0	0	500	distilled water

TABLE 3--*Details of the friction and wear experiments.*

Expt. No.	1	2	3	4	5	6	7	8	9	10	11
Alloy %C	0.05	0.05	0.2	0.2	0.05	0.05	0.2	0.2	0.05	0.05	0.05
Lubricant	L1	L1	L1	L1	L1	L1	L1	L1	L2	L2	L2
Cycles x 10^{-3}	36	36	36	36	3.6	3.6	3.6	3.6	3.6	3.6	3.6

TABLE 4--*Lubricant investigation in which the bearing surfaces from the experiments of Table 3 were subjected to additional sequential tests of 300 cycles each for various lubricants.*

Expt. No.	Lubricants					
5	L3	L4	L1			
6	L3	L4	L1	L3	L4	L1
7	L3	L4	L1	L3	L4	L1
8	L3	L4	L1	L3	L4	L1

By attaching the steel wires above the plane of the friction forces, a small "rocking motion" was induced over the cycle in that a moment balance on the sled revealed that the normal load and friction force were larger on the leading cylindrical contact compared with the trailing one[*8*]. To obtain readings from each of the friction transducers, in either direction, the steel wires were pulled into tension before testing began and thus had the same initial readings. The output voltages from the friction transducers were essentially of a "square-wave" form (with some superimposed oscillations, to be discussed later in the present paper), and were close to mirror images of each other as well as being reasonably symmetric about a common mean value. Thus, four total friction signals were available (two for the forward stroke and two for the return stroke) which, when averaged and then divided in half (because there were two contacting cylinders), gave the average friction force magnitude on a single cylindrical contact over the cycle. Signal conditioners were used (Fig. 2 - top) and a computer data acquisition system recorded the output from the two sets of strain gauges and the LVDT.

The flat test specimens (63.5 mm x 25.4 mm x 9.5 mm thick) were mounted on the lower plate (Fig. 4) and surrounded by rubber walls to retain a small quantity of lubricant during testing. The lower plate was supported by a linear bearing track and reciprocated at 1 Hz with a stroke length of 13 mm, thus having an average surface velocity of 26 mm/s.

Two cylindrical test specimens (each 25 mm in diameter and 50 mm long, with rounded ends from a crown radius of 1.27 m taking 5 mm at either end of the cylinder [*8*]) were mounted in the upper sled (Fig. 4) upon which weights were added such that the static load per cylinder was 50.5 N. The dynamic load was about 13% higher when leading, 13% lower when trailing, because of the previously mentioned "rocking motion", but the average was equal to the static value. One cylinder was fixed rigidly to the bottom of the sled but the other could tilt laterally thus ensuring even loading along the length of each cylinder.

The root mean square (RMS) surface roughness of two cylinder and two flat test specimens were measured with the profilometer (Talysurf V made by Rank Taylor Hobson, Leicester, England) at a cut-off length of 0.8 mm and the range was 19 - 36 nm with an average of 26 nm. These values were in the range of commercially available implants [*1*]. Unfortunately, further efforts to characterize the surface topography of the test specimens were not done in the present study since the full import of initial surface roughness on the subsequent wear [*9*] was not recognized at the time of testing.

The length in the direction of motion of the wear track on the cylinder was measured at a number of axial locations along the cylinder using an optical microscope and a profilometer (Talysurf V) was used to determine whether the wear track was flat. Then, the volume loss of the cylinder caused by the wear was calculated using elementary geometric formulae [*8*]. If the same wear volume was assumed to occur on the flat surface (spread out along the contact path), then wear factors (total volumetric wear in mm^3 divided by the product of load in N and sliding distance in m) could be calculated.

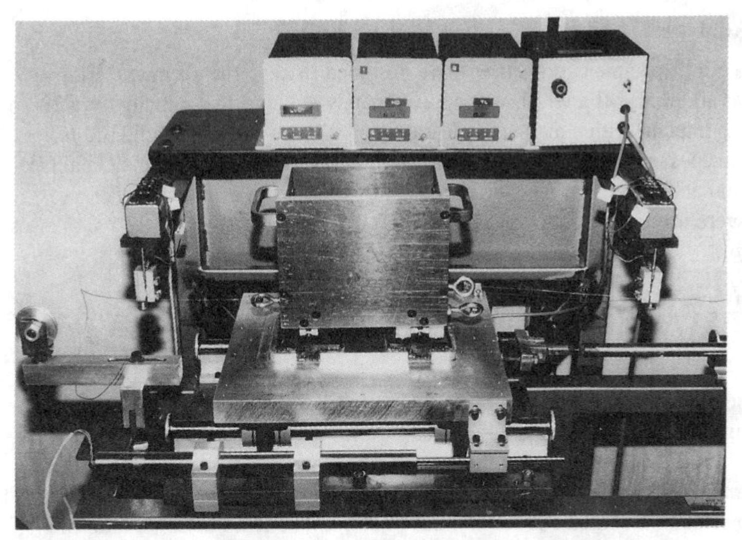

FIG. 2--*Photograph of the reciprocating cylinder-on-flat apparatus*

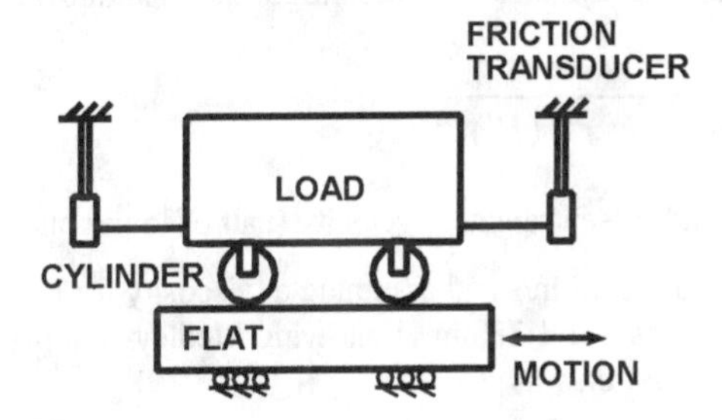

FIG. 3--*Sketch of the reciprocating cylinder-on-flat apparatus*

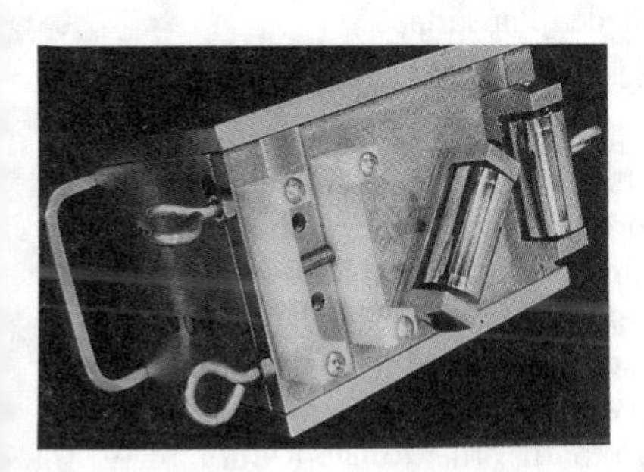

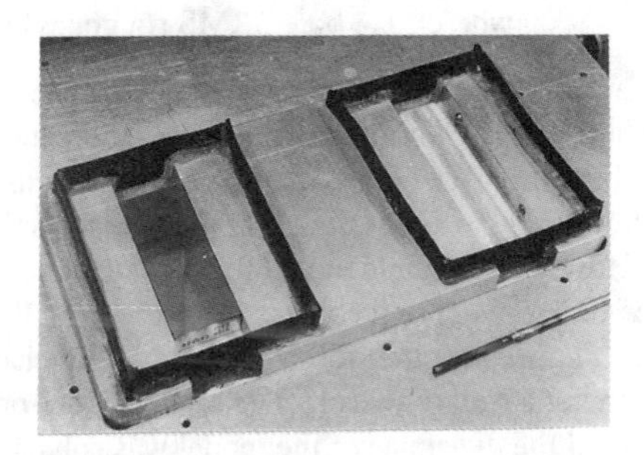

FIG. 4--*Cylindrical surfaces (left) and flat surfaces (right) with mounting fixtures.*

Preliminary Analysis

The load and specimen geometries were designed to keep the average Hertzian contact stress at about 50 MPa which was approximately equal to that initially for a 28 mm diameter hip implant with a diametral clearance of 100 μm and a load of 2100 N. This hip geometry was typical of the metal-metal hip implants tested by Medley et al [*1*]. The classic formulae for the average Hertzian contact stress for a cylinder-on-flat configuration were used in the following form:

$$\sigma_{AVG} = \sqrt{\frac{\pi F' E'}{32R}} \quad (1) \qquad \text{where} \qquad F' = \frac{F}{l_w} \quad (2), \qquad E' = \frac{E}{1 - \nu^2} \quad (3)$$

and F = load, N; l_w = length of cylinder, m; E = elastic modulus, Pa; ν = Poisson' ratio; R = cylinder radius, m

For the load of 50.5 N, the "effective" length of cylinder of 40 mm and a cylinder radius of 12.7 mm along with an assumed elastic modulus of 230 GPa and a Poisson's ratio of 0.3, the average contact stress was 49.7 MPa.

The same type of formula as given by Medley et al [*4*] was found in Herrebrugh [*10*] for central film thickness in a cylinder-on-flat configuration as follows:

$$h_c = 2.482 \frac{(\eta u R)^{0.6}}{(E')^{0.4}(F')^{0.2}} \quad (4)$$

where η =viscosity, Pa s and u =entrainment velocity (half of lower plate velocity), m/s.

For the entrainment velocity of 0.013 m/s and assuming a viscosity for a serum solution of 0.0015 Pa s, the film thickness was 1.78 nm. Following Medley et al [*4*], the lambda for the cylinder-on-flat configuration was

$$\lambda = \frac{h_c}{\sqrt{\sigma_C^2 + \sigma_F^2}} \quad (5)$$

where σ_C, σ_F = RMS roughness of cylinder, flat surface

For an average RMS roughness of 26 nm for each of the surfaces, the lambda value was 0.05 which indicated boundary lubrication conditions [*6*].

Friction force (F_f) as measured by the transducers showed some high frequency oscillations (Fig. 5) suggesting that the actual friction force magnitude varied during the cycle. However, a simple model for the tangential dynamics was assumed (Fig. 5) with a mass of 10.3 kg, a spring constant of 52.9 kN, a damping coefficient of 221 Ns/ m and a *constant* imposed friction force of 20.2 N (that changed direction instantly at the stroke ends forming a square wave). The second order ordinary differential equation that represented the dynamics of the model was solved with a fourth order Runge-Kutta numerical routine as described by Milivojevich [*11*]. The resulting "measured friction force" that was predicted by the model showed somewhat similar oscillations (Fig. 5), thus suggesting that the tangential dynamics of the apparatus might be responsible for the oscillations. In other words, the apparatus could have experienced mechanical vibrations because an essentially constant friction force drove a classical spring-mass-damper system. This was consistent with the early work of Cipera [8] in which severe signal oscillations were reduced significantly by using the thicker and thus stiffer cantilever beams of the present study for the friction transducers. Also, the previously mentioned rocking motion might have contributed to the signal oscillations.

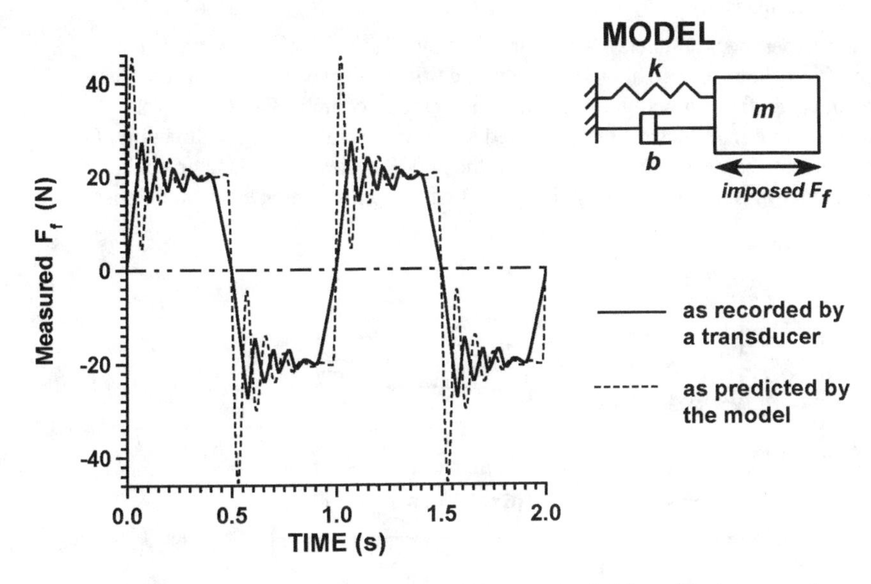

FIG. 5--*Oscillatory response of the measured F_f as recorded by a friction transducer and as predicted by the simple model with constant imposed friction force that changed instantly at the stroke ends.*

Before leaving this topic, it was noted that the measured F_f as recorded by a friction transducer did not change instantly at the stroke ends. This behavior was caused by a short period of "stick" after the relative surface velocity fell to zero near the stroke ends which continued until the friction force exceeded the maximum possible static friction force. It was possible (but not inevitable) that the friction force might have subsequently dropped once sliding was initiated and thus a higher static than dynamic friction force might have contributed to the signal oscillations. However, the assumption of a *constant magnitude* friction force in the simple model still gave a high initial peak in the oscillations (Fig. 5). Furthermore, an appropriate choice of model parameters gave a prediction of the measured F_f which showed some tendency to merge with the transducer signal at the stoke midpoint (Fig. 5). Therefore, an extension of the developed model to include "stick" alone might give a predicted oscillation pattern quite close to the actual transducer values. The exact roles of static/dynamic friction and the "stick" behavior were beyond the scope of the present study. However, it was considered valuable to simply illustrate the potential role of unwanted mechanical vibrations of the apparatus in causing some imprecision in the friction measurements.

In all of the subsequent results, a single representative value of friction was obtained for the cycle by "averaging out" the oscillations and following the procedure described in the *Methods and Materials* section to combine the signals from the two transducers.

Results and Discussion

For experiment numbers 1 - 8 using lubricant L1, the coefficients of friction increased from about 0.16 to about 0.21 over the first 3600 cycles but no difference was detected between friction with high and low alloy carbon content (Fig. 6). It was interesting to note that the specimens showed some wide scratches in the direction of motion indicating some abrasive wear during the 36000 cycles. This damage could be seen by comparing surfaces before and after testing using a scanning electron microscope (Fig. 7).

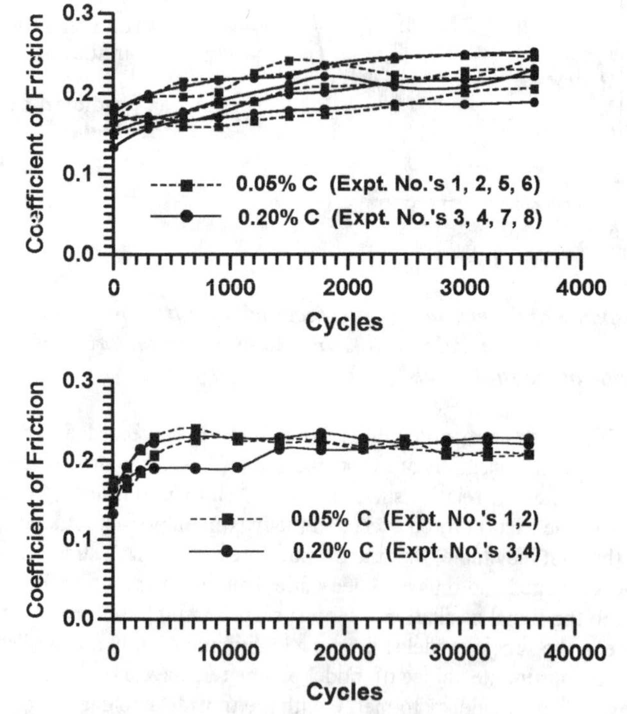

FIG. 6--*Friction over 3600 cycles (top) and 36000 cycles(bottom).*

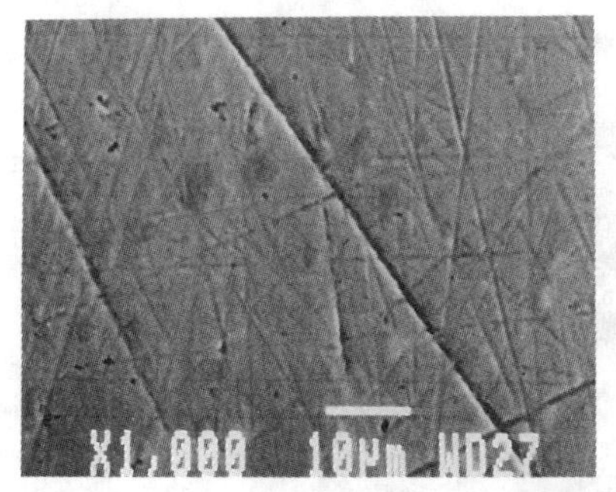

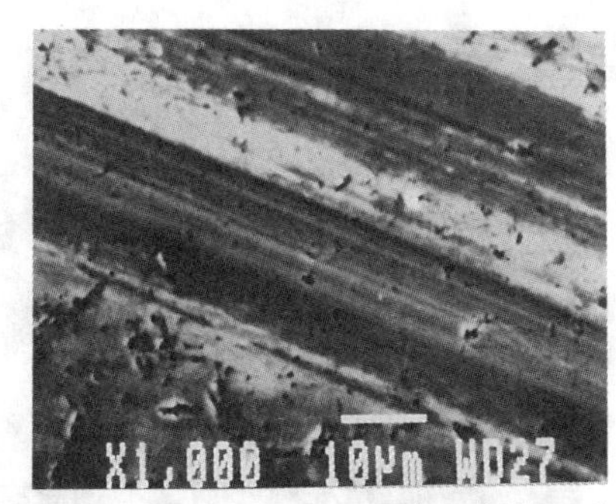

FIG. 7--*Scanning electron micrographs of 0.2% C flat specimens at 0 cycles (left) and after testing in lubricant L1 for 36000 cycles (right).*

Optical microscopy (Fig. 8 and 9), however, showed clear evidence on the cylinder surface after 3600 cycles and on the flat surface after 36000 cycles that the residual machining marks were polished out, in most cases, by the wear process. Thus, although there did seem to be additional abrasive scratching of the surfaces as shown in Fig. 7 the overall effect was to polish out surface scratches by a controlled wear process. This feature was present in alloys of both high and low carbon content and had been described as a "self-healing" process [2, *12*]. The friction did not seem much influenced by the polishing out of the scratches but perhaps the slight decline in the coefficient of friction shown in Fig. 6 after about 10000 cycles might have been a result of reducing the friction component associated with ploughing over rough surface features, by the development of the somewhat smoother surface. It should be remembered, however, that smoother surfaces in boundary lubrication conditions could have an increased friction due to more adhesion between the surfaces.

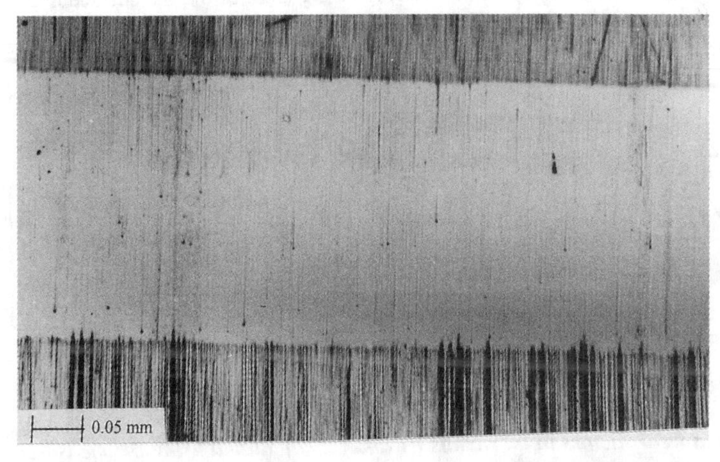

FIG. 8--Optical micrographs of the wear track on a 0.05% C cylinder after 3600 cycles.

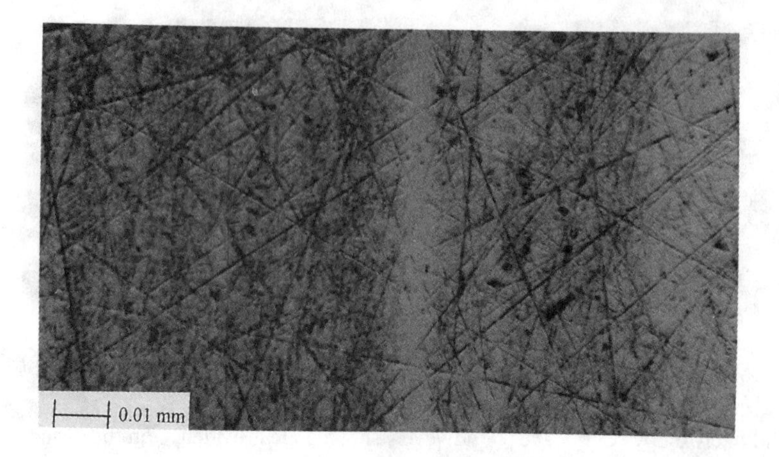

FIG. 9--*Optical micrographs of the wear track on a 0.20% C flat after 36000 cycles.*

The wear factors calculated for the experiments in the present study seemed to decrease slightly from 3600 to 36000 cycles and did not show any strong influence of alloy carbon content (Fig. 10). Wear factors seemed to be slightly higher when EDTA was not used but this result was not statistically significant. At 36000 cycles, one specimen pair had a higher wear factor than the other three specimen pairs. The RMS roughnesses of the unworn surface regions of this pair were examined in detail (eight profilometer traces of 5.6 mm at a cut-off length of 0.8 mm on each surface). The cylinder had an average RMS roughness of 20 nm but the flat surface had an average value of 37 nm. The average RMS roughness of the chosen representative surfaces mentioned previously had been 26 nm. Although the evidence was rather circumstantial, it was considered possible that the higher average RMS roughness of the flat surface might have been the factor responsible for the higher wear factor.

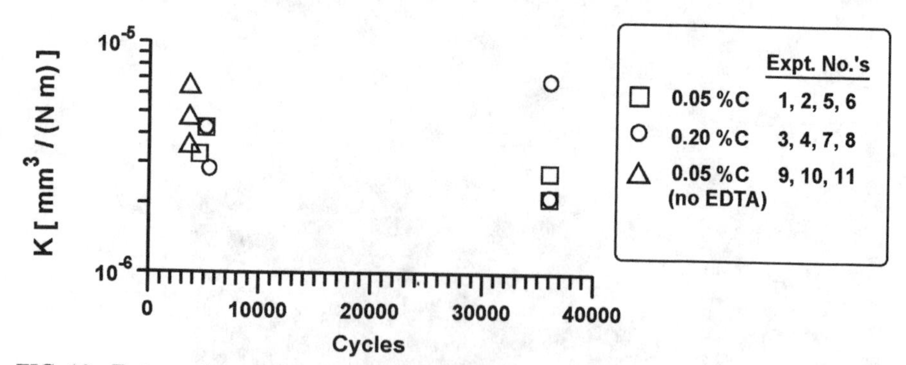

FIG. 10--*Estimated wear factors in lubricants L1 and L2 calculated using the measured volumetric wear of the cylinders and assuming the same wear for the flats.*

The limited wear data produced in the present study prevented any precise comparisons with simulator wear. However, the following calculations were performed to obtain a very approximate comparison. At 36000 cycles, the average wear factor was 3.5 x 10^{-6} mm^3/N-m . The simulator had an average load of about 891 N [*1*] and a cyclic path length of about 2 π (0.014) sin 22.5° [*4*]. Using the average wear factor from the cylinder-on-flat apparatus, simulator wear was predicted at 36000 cycles as about 3.8 mm^3 (or 31 mg) which was in the range of experiment 15 reported by Medley et al [*13*] that had the same low carbon alloy with about the same roughness as used as in the present study. It was also interesting to note that this simulator experiment, with a custom-made implant, had volumetric wear above both the linear fit of the retrievals and the tested commercial implants shown in Fig. 1. Thus, the reason that the cylinder-on-flat apparatus gave wear comparable to this particular simulator experiment might have been that they were both in a predominantly boundary lubrication regime. In any case, the cylinder-on-flat apparatus was capable of giving wear that could be related to some initial simulator wear in an approximate fashion.

The wear factors reported by Streicher et al [*7*] were about 2 x 10^{-6} mm^3/Nm for high carbon alloy (about 0.20% C) and 11 x 10^{-6} to 23 x 10^{-6} mm^3/Nm for low carbon alloy (about 0.05% C). The wear factors of the high carbon alloy were similar to those of the present study. The somewhat higher wear factors for the low carbon alloy might have been related to the very high initial contact stress (1 GPa) used by Streicher et al.

The initial wear did not seem to be much influenced by the presence or absence of EDTA as shown previously. Also, friction was not much influenced during 3600 cycles (Fig. 11) but EDTA did affect the appearance of the surfaces. When EDTA was not used (lubricant L2), deposits were found at the edges or, sometimes, in the middle of the wear track on the cylinder (Fig. 12). Unfortunately, the composition of the deposits was not examined but it was assumed that they were calcium phosphorus or perhaps calcium chromium rich. When EDTA was used, deposits were reduced significantly but not eliminated. It was interesting to note that deposits were found on retrieved metal-metal implants by McKellop et al [*2*].

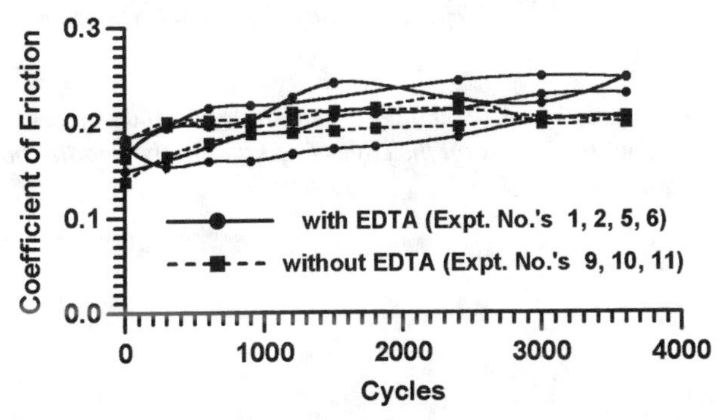

FIG. 11--*Influence of ethylene diamine tetraacetic acid (EDTA) on friction.*

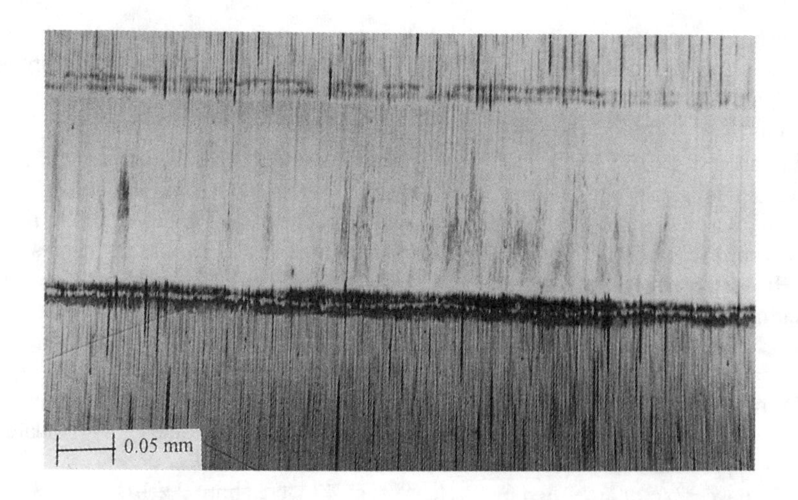

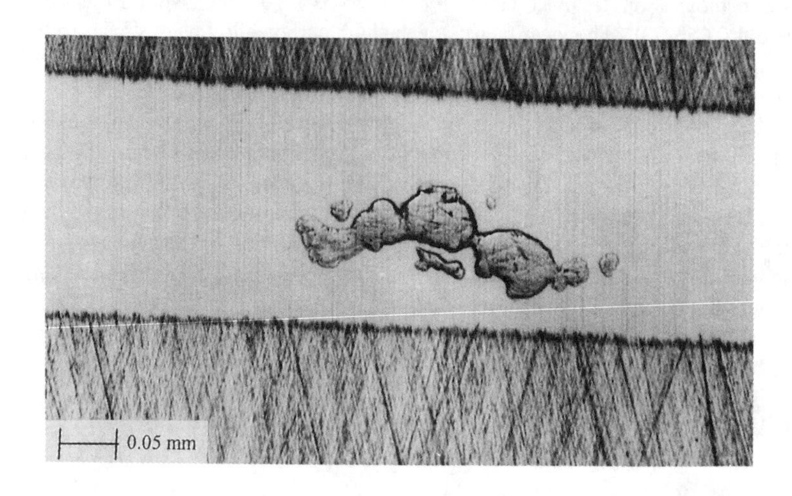

FIG. 12--*Optical micrographs for the 0.05% C cylinder after 3600 cycles testing in lubricant L2 with deposits on the edges (top) and in the middle (bottom) of the wear track on the cylinders.*

The final set of tests involved lubricants L1, L3 and L4, each having different amounts of bovine serum and thus protein content. It was found that friction increased significantly (ANOVA, post hoc contrast, $p < 0.01$) with increasing serum content (Fig. 13). This result was surprising since the protein elements in serum were expected to reduce friction and this expectation was supported by the experiments of Walker and Erkman [*3*] who found that increased protein did indeed reduce friction in their tests with cast alloy. However, Streicher et al [*7*] had found that testing wrought alloy in humid air gave lower friction on average compared with testing in a serum solution whereas when cast alloy was used no difference was detected. Thus, the present results seemed to be consistent with previous studies and suggested that humid air and distilled water gave somewhat similar tribological environments.

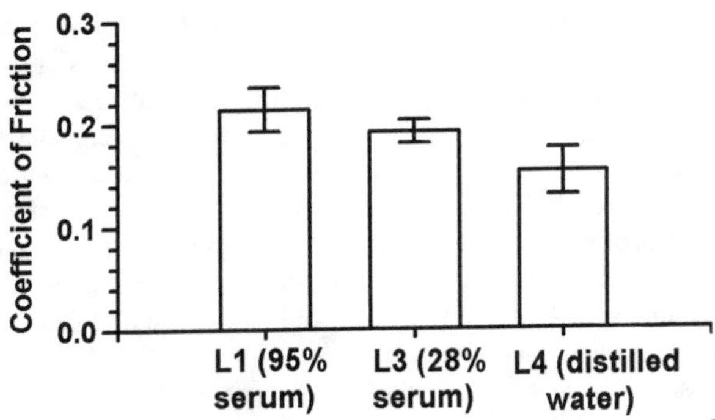

FIG. 13--*Friction in lubricants with various protein contents measured using the surfaces of experiment numbers 5, 6, 7, 8 as described in Table 3.*

Conclusions

The purpose of the present study was to investigate tribological performance of the cobalt-based alloys used in joint replacement implants under conditions of boundary as opposed to fluid film lubrication. A simplified contact was chosen and the following observations and findings were obtained from the experiments.

1. The alloy carbon content was not observed to influence the friction and wear.
2. Wrought cobalt-based alloys showed a "self-healing" type of wear in which surface scratches were gradually polished away.
3. Wear factors from the reciprocating cylinder-on-flat configuration allowed a prediction of initial simulator wear that was in the correct range.
4. Adding EDTA to the serum solution was observed to suppress surface deposits but did not change friction or wear.
5. Friction was found to increase significantly with serum content of the lubricant.

Significance

Reliable simulator protocols have not yet been established for testing metal-metal hip implants. Neither a full investigation of the many options for simulating the tribological conditions nor extensive comparison with clinical retrievals have been performed. As discussed previously, only two relevant pin-on-flat studies could be found in the literature. Therefore, the observations and findings of the present study were considered useful in streamlining the development of simulator protocols and could play a supporting role in implant design.

For example, the issue of whether or not to add EDTA to the lubricant used in simulator testing could be addressed. In the present study, adding EDTA did not seem to influence friction or wear significantly but it did provide somewhat cleaner specimen surfaces. Thus, it could be recommended for simulator studies to improve precision of wear measurements while still allowing some deposits which were found to be an *in vivo* feature [*2*]. The lack of difference between the low and high carbon versions of the cobalt-based alloy suggested that low carbon alloys might be an alternative to high carbon in metal-metal hip implants. Finally, the higher friction with increased serum content of the lubricant suggested that perhaps bovine serum had some deficiencies as a lubricant. However, the higher friction might be a result of the shearing of thick, protective layers of protein elements at the zones of intimate surface contact and thus bovine serum might be a superior lubricant for reducing wear. Clearly some components of the serum were active in the tribology and thus simulator testing protocols should take account of this behavior and select serum content of the lubricant with care.

One further point of significance was considered. In the present study, two metal surfaces were loaded together in pure sliding contact under reasonably high load with no cross-shearing action (which might be expected to hasten the self-healing behavior mentioned previously and thus reduce wear somewhat) and in a lubricant composed largely of water. Changes were made to the alloy and lubricant composition which were expected to influence the tribology in an obvious way. However, very little change was observed in the friction or the wear. Therefore, the beneficial tribology of cobalt-based alloys in orthopaedic applications might prove to be more robust than previously suspected.

Acknowledgments

The technical assistance of Ernst Huber, Victor Kiss, Steve Hitchman and Paul Renkma (all in Mech Eng at the University of Waterloo) was invaluable to this research effort. Greg Haider (Champlin Grinding Corp., Champlin, MN) performed much of the detailed specimen preparation. Robert Conta (Wright Medical Technology, Inc., Arlington, TN) facilitated the delivery of the rather complex specimens. Aleksa Milivojevich (Graduate Student, Mech Eng, University of Waterloo) provided considerable insight into the mechanical vibrations of the apparatus while working to complete his MASc Project. Editorial help from Judith Dowling improved this manuscript greatly. Financial support was provided by Wright Medical Technology, Inc., Arlington, TN and MRC Canada.

References

[*1*] Medley, J.B., Dowling, J.M., Poggie, R.A., Krygier, J.J. and Bobyn, J.D., "Simulator Wear of Some Commercially Available Metal-on-Metal Hip Implants," submitted to *Alternative Bearing Surfaces in Total Joint Replacement, ASTM STP 1346*, J.J. Jacobs and T.L. Craig, Eds., American Society for Testing and Materials, 1998.

[*2*] McKellop, H., Park, S.H., Chiesa, R., Dorn, P. Lu, B., Normand, P., Grigoris, P. and Amstutz, H. "In Vivo Wear of 3 Types of Metal-on-Metal Hip Prostheses During 2 Decades of Use," *Clinical Orthopaedics and Related Research*, No. 329S, 1996, pp. S128-S140.

[*3*] Walker, P.S. and Erkman, M.J., "Metal-on-Metal Lubrication in Artificial Human Joints," *Wear*, Vol. 21, 1972, pp. 377-392.

[*4*] Medley, J.B., Krygier, J.J., Bobyn, J.D., Chan, F.W., Lippincott, A. and Tanzer, M., "Kinematics of the MATCO™ Hip Simulator and Issues Related to Wear Testing of Metal-Metal Implants," *Proceedings of the Institution of Mechanical Engineers, Part H, Journal of Engineering in Medicine,* Vol. 211, No. H1, 1997, pp. 89-99.

[*5*] Cooke, A.F., Dowson, D. and Wright, V., "The Rheology of Synovial Fluid and Some Potential Synthetic Lubricants for Degenerate Synovial Joints," *Journal of Engineering in Medicine*, Vol. 7, 1978, pp. 66-72.

[*6*] Johnson, K.L., Greenwood, J.A. and Poon, S.Y. "A Simple Theory of Asperity Contact in Elastohydrodynamic Lubrication," *Wear*, Vol. 19, 1992, pp. 91-108.

[*7*] Streicher, R.M., Semlitsch, M., Schön, R., Weber, H. and Rieker, C. "Metal-on-Metal Articulation for Artificial Hip Joints: Laboratory Study and Clinical Results," *Proceedings of the Institution of Mechanical Engineers, Part H, Journal of Engineering in Medicine,* Vol. 210, No. H3, 1996, pp. 223-232.

[*8*] Cipera, W.M., "A Tribological Study of CoCrMo Alloys for Use in Metal-Metal Total Hip Arthroplasty," *MASc Thesis*, Dept of Mech Eng, University of Waterloo, 1996.

[*9*] Chan, F.W., Bobyn, J.D., Medley, J.B., Krygier, J.J., Yue, S. and Tanzer, M. "Wear Performance of Metal-Metal Hip Implants," *Archives of the American Academy of Orthopaedic Surgeons,* Vol. 1, No. 1, 1997, pp. 57-60.

[*10*] Herrebrugh, K., "Solving the Incompressible and Isothermal Problem in Elastohydrodynamic Lubrication Through an Integral Equation," *Transactions of the American Society of Mechanical Engineers, Journal of Lubrication Technology*, Vol. 90, 1968, pp. 262-278.

[*11*] Milivojevich, A. "The Vibrational Analysis of a Reciprocating Pin-on-Flat Friction Apparatus", *MASc Project*, Dept of Mech Eng, University of Waterloo, 1998.

[*12*] Chan, F.W., Bobyn, J.D., Medley, J.B., Krygier, J.J., Yue, S. and Tanzer, M., "The engineering issues and wear performance of metal-on-metal hip implants. *Clinical Orthopaedics and Related Research,* Vol. 333, 1996, pp. 96-107.

[*13*] Medley, J.B., Chan, F.W., Krygier, J.J. and Bobyn, J.D., "Comparison of Alloys and Designs in a Hip Simulator Study of Metal-on-Metal Implants," *Clinical Orthopaedics and Related Research*, No. 329S, 1996, pp. S160-S186.

John B. Medley[1], Judith M. Dowling [1], Robert A. Poggie [2], Jan J. Krygier [3], and J. Dennis Bobyn[3]

SIMULATOR WEAR OF SOME COMMERCIALLY AVAILABLE METAL-ON-METAL HIP IMPLANTS

REFERENCE: Medley, J. B., Dowling, J. M., Poggie, R. A., Krygier, J. J. and Bobyn, J. D., **"Simulator Wear of Some Commercially Available Metal-on-Metal Hip Implants,"** *Alternative Bearing Surfaces in Total Joint Replacement, ASTM STP 1346,* J. J. Jacobs and T. L. Craig, Eds., American Society for Testing and Materials, 1998.

ABSTRACT: Simulator wear tests were conducted for 1.5 million cycles on second generation metal-on-metal hip implants fabricated from cobalt-based alloy (ASTM F 1537-94) to compare their performance with each other and with both custom-made implants and retrieval studies published in the literature. In addition, factors controlling wear were explored. Six commercially available implants were tested (2 low carbon and 4 high carbon) for 1.5 million cycles in a MATCO™ hip simulator following previously established protocols. Volumetric wear was in the same range for all of the implants tested and much less than would be expected in comparable tests with conventional polyethylene cups. The wear of the commercial implants used in the present study was very similar to custom-made hip implants of similar diameter, clearance and surface roughness. Three of the high carbon implants of the present study had somewhat lower wear than expected when their surface roughness was taken into account but, in general, clearance, roughness and lambda (a ratio of lubricant film thickness to combined surface roughness) were factors controlling wear. The simulator wear of the present study showed some agreement with the *in vivo* wear estimated in retrieval studies in the literature.

KEYWORDS: wear, simulator, metal-on-metal, hip implants, tribology, orthopaedics

---

[1]Associate Professor and Research Associate, respectively, Department of Mechanical Engineering, University of Waterloo, Waterloo, ON N2L 3G1, Canada.

[2] Director of Applied Research, Implex Corp., 80 Commerce Dr., Allendale, NJ 07401-1600, U.S.A.

[3]Technical Coordinator and Associate Professor, respectively, Jo Miller Orthopaedic Research Laboratory, Montreal General Hospital, 1650 Cedar Ave., Montreal, PQ H3G 1A4, Canada.

Modern "second generation" versions of metal-on-metal (m-m) hip implants have been commercially available since 1988 and more than 50,000 have been implanted in Europe [*1*]. The second generation m-m hip implants have controlled clearances, low deviations from sphericity and smooth surfaces compared with the "first generation" m-m hip implants used in the 1960's and early 1970's. Also, the second generation m-m hip implants [*2*] are made from wrought cobalt-based alloy (ASTM F 1537-94) with a small grain size (ASTM No. 5 or better) rather than the cast cobalt-based alloy (ASTM F 75-92) with much coarser grains used in the first generation implants. Retrieval studies [*1, 3, 4, 5*] show much lower volumetric wear compared with the wear of conventional ultra high molecular weight polyethylene cups against metal or ceramic heads. This low wear suggests that wear particle-induced osteolysis may be reduced by using m-m hip implants. However, m-m hip implants are not approved, as yet, by the Federal Drug Administration (FDA) of the United States of America. Efforts have been made to identify the extent of the knowledge related to m-m hip arthroplasty [*6*]. One area of deficient knowledge is the simulator study of m-m hip implant wear. Simulator wear testing, with its good control and realistic representation of tribological conditions, is essential for developing improved implant design and for interpreting data from clinical retrieval studies.

The pioneering work of Streicher et al [*2, 7*] on the simulator wear of m-m hip implants, while very useful, did not examine enough implants to provide much more than a cursory preliminary investigation. Full journal papers on simulator wear of m-m hip implants have been published recently [*8, 9, 10, 11, 12*] but involved only one research group using custom-made implants rather than commercial product. Thus, the main purpose of the present study was to generate simulator wear data for m-m implants from two European manufacturers and then compare their performance with each other, with the most recent simulator study of custom-made implants [*12*] and with the *in vivo* wear estimated from implant retrievals [*4, 5, 7*]. Particular attention was focussed on the factors that have been shown to be important in the control of implant wear [*11, 12*].

Materials and Methods

Two designs of implant (Fig. 1) were tested, each from a different manufacturer, but all having diameters of 28 mm and all made from wrought cobalt-based alloy (ASTM F 1537-94). Two implants of one design were supplied by Pan Titan[4] (PT1, PT2) with a low carbon content (≈ 0.06% C) and four implants of the other design were supplied by Sulzer Orthopedics[5] (SO1, SO2, SO3, SO4) with a higher carbon content (≈ 0.20% C).

---

[4] Neustadt, Austria

[5] Winterthur, Switzerland

The geometries of all the implants were characterized (Table 1) by head diameter (D_H), diametral clearance (C_L) and combined root mean square (RMS) roughness (σ)

$$\sigma = \sqrt{R_{qH}^2 + R_{qC}^2} \quad (1)$$

where R_{qH}, R_{qC} = RMS roughness of the head, cup.

All of the measurements of geometry were conducted by the Lawrence Livermore National Laboratory (University of California, Livermore, CA).

The RMS roughness of each head and cup was obtained from a trace with a profilometer (Form Talysurf made by Rank Taylor Hobson, Leicester, UK) at 45° "latitude" with a cut-off length of 0.762 mm. The precision (or repeatability) range of the roughness measurements was estimated as about ±1.3 nm (±0.05 μin). However, the accuracy range (which was more relevant to considerations of these measurements) was difficult to quantify because a single measurement was taken away from the contact zone and the assumption made that the roughness did not vary much over the surface. This assumption dominated the estimations of accuracy. Cipera [*14*] performed measurements using a profilometer (Talysurf 5 made by Rank Taylor Hobson, Leicester, UK) on a cylinder and a flat specimen both made from wrought cobalt-based alloy (ASTM F 1537-94) and prepared by a precision grinding procedure. Eight RMS roughness measurements were made on each surface and, in both cases, they fell within the range defined by the mean value ± 15%. Assuming this range represented the implants tested in the present study, a calculus of errors analysis with Gauss's law of propagation [*13*] using average values of the RMS for the head and cup of the SO implants suggested that a combined RMS roughness (σ) based a single measurement on the head and on the cup (as given in Table 1) would be within 14% of the true average value (either higher or lower). The same calculations for the PT implants gave an accuracy range of 12 %. Without making multiple measurements over the implant surfaces, a better estimate of accuracy was not possible.

The head and cup radii were estimated for each component by averaging the radii of two best fit circles of surface coordinates obtained by a coordinate measuring machine (Sheffield Small Radius Gauge made by Sheffield Measurement, Sheffield , UK) from traces taken through the "poles" along lines of "longitude" that were 90° apart, and these radii were used subsequently to determine the head diameter and diametral clearance. The precision (or repeatability) range of the measurements was estimated as about ±12.7 nm (±0.5 μin) but once again the accuracy range was larger and more relevant to the considerations of these measurements. The maximum difference between the two radii measured on a individual SO head was 0.7 μm and thus their average value might be expected to fall with ± 0.35 μm of the true average. For SO cups the equivalent range was ± 3.1 μm . However, having only two PT implants, the range was arbitrarily increased to equal the difference between the two radii measured on an individual head or cup and thus was ±0.1 μm for the heads and ± 1.1 μm for the cups. As above, a calculus of errors analysis with Gauss's law of propagation using average values of C_L suggested that the quoted C_L values for SO head-cup combinations had and accuracy range of 7% whereas the PT head-cup combinations had an accuracy range of 2%.

In estimating the radii of curvature from best fit circles of surface coordinates, the maximum difference between the digital data and the fitted circles for either of the traces through the poles along lines of longitude was defined as the sphericity of each component (Table 1) and provided a measure of the local variation of "roundness". Sphericity was a measure of "waviness" rather than "roughness" since it recorded a larger scale variation from the nominal spherical shape of head and cup surfaces. Although sphericities were recorded to provide additional characterization of implant geometry, their influences on wear were not investigated, as yet.

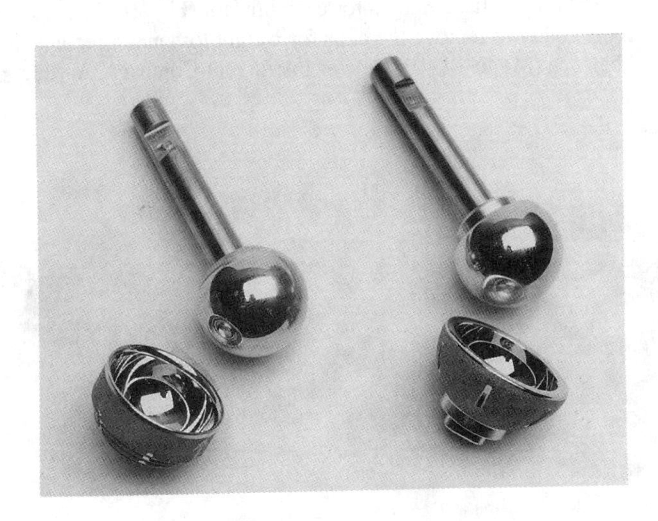

FIG. 1--*Types of implants tested; Sulzer Orthopedics(SO) (left), Pan Titan (PT) (right).*

TABLE 1--*Implants tested in the present study*

Implant	Alloy, % C	D_H, mm	C_L, μm	σ, nm	Sphericity, μm	
					Head	Cup
PT1	0.06	27.970	106	11	0.6	1.6
PT2	0.06	27.977	108	22	0.8	2.6
SO1	0.20	27.993	87	35	1.4	2.7
SO2	0.20	27.983	97	45	1.1	1.5
SO3	0.20	27.992	96	42	1.7	2.2
SO4	0.20	28.000	97	57	2.7	2.6

The MATCO™ hip simulator [*8*] was used following the protocols described previously [*10, 12*] which included mixing pure bovine serum with ethylenediamine tetraacetic acid (EDTA), an anti-fungal agent and streptomycin to make a 95% bovine serum mixture. The PT and SO implants had polyethylene shells attached to the back faces of the cups and because this material absorbed fluids, it was removed to improve the accuracy of the gravimetric assessment of the wear. Initially, soft mounting in the simulator was attempted with large polyurethane molds as used in previous work [*8, 9, 10, 11, 12*] but fixation was not secure and a metal insert with a much smaller sized polyurethane mold was employed (Fig. 2). It was also necessary to cut "anti-rotation" grooves in the back faces of the cups (Fig. 1) and develop a molding apparatus to allow custom fabrication of the polyurethane molds for each implant (Fig. 2). The result was a secure fixation with the ability to remove the cups for weight loss measurements using a precision analytical balance (Model M310, Denver Instrument Company, Arvada, CO).

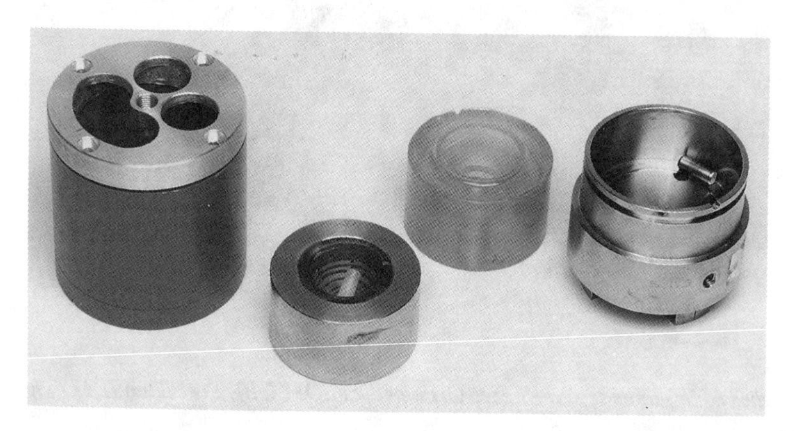

FIG. 2--*Polyurethane molding apparatus (far left), metal insert containing polyurethane mold (left), old full-sized polyurethane mold (right), simulator mounting chamber (far right).*

To check the fidelity of the applied load, a load monitoring apparatus (Fig. 3) was developed. This apparatus replaced a normal test chamber and had a ball bearing mounted on the rotating shaft to allow central location of a stationary aluminium block which supported a load cell. The test chamber geometry was copied with a large polyurethane mould and a custom-made 28 mm diameter cup was mounted. The load was found to vary somewhat during testing (about ±25 N) and had a minimum load of about 176 N during the swing phase (last 40% or so of the cycle) which was higher than specified by the ideal "Paul" curve. A typical measured load curve indicated an average value of 891.2 N (Fig. 3). Also, the average cycle period was determined over two 10 hour periods and averaged to give a value of 0.8783 s which was slightly below the previously used value of 0.882 s [*8, 9*].

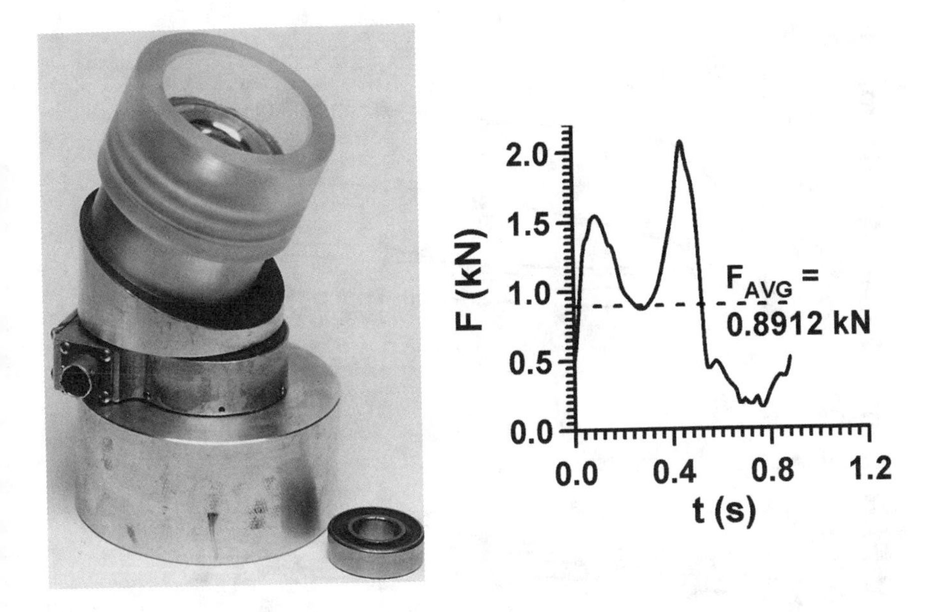

FIG. 3--*Load cell (central section with electrical connector) in a stationary chamber fixture with old full-sized polyurethane mold and large custom cup (left) along with a typical load trace (right).*

Each implant was tested for 1.514 million cycles. After about every 0.25 million cycles, the test was interrupted for cleaning and weighing of all the heads and cups, and changing of the bovine serum mixture. The cumulative weight loss for each component was converted to volume loss by dividing by the alloy density of 8.28 mg/mm^3. The volumetric wear data were then compared with some available data for both custom-made [*12*] and retrieved implants [*4, 5, 7*].

Results and Discussion

In general, both PT and SO implants (Fig. 4) showed similar wear behavior. After 1.514 million cycles, the wear lay in the range 0.3 to 0.8 mm^3. Under very similar conditions and in the same type of simulator, the wear of polyethylene cups against metal heads was about 30 mm^3 [*15*]. Thus, m-m implants reduced the volume of wear debris by at least 97%. Furthermore, the wear rate of the m-m implants decreased as the test proceeded, whereas the wear rate of conventional polyethylene cups remained relatively constant [*15*]. Consequently, the percent reduction in volumetric wear of the m-m implants compared with that of conventional polyethylene would be likely to increase over time.

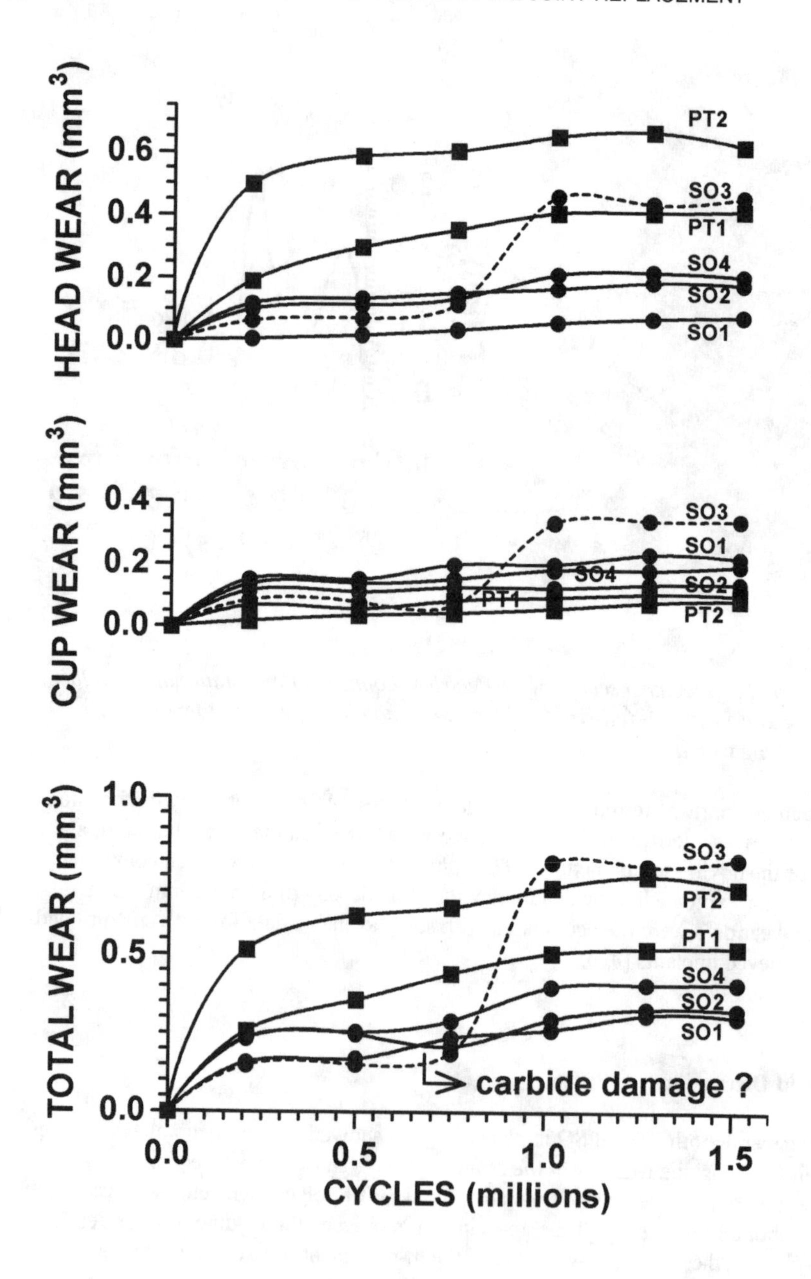

FIG. 4-- *Volumetric wear over 1.514 million cycles.*

The low carbon PT implants had slightly higher wear except for implant SO3 which sustained an increased wear rate at about 1 million cycles. Visual observation of the cup of implant SO3 revealed a groove cut in a circular path on the cup surface which followed the center of the predicted wear path. Separate examination of head and cup wear of implant SO3 (Fig. 4) revealed that both sustained a similar increase at 1 million cycles. Perhaps a large carbide in the head caused abrasive damage to the cup surface, and was dislodged subsequently. Some observations of the head of implant SO3 in the scanning electron microscope after 1.017 million cycles (Fig. 5) revealed holes in the surface from which a large carbide could have been removed. It was also interesting to observe smaller holes in the surface in quite extensive regions of micro-pitting. However, since a rigorous microscopy study had not been performed, the tribological significance of both the larger and smaller holes remained open to speculation.

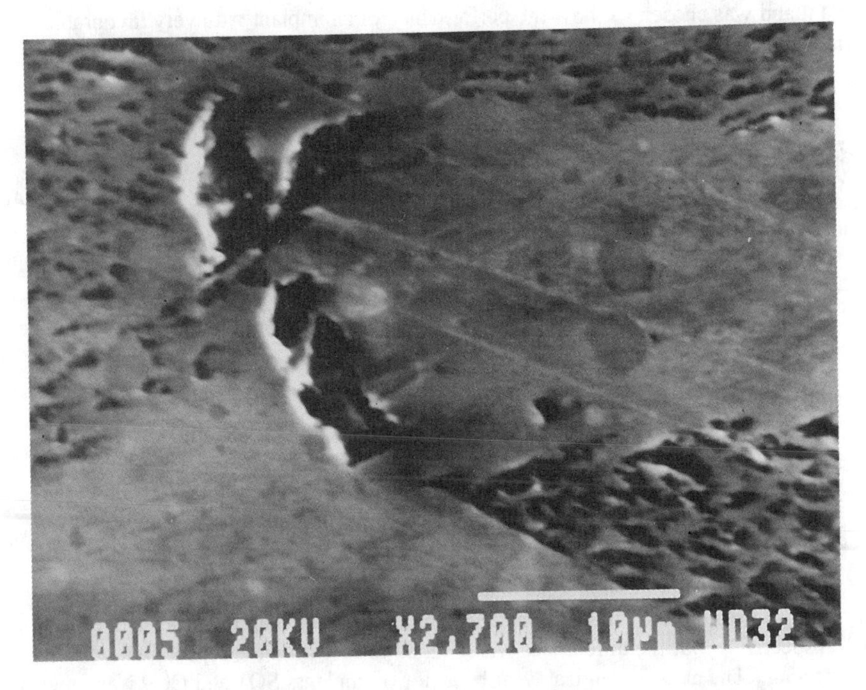

FIG. 5--*Surface of the head of implant SO3 after 1.017 million cycles.*

If implant SO3 was treated as a maverick data point, close examination of head and cup wear of the remaining implants (Fig. 4) revealed that the SO implants tended to have similar head and cup wear while the PT implants had lower cup wear than the SO implants, but higher head wear. It was interesting to note that the alloy used by Pan Titan for their heads was provided by a different supplier than the alloy for the cups. This suggested that some difference in the alloy might have been responsible for this higher head wear. Furthermore, the slightly higher wear of the PT implants compared with the

SO implants suggested that the higher carbon content of the SO implant material might improve wear performance. However, such an inference could not be made with certainty until the factors controlling wear were examined. Furthermore, only 6 implants were tested in the present study and thus to assess the significance of the findings, comparison with other similar research was warranted.

A comparison of the results of the present study was made with those of Chan et al [*12*] who used custom-made (CU) implants (fabricated by Wright Medical Technology, Arlington, TN). A number of CU implants, with numbers corresponding to those in Chan et al [*12*], were chosen for direct scrutiny (Table 2) because they matched specific PT and SO implants of the present study in alloy percent carbon, diametral clearance and combined RMS roughness. Comparison with the geometric characterization present in Table 1 revealed the following implant pairs had similar geometries: (PT1, CU2), (PT2, CU5) and (SO1, CU9). The CU13 implant had a lower clearance and roughness than the SO1 implant and was chosen to show the performance of an implant with very favourable geometric features.

TABLE 2--*Some custom-made (CU) implants from Chan et al [12].*

Implant	Alloy, % C	D_H , mm	C_L , μm	σ, nm	Sphericity, μm	
					Head	Cup
CU2	0.05	27.898	102	11	0.9	1.5
CU5	0.05	27.893	107	17	0.6	1.2
CU9	0.20	27.929	71	35	1.3	0.7
CU13	0.20	27.934	66	4	1.2	0.8

Geometrically similar commercial and custom-made implants showed similar wear behavior (Fig. 6). Both CU2 and CU5 implants had higher wear than their partners PT1 and PT2, respectively, but the differences were judged to be within the repeatability of simulator testing. The almost identical wear behavior of implants SO1 and CU9 was considered fortuitous. The very low wear of implant CU13 suggested that with favorable geometric features, the initial high wear at the beginning of the simulator testing could be reduced significantly. Overall, the comparison presented in Fig. 6 suggested that CU implants could represent commercial product.

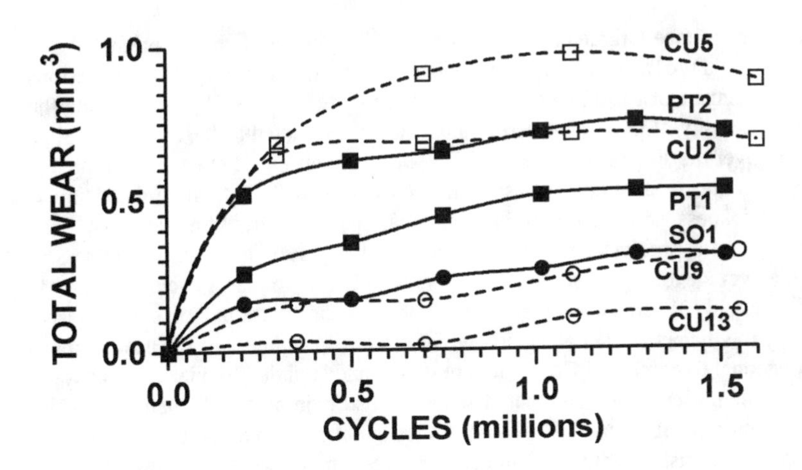

FIG. 6--*Comparison of the total volumetric wear for some of the commercial (SM and PT) implants of the present study with selected custom-made (CU) implants from Chan et al [12].*

Analysis

Factors Controlling Wear

Diametral clearance, combined RMS surface roughness and lambda were calculated following Medley et al [*8*]. Lambda was defined as

$$\lambda = \frac{h_c}{\sigma} \tag{2}$$

where h_c = elastohydrodynamic central film thickness
σ = combined RMS roughness defined previously in eqn. (1)

and gave an approximate assessment of whether the lubricant film thickness was sufficient to separate the surface asperities. Full separation was considered to occur at about $\lambda = 3$ and such separation would eliminate virtually all abrasive and adhesive wear (although some wear from surface fatigue could still occur). The lubricant film was predicted by a theoretical formula [*16*] which was a correlation of numerical solutions of the equations of elastohydrodynamic lubrication theory as discussed by Medley et al [*8*]. In applying the formula, the viscosity of the bovine serum mixture was estimated as 0.015 Pa s. Also, an average load over the simulator cycle of 891.2 N (Fig. 3) was used even though the formula was for steady state conditions because Chan et al [*17*], in their study of time varying film thickness, showed that the average load gave a central film thickness corresponding to the predicted minimum value over the cycle. Thus, a film thickness based on the average load gave a minimum lambda over the simulator cycle.

Chan et al [*12*] had shown that the volumetric wear after 3 million cycles was controlled by the diametral clearance, centre line average roughness of the head (expected to be proportional to combined RMS roughness [*8*]) and lambda. Similar analysis was performed in the present study and included all the custom implants of Chan et al [*12*] with the exception of CU6 and CU7. Both of these implants exhibited unusually high wear which was consistent with their higher clearances and roughness. However, their inclusion required graphs which obscured the behavior of the implants of the present study because of the reduced scale of the wear axes and thus they were excluded. To separate the influences of diametral clearance and combined RMS roughness, a selection of implants of similar roughness was used to plot wear versus clearance and a selection of implants of similar clearance was used to plot wear versus roughness. However, all implants were used to plot of wear versus lambda because lambda incorporated both roughness and clearance.

The resulting graphs (Fig. 7) all showed total wear after 1.514 million cycles, which was either estimated from the graphs of Chan et al [*12*] or measured directly in the present study. As expected from previous observations (Fig. 6), the results of the present study fell within the scatter of the results of Chan et al with the exception of the combined RMS roughness of the SO2, SO3 and SO4 implants. These implants were quite rough yet did not wear as much as the trends of the PT and CU implants suggested. Further investigation would be required to determine reasons for the wear behavior of these SO implants. In any case, the very low wear of CU13 (lambda of about 10) showed that implants of lower roughness than the SO implants could give even lower wear in a simulator.

The wear of high and low carbon alloys shown in Fig. 7 seemed similar but Chan et al [*12*] had found a slightly higher wear of the low carbon alloys using a statistical treatment of their data. Once again, further testing would be required to determine whether alloy carbon content was important for the types of commercial implant examined in the present study.

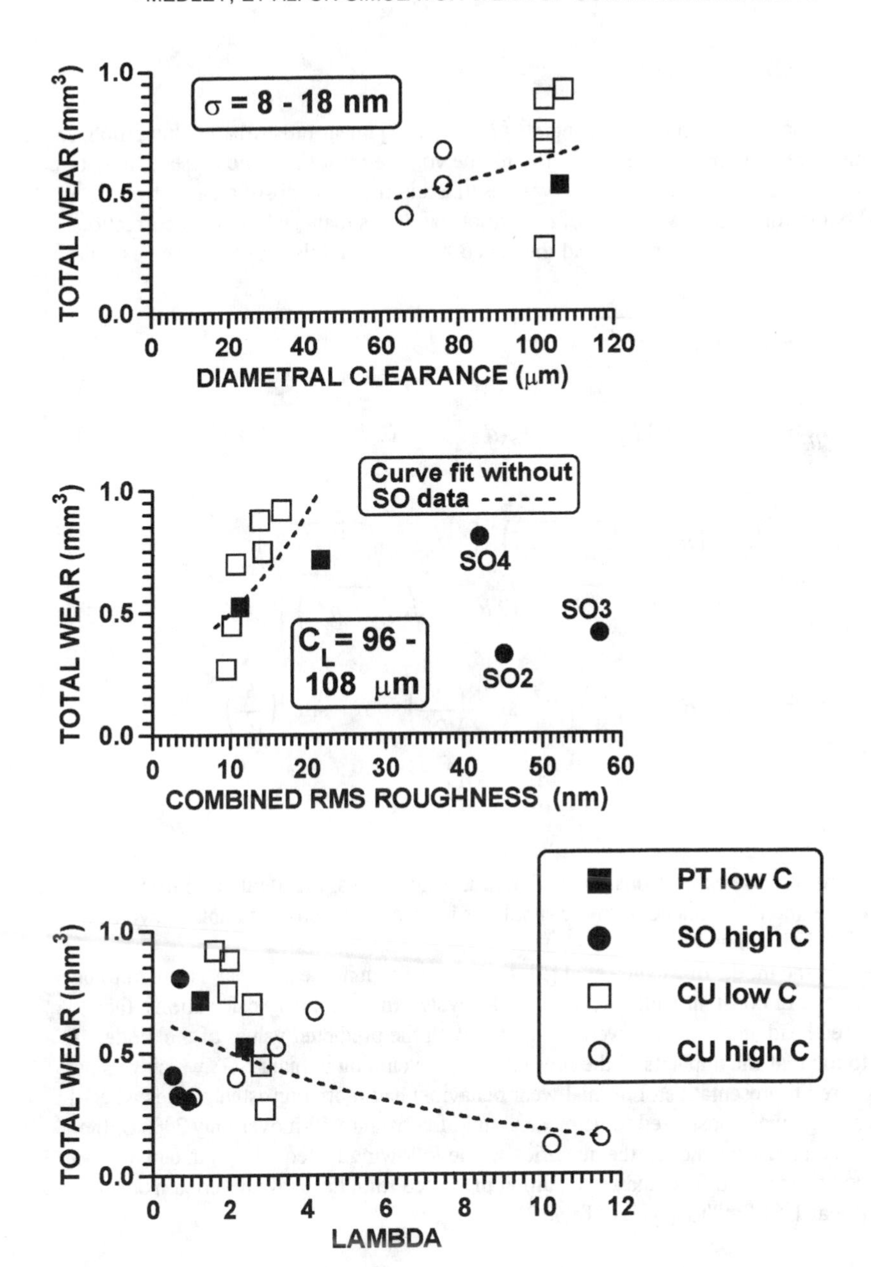

FIG. 7--*Factors controlling wear; clearance, roughness, lambda after 1.514 million cycles for implants from the present study (PT, SO) and from Chan et al [12] (CU).*

Prediction of Total Linear Wear

In many of the retrieved implants [*1, 3, 4, 5, 7*] linear rather than volumetric wear was measured and thus it was useful to link the volumetric wear of the present study to a predicted linear wear. A procedure was described in the appendix of a paper by Medley et al [*9*] but unfortunately a number of typographical errors managed to avoid correction. The correct versions of eqn. (2) and the next 3 equations in this appendix were as follows:

$$d = R_H - \sqrt{R_H^2 - b^2} \tag{3}$$

$$m_H = \frac{\pi\rho}{3}\left[d^2\,(3R_H - d) - (d - \delta)^2\,(3R_C - d + \delta)\right] \tag{4}$$

$$m_H = \frac{\pi\rho}{3}\left[\left(R_H - \sqrt{R_H^2 - b^2}\right)^2\left(2R_H + \sqrt{R_H^2 - b^2}\right) - \left(R_C - \sqrt{R_C^2 - b^2}\right)^2\left(2R_C + \sqrt{R_C^2 - b^2}\right)\right] \tag{5}$$

$$m_C = 0.8\,\pi\rho R_C \sin\left(\frac{\pi}{8}\right)\left[R_H^2 \sin^{-1}\left(\frac{b}{R_H}\right) - R_C^2 \sin^{-1}\left(\frac{b}{R_C}\right) + b\left(\sqrt{R_C^2 - b^2} - \sqrt{R_H^2 - b^2}\right)\right] \tag{6}$$

The terms in these expressions, the underlying assumptions, the iterative solution procedure and the application to the simulator wear of some custom implants were all described in Medley et al [*9*].

In the model of Medley et al [*9*], the wear trough in the cup was assumed to be present and of constant width for 40% of the cycle. In preliminary calculations, the measured head and cup wear were compared with the predicted values of the model. It was found that the implants of the present study (excluding implant SO3 which was not considered representative of normal wear behavior) had more consistent values when the wear trough was considered to be present and of constant width over only 23% of the cycle. To adjust the model, the numerical value following the equal sign in eqn. (6) was changed from 0.8 to 0.46 and the resulting predicted total linear wear varied from about 5 to 9 μm at 1.514 million cycles (Table 3).

TABLE 3--*Using the procedure described by Medley et al [9] to predict total linear wear at 1.514 million cycles in the simulator with the assumption of cup wear only over 23% of the cycle.*

Specimen	Total wear, mm^3	Head wear, mm^3	Predicted total linear wear, μm
PT1	0.525	0.420	7.2
PT2	0.716	0.625	8.6
SO1	0.305	0.082	4.8
SO2	0.326	0.184	5.2
SO3	0.806	0.462	7.5
SO4	0.411	0.212	6.0

Without actually measuring total linear wear, it was not known whether the model provided a good approximation. However, McKellop et al [*4*] in their retrieval study of m-m hip implants had measured total linear wear and volumetric head wear. For the lower wear cases (numbers 1,2, 9, 10, 11, 20 of Table 1 from McKellop et al [*4*]), which were considered comparable with implants worn in the simulator, a correlation of total linear wear versus volumetric head wear was apparent (Fig. 8). It was unfortunate that McKellop et al had been unable to ascertain the volumetric wear of the cups because a correlation of total linear wear versus total volumetric wear would have been more appropriate. However, the correlation of total linear wear versus volumetric *head* wear was not illogical because total volumetric wear was likely to have been split between head and cup in an approximately fixed ratio.

The predicted total linear wear of the model versus the measured volumetric head wear in the present simulator study was plotted along with the selected implants from the retrieval study of McKellop et al [*4*] (Fig. 8). An extrapolation of a linear least squares fit of the "model" data came quite close to a linear least squares fit of the measured retrieval values. This comparison provided some support for the model predictions but without actually measuring the linear wear of the implants tested in the simulator, the accuracy of the predicted total linear wear values could not be determined with certainty. However, as mentioned previously, having some prediction of linear wear allowed comparisons with retrieval studies which quoted exclusively in terms of linear wear.

For example, the total linear wear of one "typical" second generation m-m implant (with a 28 mm diameter and "appropriate" or "optimal" clearance) in a Stanmore Mk 3 hip simulator was reported by both Schmidt et al [*5*] and by Streicher et al [*7*] to have a value of about 30 μm at 1.514 million cycles. When compared to the wear of the retrieved implants, this linear wear was somewhat higher according to Fig. 6 of Streicher et al [*7*] or within the scatter according to Fig. 7 of Schmidt et al [*5*]. The linear wear predicted in Table 3 for the present study would place the simulator wear of the present study below the average retrieval wear, but well within the scatter of values. It was considered relevant to note that many early retrievals were loose and might have sustained higher wear as a result.

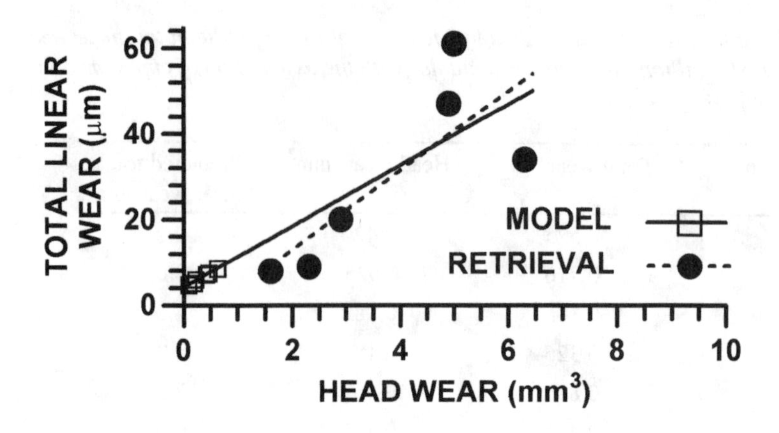

FIG. 8--*Total linear wear versus volumetric head wear measured in the retrieval study of McKellop et al [4] compared with the predicted total linear wear versus measured volumetric head wear in the present simulator study.*

Direct Comparison with In Vivo Wear of McKee-Farrar Implants

Although the present study tested second generation m-m implants, it was still considered relevant to compare the simulator wear with the *in vivo* wear of a subset of the first generation m-m implants examined by McKellop et al [*4*]. To be classified in this subset, the implants had to have an effective radius [*8, 9*] greater than 4 m, which was a feature of the second generation m-m implants with their controlled clearances. The subset of implants were all of the McKee-Farrar type (numbers 1, 2, 8, 10, 11 of Table 1 in McKellop et al [*4*]) and had their volumetric head wear assessed by a coordinate measuring machine.

The simulator head wear of the present study was compared with that of these retrieved implants (Fig. 9) assuming that 1 million cycles was equivalent to 1 year *in vivo*. An extrapolation of a linear least squares fit of the simulator data (excluding the origin as a data point) came reasonably close to a linear least squares fit of the retrieval data (also excluding the origin as a data point). The simulator did predicted wear below that of the retrieved implants as found in the previous section when comparisons were made to the retrieval data for modern m-m implants [*5, 7*]. As stated previously, the retrieved implants were often removed because of loosening and might thus have somewhat higher wear than well functioning implants *in vivo* and also the McKee Farrar implants might have had higher initial surface roughness compared with the implants tested in the simulator.

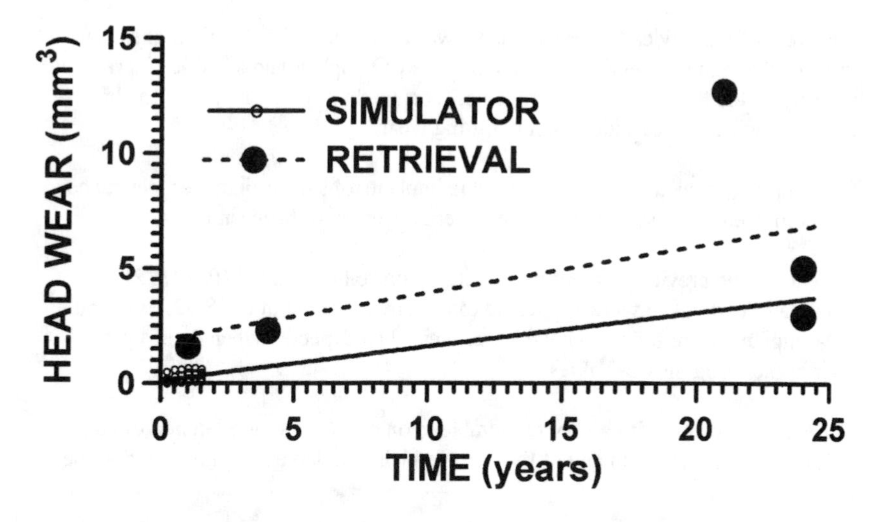

FIG. 9--*Comparison of retrieved McKee-Farrar implants with effective radii greater than 4 m from McKellop et al [4] with simulator wear of the present study (except SO3) assuming that 1 million cycles was equivalent to 1 year in vivo.*

The above comparison of the wear from the present simulator study to that of retrieved implants from McKellop et al [*4*] was not very precise because of the extensive extrapolation of the linear least squares fit of the simulator data, because of the many unknown variables in the retrieval study (such as starting implant geometry, patient activity levels, etc.) and because of the different implants used in the simulator compared with those retrieved. However, in the absence of any alternative retrieval data or alternative simulator data in the literature, there was little choice but to use the data available. Making such comparisons was considered an essential part of the *engineering* of metal-on-metal hip implants because making design decisions based on simulator data, without some understanding of the relationship of the simulator data to *in vivo* wear performance, would introduce distortion and uncertainty. It was also considered important to note that since metal-on-metal hip implants were a commercial reality in Europe, design decisions and product development could conceivably follow from research such as that of the present study.

Conclusions

1. The volumetric wear of all of the commercially available m-m hip implants in the simulator was found to be quite similar, and it was much less than that found previously [*15*] for conventional polyethylene against metal heads.

2. The wear of the low carbon PT implants was observed to be slightly higher than three of the high carbon SO implants, but one SO implant had a sudden increase in wear up to the levels of the PT implants. This might have been related to abrasive damage caused by "carbide pullout" during wear.

3. Commercially available and custom-made implants of similar diameter, clearance and combined RMS surface roughness were observed to have similar wear.

4. In general, the previously identified "factors controlling wear" [*10, 11, 12*] (lambda in particular) were applicable to the present data but the SO2, SO3 and SO4 implants were found to have lower wear than expected when considering their higher roughnesses values.

5. The CU13 implant, with a very favourable geometry (and thus a lambda of about 10), had lower wear than any of the commercially available implants tested in the present study.

6. A prediction of linear wear was made from the volumetric wear of the present simulator tests and it was less than the simulator wear of a modern second generation m-m implant reported in other studies [*5, 7*] and in the low region of the scatter in their reported wear of retrieved implants.

7. A direct comparison of volumetric head wear from the present study and from a previous study [*4*] of retrieved McKee-Farrar implants (with effective radii and thus clearances similar to second generation implants) showed simulator wear below the average of retrieved implants but within their scatter.

Acknowledgements

Mr. Michael Prokosch of the Lawrence Livermore National Laboratory measured the implant geometry with considerable skill and invaluable technical assistance was provided by Mr. Ernst Huber at the University of Waterloo. Mr. Frank Chan, a colleague from the Jo Miller Orthopaedic Research Laboratory, provided data from a submitted paper for comparison purposes. Financial support was provided by Implex Corp., Allendale, NJ.

References

[*1*] Semlitsch, M. and Willert, H.G., "Clinical Wear Behaviour of Ultra High Molecular Weight Polyethylene Cups Paired with Metal and Ceramic Ball Heads in Comparison to Metal-on-Metal Pairings of Hip Joint Replacements," *Proceedings of the Institution of Mechanical Engineers, Part H, Journal of Engineering in Medicine,* Vol. 211, No. H1, 1997, pp. 73-88.

[*2*] Streicher, R.M., Schön, R. and Semlitsch, M.F., "Investigation of the Tribological Behaviour of Metal-on-Metal Combinations for Artificial Hip Joints," *Biomedizinische Technik.,* Vol. 35, No. 5, 1990, pp. 107-111.

[*3*] Semlitsch, M., Streicher, R.M. and Weber, H., "Wear Behaviour of Cast CoCrMo Cups and Balls in Long-Term Implanted Total Hip Prostheses," *Orthopäde,* Vol. 18, 1989, pp. 377-381.

[*4*] McKellop, H., Park, S.H., Chiesa, R., Dorn, P. Lu, B., Normand, P., Grigoris, P. and Amstutz, H. "In Vivo Wear of 3 Types of Metal on Metal Hip Prostheses During 2 Decades of Use," *Clinical Orthopaedics and Related Research,* No. 329S, 1996, pp. S128-S140.

[*5*] Schmidt, M., Weber, H. and Schön, R., "Cobalt Chromium Molydenum Metal Combination for Modular Hip Prostheses" *Clinical Orthopaedics and Related Research,* No. 329S, 1996, pp. S35-S47.

[*6*] Amstutz, H.C., Campbell, P., McKellop, H., Schmalzried, T.P., Gillespie, W.J., Howie, D., Jacobs, J., Medley, J.B. and Merritt, K., "Metal on Metal Total Hip Replacement Workshop Consensus Document," *Clinical Orthopaedics and Related Research,* No. 329S, 1996, pp. S297-S303.

[*7*] Streicher, R.M., Semlitsch, M., Schön, R., Weber, H. and Rieker, C. "Metal-on-Metal Articulation for Artificial Hip Joints: Laboratory Study and Clinical Results," *Proceedings of the Institution of Mechanical Engineers, Part H, Journal of Engineering in Medicine,* Vol. 210, No. H3, 1996, pp. 223-232.

[*8*] Medley, J.B., Krygier, J.J., Bobyn, J.D., Chan, F.W., Lippincott, A. and Tanzer, M., "Kinematics of the MATCO™ Hip Simulator and Issues Related to Wear Testing of Metal-Metal Implants," *Proceedings of the Institution of Mechanical Engineers, Part H, Journal of Engineering in Medicine,* Vol. 211, No. H1, 1997, pp. 89-99.

[*9*] Medley, J.B., Chan, F.W., Krygier, J.J. and Bobyn, J.D., "Comparison of Alloys and Designs in a Hip Simulator Study of Metal-Metal Implants," *Clinical Orthopaedics and Related Research,* No. 329S, 1996, pp. S160-S186.

[*10*] Chan, F.W., Bobyn, J.D., Medley, J.B., Krygier, J.J., Yue, S. and Tanzer, M., "Engineering Issues and Wear Performance of Metal-on-Metal Hip Implants. *Clinical Orthopaedics and Related Research,* No. 333, 1996, pp. 96-107.

[*11*] Chan, F.W., Bobyn, J.D., Medley, J.B., Krygier, J.J., Yue, S. and Tanzer, M. "Wear Performance of Metal-Metal Hip Implants," *Archives of the American Academy of Orthopaedic Surgeons,* Vol. 1, No. 1, 1997, pp. 57-60.

[*12*] Chan, F.W., Bobyn, J.D., Medley, J.B., Krygier, J.J., Podgorsak, G.F. and Tanzer, M., "Metal-Metal Hip Implants: Optimization of Design Parameters That Control Wear," submitted to *Clinical Orthopaedics and Related Research*, 1997.

[*13*] Gellert, W., Küstner, Hellwich, M. and Kästner, H. *The VNR Concise Encyclopedia of Mathematics,* Van Nostrand Reinhold, New York, 1977, pp. 612-616.

[*14*] Cipera, W.M., "A Tribological Study of CoCrMo Alloys for Use in Metal-Metal Total Hip Arthroplasty," *MASc Thesis*, Dept of Mech Eng, University of Waterloo, 1996.

[*15*] McKellop, H., Lu, B. and Li, S., "Wear of Acetabular Cups of Conventional and Modified UHMW Polyethylene Compared on a Hip Joint Simulator," *Transactions of the Orthopaedic Research Society*, 1992, pp. 356.

[*16*] Hamrock, B.J., *Fundamentals of Fluid Film Lubrication,* McGraw-Hill, New York, 1994, pp. 502-508.

[*17*] Chan, F.W., Medley, J.B., Bobyn, J.D. and Krygier, J.J., "Time-Varying Fluid Film Lubrication of Metal-Metal Hip Implants in Simulator Tests," *Alternative Bearing Surfaces in Total Joint Replacement, ASTM STP 1346*, J.J. Jacobs and T.L. Craig, Eds., American Society for Testing and Materials, 1998.

Frank W. Chan,[1] John B. Medley,[2] J. Dennis Bobyn,[3] and Jan J. Krygier[4]

NUMERICAL ANALYSIS OF TIME-VARYING FLUID FILM THICKNESS IN METAL-METAL HIP IMPLANTS IN SIMULATOR TESTS

REFERENCE: Chan, F. W., Medley, J. B., Bobyn, J. D., and Krygier, J. J., "**Numerical Analysis of Time-Varying Fluid Film Thickness in Metal-Metal Hip Implants in Simulator Tests,**" *Alternative Bearing Surfaces in Total Joint Replacement, ASTM STP 1346*, J. J. Jacobs and T. L. Craig, Eds., American Society for Testing and Materials, 1998.

ABSTRACT: *In vitro* testing of metal-metal hip implants has shown that metal-metal wear can be up to two orders of magnitude less than the wear of conventional metal-polyethylene articulations. This low wear may be related, in part, to fluid film lubrication at the bearing surfaces. A transient, elastohydrodynamic lubrication model incorporating both squeeze and entraining actions in the hip was developed to predict fluid film thickness for metal-metal hip implants during simulator testing. For a typical case, the model showed that cyclic steady state, with film thickness variations from 38 to 70 nm, was reached in about 3 cycles. Decreased diametral clearance, increased lubricant viscosity, and increased cycle frequency resulted in increased film thicknesses. However, film thickness did not change markedly for different load magnitudes. In all cases, steady state film thickness values calculated using the average load during the cycle corresponded to minimum cyclic steady state values, indicating that this may be a simplified method to predict minimum film thickness. Lambda ratio (ratio of fluid film thickness to combined surface roughness of articulating components) decreased as surface roughness increased, indicating a transition from full fluid film lubrication to boundary lubrication. Steady state lambda ratios were related to the total wear of simulator-tested implants with wear decreasing significantly with increasing lambda ratio. With proper selection of low clearance and low surface roughness values, lambda ratios that predict full fluid film lubrication and possibly further improved wear performance can be obtained, making lambda ratio a potentially useful tool in the design of metal-metal hip implants.

[1] Ph.D. candidate, Department of Biomedical Engineering, McGill University, Jo Miller Orthopaedic Research Laboratory, Montreal General Hospital, 1650 Cedar Avenue, Montreal, Quebec, Canada H3G 1A4.

[2] Associate professor, Department of Mechanical Engineering, University of Waterloo, 200 University Avenue West, Waterloo, Ontario, Canada N2L 3G1.

[3] Associate professor, Departments of Surgery and Biomedical Engineering, McGill University, Jo Miller Orthopaedic Research Laboratory, Montreal General Hospital, 1650 Cedar Avenue, Montreal, Quebec, Canada H3G 1A4.

[4] Technical coordinator, Jo Miller Orthopaedic Research Laboratory, Montreal General Hospital, 1650 Cedar Avenue, Montreal, Quebec, Canada H3G 1A4.

KEYWORDS: fluid film lubrication, tribology, hip implant, hip implant design, transient elastohydrodynamic lubrication, orthopaedics, wear

Nomenclature

a	Radius of Hertzian contact area [m]
E	Modulus of elasticity [Pa or N/m^2]
E'	Effective modulus of elasticity [Pa or N/m^2]
F	Total load [N]
F_E	Force due to entraining action [N]
F_S	Force due to squeeze action [N]
h_C	Central film thickness [nm]
p	Pressure [Pa or N/m^2]
R	Effective (or reduced) radius [m]
R_C	Radius of acetabular cup [m]
R_H	Radius of femoral head [m]
t	Time [s]
u	Entrainment velocity [m/s]
η	Viscosity [Pa•s or N•s/m^2]
λ	Lambda ratio
ν	Poisson's ratio
σ_C	Root mean square (rms) surface roughness of acetabular cup [nm]
σ_H	Root mean square (rms) surface roughness of femoral head [nm]
ω	Angular velocity of simulator [rad/s]

A major concern in total hip arthroplasty is peri-implant osteolysis caused by the generation of polyethylene wear particles at the articulating surfaces. There has been renewed interest in metal-metal bearings as a solution to this problem in view of their potential for improved wear performance. Retrieval analyses of modern metal-metal implants originating primarily from Europe over the past decade have indicated good clinical results and low wear [1,2,3,4]. *In vitro* testing of metal-metal implants using hip simulators has shown that metal-metal wear can be up to two orders of magnitude less than the wear of conventional metal-polyethylene articulations [5,6,7,8,9,10,11].

With current manufacturing techniques, components can generally be made with stringent dimensional tolerances and quality control that may produce conditions favorable for fluid film lubrication to occur to some degree [5,9,10,12]. Therefore, it has been suggested that the low wear of these modern metal-metal components is partially a result of fluid film lubrication at the articulation [5,9]. A comparative lubrication analysis of metal-metal, ceramic-ceramic, and metal-polyethylene hip bearings under *in vivo* conditions suggested that full fluid film lubrication is unlikely in metal-polyethylene articulations but can, indeed, occur in hard bearing combinations [13]. This analysis, however, was carried out for steady state conditions while a more realistic approach would be to examine fluid film lubrication with time-varying loads and velocities taken into account. Such an analysis is more complicated but an analytical approach has been applied to natural hip joints [14]. Although a study of time-varying fluid film lubrication under *in vivo* conditions is useful, the wear of metal-metal hip implants under controlled conditions has been established only for simulators [5,8,9,10,12]. Therefore, a study of the time-varying fluid film lubrication of these implants during simulator testing would be tremendously useful.

The purpose of the present study was to develop a transient, elastohydrodynamic lubrication (ehl) model incorporating time-varying conditions suitable for predicting the fluid film thickness at the head-cup articulation of metal-metal hip implants tested in hip simulators and to illustrate the effects on film thickness of design and testing parameters including head-cup clearance, lubricant viscosity, load magnitude, and cycle frequency.

Methods

The metal-metal head-cup articulation was approximated by classical Hertzian theory in which the radius of the contact area was determined by

$$a = \left(\frac{3FR}{2E'}\right)^{\frac{1}{3}} \tag{1}$$

where

$$R = \frac{R_C R_H}{R_C - R_H} \tag{2}$$

$$E' = \frac{E}{1-\nu^2} \tag{3}$$

Hertzian theory was considered appropriate for the thick-walled, 28 mm diameter cups in some previous investigations [5,10] but may underestimate contact areas for thin-walled cups [6,9].

A modulus of elasticity, E, of 210 GPa and Poisson's ratio, ν, of 0.3 [15] were selected as typical values for metal-metal hip implants manufactured from ASTM medical grades of cobalt-chromium-molybdenum (CoCrMo) alloy (F1537-94 and F75-92). For the present study, only implants with a nominal radius of 14 mm were considered.

For hip simulator testing, bovine serum is typically used as the lubricating medium. In the present study, a value for viscosity, η, of 0.002 Pa•s was used, which was higher than the viscosity of water (0.001 Pa•s) but lower than the value assumed for synovial fluid (0.005 Pa•s) in a previous investigation [13]. Bovine serum was assumed to be an isoviscous, Newtonian fluid, similar assumptions to what were made for synovial fluid in replaced hip joints [13].

The lubrication mechanics of a hip simulator include both squeeze and entraining actions. Squeeze action is a result of the relative normal motion between the surfaces due to the applied normal load acting on the articulation (Figure 1). The load profile used in the current analysis was based on normal gait [16] with a peak of 2100 N (three times body weight (BW), 1 BW ≡ 700 N) and a frequency of 1 Hz. Entraining action is a result of the tangential motion of the surfaces, pulling lubricant into the contact zone (Figure 1). Because much of the recent published work on simulator wear testing of metal-metal implants has been carried out with the model EW08 MMED hip simulator (MATCO, La Canada, CA) [5,6,7,8,9,10,17,18], the kinematics of the transient ehl model was based on this simulator. Following Medley et al. [12], entrainment velocity was considered to be constant over the gait cycle.

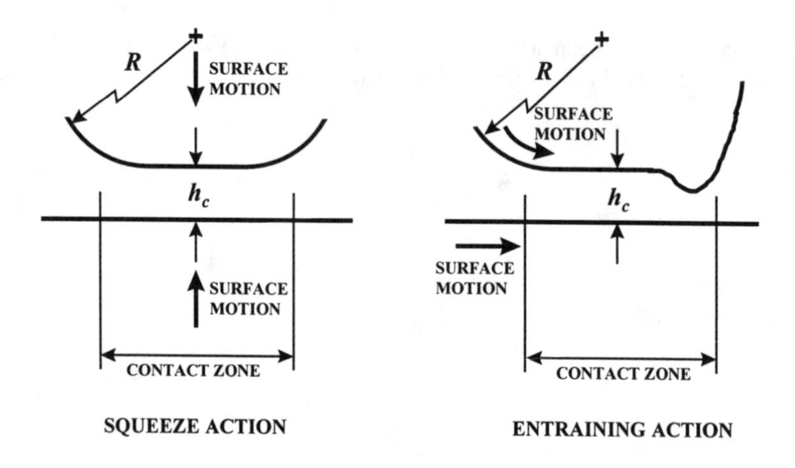

FIGURE 1 – *Squeeze and entraining actions in the hip.*

Fluid Film Thickness under Squeeze Action

The formula for transient fluid film thickness under pure squeeze motion was derived from Reynold's equation in cylindrical coordinates [14]

$$\frac{1}{r}\frac{\partial}{\partial r}\left(r\frac{h_c^{\ 3}}{\eta}\frac{\partial p}{\partial r}\right) = 12\frac{\partial h_c}{\partial t} \tag{4}$$

with the following boundary conditions,

$$\begin{aligned} p &= 0 \quad @ \quad r = a \\ \frac{\partial p}{\partial r} &= 0 \quad @ \quad r = 0 \end{aligned} \tag{5}$$

Equation (4) was solved for pressure, p,

$$p = \frac{3\eta}{h_c}\frac{dh_c}{dt}\left(r^2 - a^2\right) \tag{6}$$

and integrated over the contact area to obtain the force due to the squeeze action, F_S,

$$F_S = -\frac{3\pi\eta a^4}{2h_c^{\ 3}}\frac{dh_c}{dt} \tag{7}$$

Fluid Film Thickness under Entraining Action

A formula for pure entraining action, based on extensive numerical analysis by Hamrock [19], was adapted by Medley et al. [12] to give the central film thickness, h_C,

$$h_c = 5.083\frac{(\eta u)^{0.660} R^{0.767}}{(E')^{0.447} F^{0.213}} \tag{8}$$

Equation (8) was rearranged to include the radius of the contact area, a and solved for the force, F, which was defined as the force due to the entraining action, F_E,

$$F_E = 8.9259(\eta u)\frac{R^{0.4848} a^{2.9393}}{h_c^{\ 1.5152}} \tag{9}$$

where the entrainment velocity, u, was determined from the kinematics of the simulator,

$$u = \frac{1}{2}\left[\omega R_C \sin\left(\frac{\pi}{8}\right)\right] \tag{10}$$

Transient Elastohydrodynamic Model

The expressions for force under squeeze and entraining actions separately were combined by superposition following Jin et al. [14] to obtain an expression for total force, F,

$$F = F_S + F_E \tag{11}$$

The contact areas for both squeeze and entraining actions were assumed to be equal following the approaches of previous studies [20,21] but differing in this respect to the work of Jin et al. [14]. Equation (11) was rearranged with the use of equation (1) to obtain an expression for the time differential of fluid film thickness, dh_C/dt,

$$\frac{dh_c}{dt} = 1.4514\frac{h_c^{\ 1.4848}(E')^{0.6566}u}{F^{0.6566}R^{0.1717}} - 0.1236\frac{h_c^{\ 3}(E')^{1.3333}}{\eta F^{0.3333}R^{1.3333}} \tag{12}$$

Equation (12), a first order, nonlinear, ordinary differential equation, was solved for fluid film thickness, h_C, using a fourth-order Runge-Kutta numerical routine with code written in the MatLab (MathWorks, Inc., Natick, MA) programming language. To reduce the effects of round-off errors, double precision values were used in the calculations. To reduce the effects of truncation errors, the model was run consecutively with time steps decreased by half until a difference of less than 0.01% occurred between values at one time step and the values at corresponding times for the next larger time step. The smaller time step was used for all subsequent runs of the model.

The model was initially run for what was defined in this study to be the "set point" or reference conditions (Case 1 - Set Point in Table 1) to represent mid-range values in the current state-of-the-art for the design and testing of metal-metal hip implants. The various input parameters such as head-cup diametral clearance ($2[R_C-R_H]$), lubricant viscosity, load magnitude, and cycle frequency were varied for subsequent runs (Table 1) to determine the independent effects of these parameters on fluid film thickness. Different values for clearance, which has been shown to affect metal-metal implant wear [5,8,9,17,18], were selected (Table 1) to represent the general range in current experimental and clinical metal-metal implants [3,5,6,7,8,9,10,22]. Compared with the set point viscosity, lower and higher viscosities (Table 1) were used to represent water and the value used previously in a steady state lubrication analysis of artificial hip joints [13], respectively. The effect on film thickness of different load magnitudes and cycle frequencies (Table 1) which have been used in other hip simulator testing protocols was also evaluated [11,23].

For each combination of input parameters, the transient ehl model was run until cyclic steady state was achieved where differences between consecutive cycles at corresponding points within each period did not exceed 0.01%. For all combinations of input parameters, the cyclic, steady state fluid film thickness was plotted against time.

TABLE 1 – *Input parameters.*

CASE*	DIAMETRAL CLEARANCE (μm)	VISCOSITY (Pa.s)	PEAK LOAD (BW)†	FREQUENCY (Hz)
1 – SET POINT	**90**	**0.002**	**3**	**1**
2	45	0.002	3	1
3	120	0.002	3	1
4	90	0.001	3	1
5	90	0.005	3	1
6	90	0.002	2	1
7	90	0.002	5	1
8	90	0.002	3	0.5
9	90	0.002	3	2

* Graphs in "Results" refer to case numbers described here.
† BW = body weight, 1 BW ≡ 700 N.

Steady State Formulation to Predict Film Thickness

Equation (8) for elastohydrodynamic lubrication due to entraining action alone was used with a constant load to obtain a simplified, steady state value for film thickness. Calculated using loads set to the minimum, maximum, and average loads within one gait cycle, the steady state results were compared with the time-varying film thickness values from the transient ehl model to determine any correlation between methods.

Lambda Ratio

A common tribological method of assessing the mode of fluid film lubrication is the use of lambda ratio, λ,

$$\lambda = \frac{h_c}{\sqrt{\sigma_H^2 + \sigma_C^2}} \tag{13}$$

Described as the ratio of fluid film thickness to the combined root mean square (rms) surface roughness of the articulating components, lambda ratio is a convenient way to describe the extent of separation between the head and cup. In general terms, lambda ratios greater than about three suggest that full fluid film lubrication may be the predominant mode and that surfaces are essentially separated by a continuous lubricant film where the applied load is carried by the film itself [24]. Lambda ratios less than about one suggest the mode of boundary lubrication where more localized surface interaction (including the likelihood of direct surface contact) occurs and the load is carried primarily by asperity tips alone [25]. Lambda ratios between about one and three suggest mixed film lubrication where the load may be shared between the lubricant film and direct asperity interaction.

Lambda ratios were calculated from the time-varying fluid film thickness results for the implant with the set point conditions (Case 1). A range of surface roughness values (5, 10, 25, and 50 nm) was used to evaluate the effect on lubrication of common roughness values obtained by manufacturing techniques for modern experimental and clinical metal-metal implants [5,6,7,8,9,10]. Lambda ratios were plotted against time for the different surface roughness values.

To illustrate the relationship between fluid film lubrication and implant wear, the lambda ratios for previously tested implants [5,8] were calculated from the steady state film thickness equation (using a particular constant load) and plotted against total volumetric wear. The surface roughness values measured at the beginning of the tests were used in the calculations of lambda ratio.

Results and Discussion

The analysis for the set point condition was carried out using progressively finer (smaller) time steps (0.01, 0.005, 0.001, 0.0005 s, etc.). The appropriate time step yielding differences of 0.01% between results for consecutive time steps was 0.0001 s which was used for all subsequent runs.

The use of different initial film thickness values did not noticeably affect the convergence of the transient ehl model to a cyclic steady state (less than 0.01% difference between consecutive cycles). For all combinations of input parameters, cyclic steady state was achieved within the first three cycles of iteration (Figure 2).

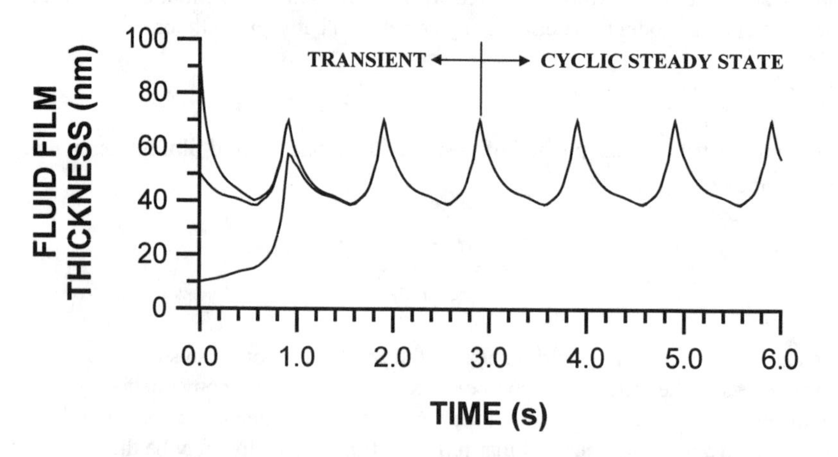

FIGURE 2 – *Time-varying fluid film thickness for set point conditions (Case 1) using different initial film thickness values. The transient elastohydrodynamic model reached cyclic steady state within the first three cycles of iteration.*

Set Point Conditions

The time-varying film thickness for the set point condition for one cycle within cyclic steady state is shown along with the corresponding force over time (Figure 3). With an overall variation in applied load from 36 to 2100 N, the film thickness experienced changes from about 38 to 70 nm, the minimum film thickness occurring immediately after the point of maximum load. The relatively small effect of load on film thickness within a gait cycle may be explained by the powerful squeeze action which maintained the lubricant film generated by the entraining action from the previous cycle. It is interesting to note that the low cyclic variation in fluid film thickness has been shown to occur in transient fluid film lubrication models for the natural hip and ankle joints [14,26,27].

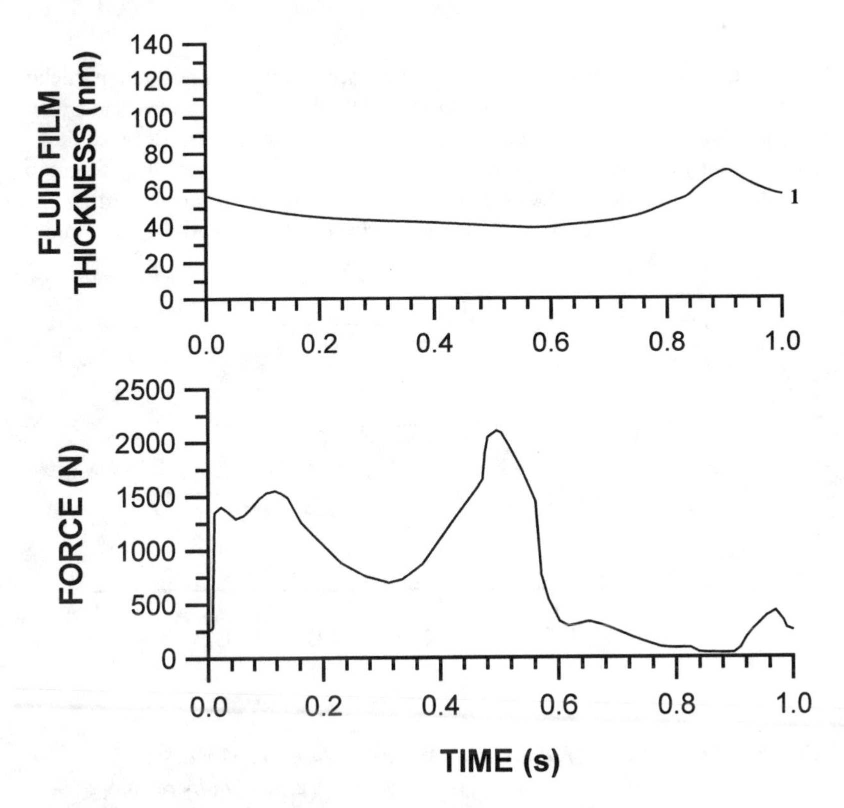

FIGURE 3 – *Time-varying fluid film thickness for set point conditions for one cycle within cyclic steady state along with corresponding force. Large changes in load did not markedly influence fluid film thickness. The minimum film thickness occurred immediately after the maximum load.*

Head-Cup Diametral Clearance

Head-cup diametral clearance influenced fluid film thickness with decreasing clearance resulting in increasing film thickness values (Figure 4). Decreasing clearance results in larger contact areas and smaller contact pressures. The edge inlet zone converges more gradually, resulting in more favorable conditions for an increase in film thickness. It should be cautioned that although decreased clearance may result in increased film thickness and possibly decreased implant wear, there may be a minimum clearance below which further improvement in wear performance may not occur [5,9]. Excessively small clearances with large contact areas may reduce the inlet zone, thus impairing lubricant entrainment.

Lubricant Viscosity

Increasing the value for viscosity of the bovine serum lubricant resulted in thicker fluid films (Figure 5) with the high viscosity value (0.005 Pa·s) causing more than a two-fold increase in film thickness compared with the low value (0.001 Pa·s). Because film thickness was strongly affected by viscosity, the selection of this parameter was found to be very important. Application of the present model to specific hip simulator testing protocols would require accurate measurement of lubricant viscosity under appropriate shear rates.

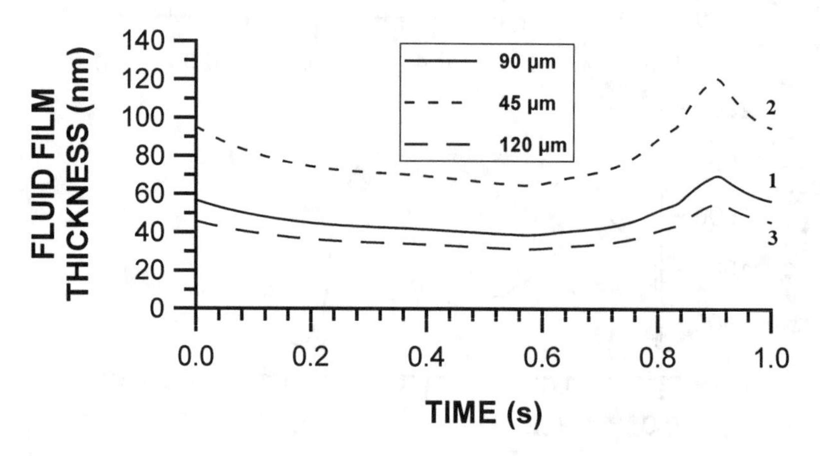

FIGURE 4 – *Time-varying fluid film thickness as a function of head-cup diametral clearance. Decreasing clearance resulted in increasing film thickness.*

Load Magnitude

Despite changes in the magnitude of applied load from peaks of 2 to 5 BW, the fluid film thickness varied slightly within one gait cycle from an average value of about 44 to 51 nm, a 16% increase (Figure 6). The small change in film thickness with greater than twice the applied load may be attributed to the increase in contact area with load. The larger contact area enhances both entraining and squeeze actions enough to counteract, to a large extent, the expected tendency of increasing load to reduce film thickness. The insensitivity of film thickness to load magnitude suggested that neither the values nor the exact form of the load curve was very important.

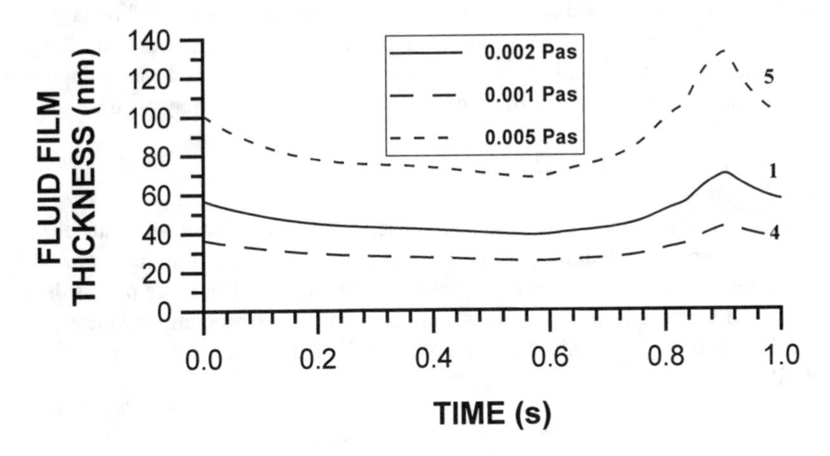

FIGURE 5 – *Time-varying fluid film thickness as a function of lubricant viscosity. Film thickness more than doubled for a viscosity of 0.005 Pa•s compared with a value of 0.001 Pa•s.*

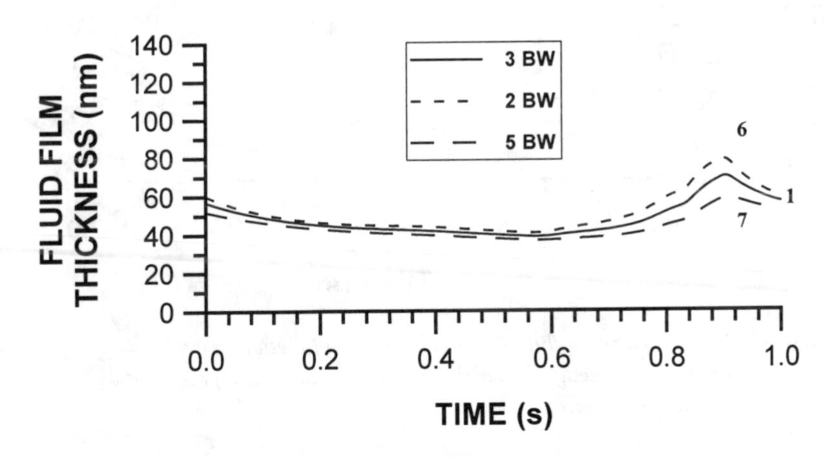

FIGURE 6 – *Time-varying fluid film thickness as a function of load magnitude. A small 16% increase in average film thickness resulted from an increase in peak load from 2 to 5 BW.*

Cycle Frequency

The cycle frequency influenced the fluid film lubrication with increased frequency resulting in larger film thickness values (Figure 7). An increase in cycle frequency increased both the entraining velocity and frequency with which the load was applied. Given the insensibility of film thickness to load variations (shown previously), the effects shown here could only be caused by the increase in entrainment velocity. While higher frequencies might be acceptable for conventional metal-polyethylene articulations [23], these results indicate that it would probably be inappropriate to test metal-metal implants at higher frequencies since thicker films and unrealistically low wear may occur.

Steady State Formulation to Predict Film Thickness

Using the average force within the gait cycle, equation (8), the steady state ehl formula for entraining action alone, yielded a value very close to the minimum value from the transient ehl model for each case (Table 2). An average difference of less than 3% was obtained for the steady state values compared with those predicted by the transient model, making the steady state method a useful, simplified method to predict minimum film thickness.

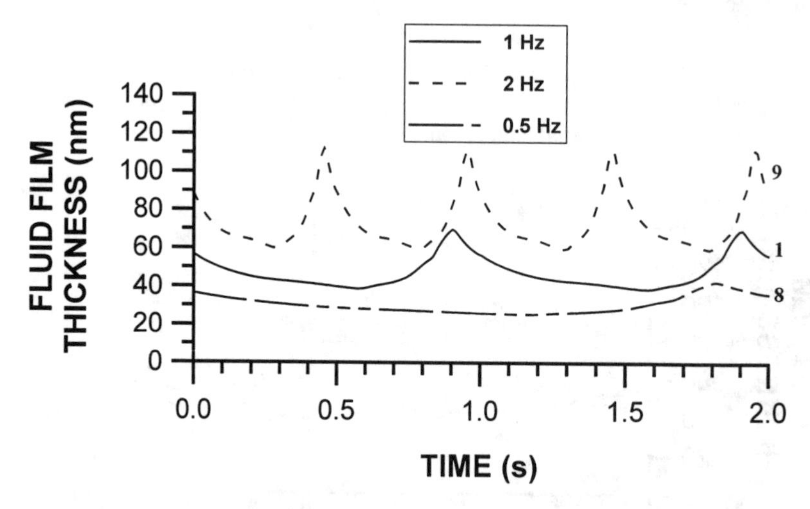

FIGURE 7 – *Time-varying fluid film thickness as a function of cycle frequency. Markedly higher film thickness values are predicted as frequency is increased.*

Lambda Ratio

The lambda ratio calculated from the time-varying film thickness for the set point condition was determined for different values of combined rms surface roughness (5, 10, 25, 50 nm) (Figure 8). For example, from equation (13), a combined roughness of 10 nm could represent an actual rms surface roughness of each component of 7.07 nm (assuming equal roughnesses). In general, lambda ratio decreased as surface roughness increased. For the set point condition with a diametral clearance of 90 μm, full fluid film lubrication could be expected if the combined roughness of the components was below approximately 10 nm. With a combined roughness of 25 nm, the implant would operate in the mixed film lubrication mode. With a combined roughness of 50 nm, boundary lubrication may occur along with the possibility of increased wear. Because lower clearances give rise to larger film thickness values (Figure 4) and thus higher lambda ratios for a given surface roughness, implants with lower clearances may tolerate greater surface roughness values and still operate within the full fluid film lubrication mode.

TABLE 2 – *Steady state prediction of minimum film thickness at cyclic steady state.*

CASE #	AVERAGE LOAD (N)	STEADY STATE FILM THICKNESS WITH AVERAGE FORCE (nm)	MINIMUM FILM THICKNESS FROM TRANSIENT MODEL (nm)	PERCENT DIFFERENCE (%)
1 (SET POINT)	797	38.3	38.7	1.2
2	797	65.0	64.6	0.6
3	797	30.7	31.3	1.9
4	797	24.2	25.3	4.3
5	797	70.0	68.3	2.5
6	531	41.7	40.6	2.7
7	1328	34.3	36.8	6.8
8	797	60.4	59.5	1.6
9	797	24.2	25.3	4.3
	AVERAGE PERCENT DIFFERENCE (%)			**2.9**

The steady state lambda ratio was calculated using the entraining action expression, equation (8), with the average load of 891 N in a simulator test cycle. The lambda ratio was plotted against the total volumetric wear of 19 metal-metal implants from a recent study [5] and tested in a hip simulator to three million cycles (approximately equivalent to three years of *in vivo* service) (Figure 9). In general, the wear decreased as the lambda ratio increased (film thickness became progressively larger than the surface roughness). Analysis of variance indicated that the greater than two-fold increase in average volumetric wear of 0.89 mm^3 ($n=6$, 0.34 to 1.45 mm^3) for implants with lambda ratio less than one compared with 0.36 mm^3 ($n=6$, 0.15 to 0.74 mm^3) for implants with lambda ratio greater than three was statistically significantly ($p=0.014$). While the scatter in volumetric wear as a function of lambda ratio suggested the influence of other factors, these results still indicated that the steady state lambda ratio was a useful predictor of wear performance and a potentially valuable tool for implant design. Furthermore, because both clearance and surface roughness are important parameters affecting film thickness and lambda ratio, it is fortuitous that they are directly controlled by implant design and manufacturing.

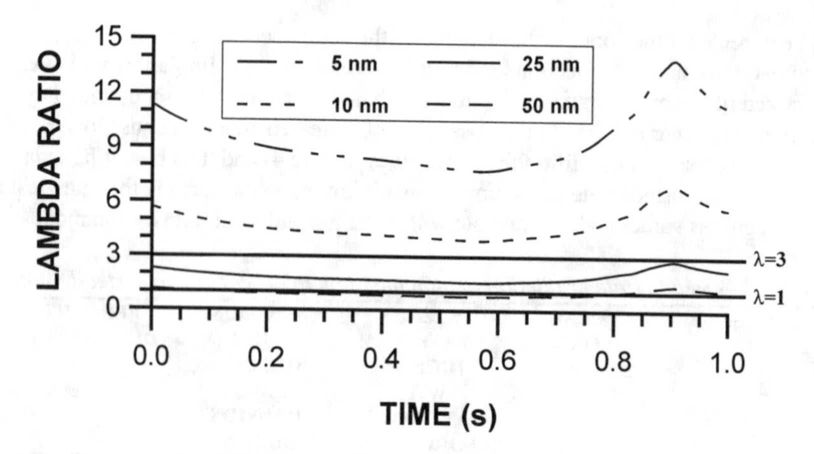

FIGURE 8 – *Time-varying lambda ratio as a function of combined surface roughness. Lambda ratio decreased as surface roughness increased, indicating a transition from full fluid film lubrication (λ>3) to boundary lubrication (λ<1).*

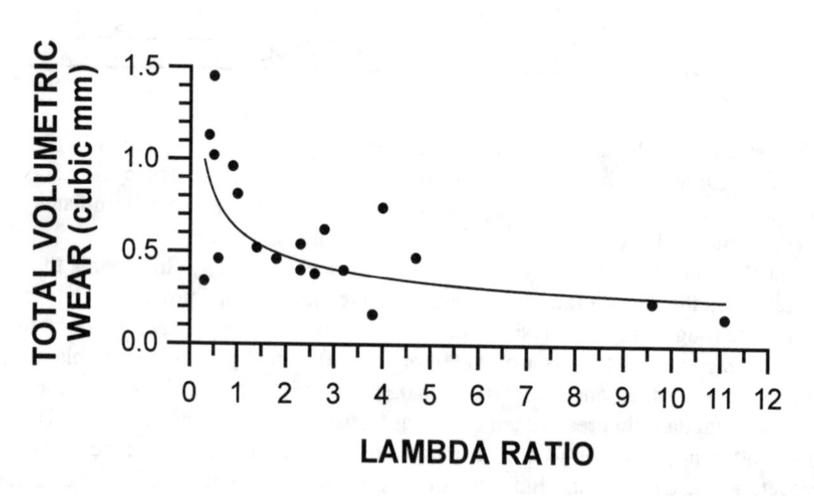

FIGURE 9 – *Total volumetric wear after three million cycles of simulator testing plotted against steady state lambda ratio. Wear decreased as lambda ratio increased (as head-cup separation increased).*

Conclusions

1. Cyclic steady state was reached quickly in the transient ehl model.
2. Fluid film thickness did not vary markedly within each cycle.
3. Clearance, lubricant viscosity, and cycle frequency were important parameters that influenced film thickness.
4. Load magnitude did not markedly influence film thickness.
5. The steady state ehl expression for film thickness due to entraining action calculated using the average load within each cycle was a simplified method to predict minimum transient film thickness.
6. Wear decreased with increasing lambda ratio, suggesting that fluid film lubrication influenced the wear of metal-metal hip implants.

Acknowledgments

The authors gratefully acknowledge the support of the Medical Research Council (MRC) of Canada.

References

[1] McKellop, H., Park, S.-H., Chiesa, R., Doorn, P., Lu, B., Normand, P., Grigoris, P., and Amstutz, H., "In vivo wear of 3 types of metal on metal hip prostheses during 2 decades of use," *Clinical Orthopaedics and Related Research*, Vol. 329S, 1996, pp. S128-S140.

[2] Door, L.D., Hilton, K.R., Wan, Z., Markovich, G.D., and Bloebaum, R., "Modern metal on metal articulations for total hip replacements," *Clinical Orthopaedics and Related Research*, Vol. 333, 1996, pp. 108-117.

[3] McKellop, H., Campbell, P., Lu, B., Park, S.-H., Doorn, P., and Dorr, L., "Clinical wear performance of modern metal-on-metal hip arthroplasties," *Alternative Bearing Surfaces in Total Joint Replacement, ASTM STP 1346*, Jacobs, JJ and Craig, TL, Eds., American Society for Testing and Materials, 1998.

[4] Rieker, C.B., Köttig, P., Schön, R., Windler, M., and Wyss, U.P., "Clinical wear performance of metal-on-metal hip arthroplasties," *Alternative Bearing Surfaces in Total Joint Replacement, ASTM STP 1346*, Jacobs, JJ and Craig, TL, Eds., American Society for Testing and Materials, 1998.

[5] Chan, F.W., Bobyn, J.D., Medley, J.B., Krygier, J.J., Podgorsak, G.F., and Tanzer, M., "Metal-metal hip implants: investigation of design parameters that control wear," submitted to *Clinical Orthopaedics and Related Research*, 1997.

[6] Medley, J.B., Dowling, J.M., Poggie, R.A., Krygier, J.J., and Bobyn, J.D., "Simulator wear of some commercially available metal-on-metal hip implants," *Alternative Bearing Surfaces in Total Joint Replacement, ASTM STP 1346*, Jacobs, JJ and Craig, TL, Eds., American Society for Testing and Materials, 1998.

[7] Schmidt, M.B. and Farrar, R., "Characterization of the wear behavior of metal-on-metal hip components using a joint simulator," *Alternative Bearing Surfaces in Total Joint Replacement, ASTM STP 1346*, Jacobs, JJ and Craig, TL, Eds., American Society for Testing and Materials, 1998.

[8] Chan, F.W., Bobyn, J.D., Medley, J.B., Krygier, J.J., Yue, S., and Tanzer, M., "Wear performance of metal-metal hip implants," *Archives of the American Academy of Orthopaedic Surgeons*, Vol. 1, No. 1, 1997, pp. 57-60.

[9] Chan, F.W., Bobyn, J.D., Medley, J.B., Krygier, J.J., Yue, S., and Tanzer, M., "Engineering issues and wear performance of metal on metal hip implants," *Clinical Orthopaedics and Related Research*, Vol. 333, 1996, pp. 96-107.

[10] Medley, J.B., Chan, F.W., Krygier, J.J., and Bobyn, J.D., "Comparison of alloys and designs in a hip simulator study of metal on metal implants," *Clinical Orthopaedics and Related Research*, Vol. 329, 1996, pp. S148-S159.

[11] Streicher, R.M., Semlitsch, M., Schön, R., Weber, H., and Rieker, C., "Metal-on-metal articulation for artificial hip joints: laboratory study and clinical results," *Proceedings of the Institution of Mechanical Engineers, Journal of Engineering in Medicine*, Vol. 210, 1996, pp. 223-232.

[12] Medley, J.B., Krygier, J.J., Bobyn, J.D., Chan, F.W., Lippincott, A., and Tanzer, M., "Kinematics of the MATCO hip simulator and issues related to wear testing of metal-metal implants," *Proceedings of the Institution of Mechanical Engineers, Journal of Engineering in Medicine*, Vol. 211, 1997, pp. 89-100.

[13] Jin, Z.M., Dowson, D., and Fisher, J., "Analysis of fluid film lubrication in artificial hip joint replacements with surfaces of high elastic modulus," *Proceedings of the Institution of Mechanical Engineers, Journal of Engineering in Medicine*, Vol. 211, 1997, pp. 247-256.

[14] Jin, Z.M., Dowson, D., and Fisher, J., "Fluid film lubrication in natural hip joints," *Thin Films in Tribology*, Dowson, D., Taylor, C.M., and Godet, M., Eds, Elsevier Science Publishers, Amsterdam, 1993, pp. 545-555.

[15] Swanson, S.A.V. and Freeman, M.A.R., *The Scientific Basis of Joint Replacement*, Pitman Medical, London, 1977, p.11.

[16] Paul, J.P., "Forces transmitted by joints in the human body," *Proceedings of the Institution of Mechanical Engineers*, Vol. 181F, 1967, pp. 8-15.

[17] Farrar, R. and Schmidt, M.B., "The effect of diametral clearance on wear between head and cup for metal on metal articulations," *Transactions of the Orthopaedic Research Society 43rd Annual Meeting*, Vol. 22, 1997, p. 71.

[18] Scott, R.A. and Schroeder, D.W., "The effect of radial mismatch on the wear of metal on metal hip prosthesis: a hip simulator study," *Transactions of the Orthopaedic Research Society 43rd Annual Meeting*, Vol. 22, 1997, p. 764.

[19] Hamrock, B.J., *Fundamentals of Fluid Film Lubrication*, McGraw-Hill, New York, 1994.

[20] Gladstone, J.R. and Medley, J.B., "Comparison of theoretical and experimental values for friction of lubricated elastomeric surface layers under transient conditions," *Tribology Series 17*, Elsevier Science Publishers: London, 1990, pp. 241-250.

[21] Smith, T.J. and Medley, J.B., "Development of transient elastohydrodynamic models for synovial joint lubrication," *Tribology Series 11*, Elsevier Science Publishers: London, 1986, pp. 369-374.

[22] Semlitsch, M., Streicher, R.M., and Weber, H., "Wear behaviour of cast CoCrMo cups and balls in long-term implanted total hip prostheses," *Orthopaede*, Vol. 18, 1989, pp. 377-381.

[23] Bragdon, C.R., O'Connor, D.O., Lowenstein, J.D., Jasty, M., and Syniuta, W.D., "The importance of multidirectional motion on the wear of polyethylene," *Proceedings of the Institution of Mechanical Engineers, Journal of Engineering in Medicine*, Vol. 210, 1996, pp. 157-165.

[24] Yu, H. and Medley, J.B., "Influence of lubricant additives on friction in a disc machine," *Tribology Series 32*, Elsevier Science Publishers, London, 1997, pp. 475-486.

[25] Johnson, K.L., Greenwood, J.A., and Poon, S.Y., "A simple theory of asperity contact in elastohydrodynamic lubrication," *Wear*, Vol. 19, 1972, pp. 91-108.

[26] Medley, J.B., Dowson, D., and Wright, V., "Transient elasto-hydrodynamic lubrication models for the human ankle joint," *Engineering in Medicine*, Vol. 13, 1984, pp. 137-151.

[27] Jin, Z.M., "The micro-elastohydrodynamic lubrication of synovial joints," Ph.D. thesis, University of Leeds, 1988.

Sang-Hyun Park,[1] Harry McKellop,[1] Bin Lu,[1] Frank Chan,[2] Roberto Chiesa[3]

WEAR MORPHOLOGY OF METAL-METAL IMPLANTS: HIP SIMULATOR TESTS COMPARED WITH CLINICAL RETRIEVALS

REFERENCE: Park, S. –H., McKellop, H., Lu, B., Chan, F., and Chiesa, R., **"Wear Morphology of Metal-Metal Implants: Hip Simulator Tests Compared with Clinical Retrievals,"** *Alternative Bearing Surfaces in Total Joint Replacement, ASTM STP 1346*, J. J. Jacobs and T. L. Craig, Eds., American Society for Testing and Materials, 1998.

ABSTRACT: This study compared the bearing surfaces of modern-generation metal-metal implants worn in five different hip joint simulators and worn in vivo. Comparable wear morphology was found between in vitro and in vivo worn implants. The non-contact zones displayed fine residual scratches from the original polishing, and carbide bumps that were either rounded or irregular. In the main bearing zones, the polishing marks and third-body scratches were worn smooth. Moreover, there were flat-bottomed depressions, apparently carbides that had been dissolved below the level of surrounding matrix. Localized numerous micropits were found in the smoothly worn area on most of simulator tested specimens and on some of the retrieved implants. Surrounding the main wear zone was a transition zone containing dense third-body scratches, and thin deposits containing calcium phosphate. The comparable wear morphology suggested that in vitro wear simulators can provide an accurate model of the wear in vivo of modern-generation metal-metal total hip replacements.

KEYWORDS: metal-on-metal, hip prosthesis, wear, morphology, hip joint simulator, clinical retrievals

---

There is growing interest in metal-metal hip prostheses as a potential solution to the problem of osteolysis induced by polyethylene wear debris. Although some of the first-generation metal-metal hips experienced a high failure rate, many metal-metal implants have survived twenty years or more of active use without apparent wear-related problems [1,4,6]. For the second-generation metal-metal implants now being developed, joint simulator wear tests can be used to evaluate new materials and designs prior to their

[1]Assistant and Associate Professor, and Laboratory Manager, respectively, The J. Vernon Luck Sr., M.D., Orthopaedic Research Center, Orthopaedic Hospital / Dept. of Orthopaedic, University of Southern California, Los Angeles, CA 90007.

[2]Ph.D. candidate, Jo Miller Orthopaedic Research Laboratory, McGill University, Montreal, Quebec H3G 1A4.

[3]Ph.D., Dipartimento di Chimica Fisica Applicata, Politecnico di Milano, Italy.

clinical use. However, care must be taken that the wear produced in the laboratory is the same as that which will occur in vivo. This study compared the bearing surfaces of modern-generation metal-metal implants worn in five different hip joint simulators with those of metal-metal implants worn in vivo.

Experimental Method

Hip Simulator Wear Tests

The seventeen modern-generation, metal-metal total hip replacements examined in this study had been tested up to three million cycles in five different joint simulators, manufactured by three companies and located in five different laboratories (Table 1). The cobalt-chromium alloys included those satisfying ASTM F75 (cast, high carbon) and ASTM F1537 (wrought, low and high carbon). Five pairs of implants were tested in the "anatomical" position, i.e., with the cup mounted in the simulator above the ball, and twelve pairs were tested in the inverted position with the cup below the ball. Bovine serum was used as the lubricant in each case, but with varying concentrations and with additives (Table 2) that included antibiotics to retard bacterial degradation and, in some cases, ethylenediaminetetraacetic acid (EDTA) to minimize precipitation of calcium phosphate on the bearing surfaces [5]. Wear morphology analysis was performed after finishing the wear simulation. However, implants tested at the J. Vernon Luck Orthopaedic Research Center were analyzed after every million cycles of wear simulation.

TABLE 1--*Summary of simulators and specimens tested.*

LABORATORY	TYPE SIMULATOR	TEST POSITION	IMPLANT MANUFACTURER & ASTM SPECIFICATION
J. Vernon Luck Orthop. Res. Center	MMED	anatomical & inverted	Sulzer Orthopaedics (Metasul™) F1537 (high carbon, wrought)
Jo Miller Laboratory	MMED	inverted	Wright Medical F75 (high carbon, cast) F1537 (low carbon, wrought)
Intermedics Orthopaedics	MMED	inverted	Sulzer Orthopaedics (Metasul™) F1537 (high carbon, wrought)
Sulzer Medical Technology	STANMORE MK III	anatomical	Sulzer Orthopaedics (Metasul™) F1537 (high carbon, wrought)
Massachusetts General Hospital	AMTI	anatomical	Sulzer Orthopaedics (Metasul™) F1537 (high carbon, wrought)

TABLE 2--*Summary of test conditions.*

LABORATORY	LUBRICANT	ANTIBIOTIC	EDTA	TEST DURATION
J. Vernon Luck Orthopaedic Research Center	bovine serum 90%	sodium azide or Proxel GXL*	added	3×10^6
Jo Miller Laboratory	bovine serum 90%	penicillin, fungizone	added or without	3×10^6
Intermedics Orthopaedics	bovine serum 90%	sodium azide	added	3×10^6
Sulzer Medical Technology	bovine serum 33%	propylene-phenoxetol	without	2×10^6
Massachusetts General Hospital	bovine serum 90%	sodium azide	added	1×10^6

* Zenaca Inc., Wilmington, DE.

Retrieved Implants

The clinically retrieved implants included eight Metasul™ (Sulzer Orthopaedics Ltd., Switzerland) cobalt-chromium alloy ASTM F1537 (ISO5832-12, wrought, 0.2% C) metal-metal total hip replacements. These were retrieved from five male and three female patients, 52 to 84 years of age. The implants were revised after 19 to 58 months *in situ*, two for aseptic loosening, two for infection, and one for dislocation, and three were obtained post-mortem.

Wear Morphology Analysis

Each of the simulator-tested and clinical retrieved implants was inspected with a light microscope for mapping of the original surfaces and worn areas. The components were then ultrasonically cleaned in a detergent solution and dried with filtered nitrogen gas. The surface morphologies were then characterized on a Zeiss DSM 960 scanning electron microscope, using a GW backscattered electron detector in the topographic mode.

Results

Wear Morphology of Simulator-tested Implants

There were three distinct zones on the surfaces of the simulator-tested specimens: the non-contact zone showing the original polishing marks, the main wear zone, and the transition zone in the form of a roughly circular band around the main wear zone. The main wear zones were concentrated near the load axis on a component that was fixed relative to the load axis, and were more distributed on the moving component. These

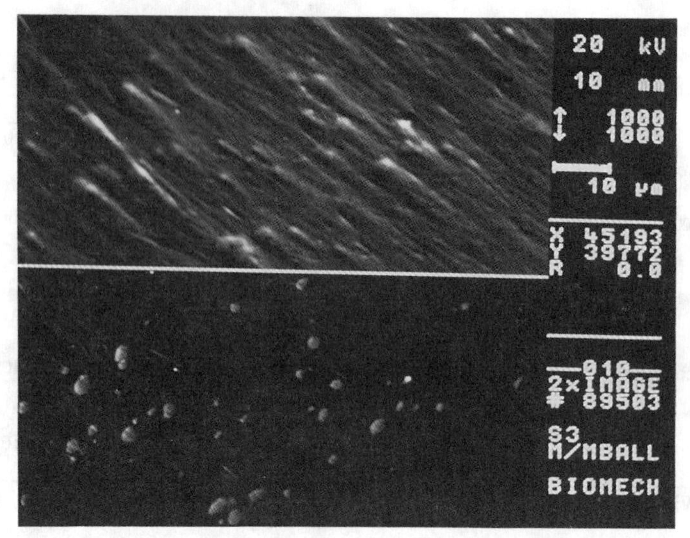

Figure 1: *Non-contact area of a Metasul™ ball. The surface was covered with polishing scratches on the soft matrix, and smeared round bumps (top: X1000). Atomic number contrast mode of the same field revealed that the round bumps were chromium carbides (bottom: X1000).*

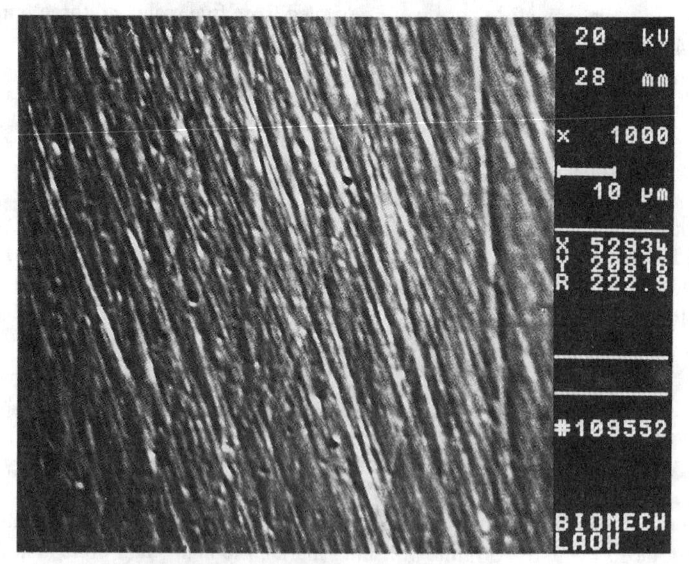

Figure 2: *Non-contact area of a Wright Medical high carbon ball (X1000). Surface was covered with polishing scratches, but without visible carbide bumps.*

features were comparable regardless of whether the implants had been tested in the anatomical or inverted position.

The non-contact zone of the Metasul™ implants displayed fine finishing scratches on the soft matrix, and round chromium carbide bumps averaging 5 μm in diameter (Figure 1). In contrast, the non-contact zone of the Wright implants, (whether cast high carbon or wrought low carbon alloy), included only finishing scratches without any obvious surface carbides (Figure 2).

In the main wear zone, the surface had been polished smoother than the original, non-contact zone. Residual polishing scratches and larger scratches were worn away, leaving a smooth surface with only fine scratches (Figure 3). Early in the wear test (i.e., less than one million cycles), dislodged surface carbides on the Metasul™ implants had apparently produced large, third-body scratches (carbide "comets", Figure 4). In contrast, after the initial wear-in, dislodging of the carbide was stopped, and most of the large third-body scratches had been polished smooth, leaving only fine scratches. In addition, in the main wear zone, there were numerous shallow, flat-bottomed, round craters or depressions, less than 1 μm deep and an average 5 μm in diameter (Figures 3 and 5). These depressions contained elevated concentrations of chromium and carbon (i.e., consistent with carbides), and were comparable in size and distribution to the original carbide bumps. The surfaces of the Wright F75 high carbon implants also showed these shallow carbide depressions but, in this case, they were more irregularly shaped, up to 20 μm in the largest dimension. Some areas of the F75 surfaces contained etched grain boundaries, as well as a few pits around the carbides (Figure 6). The carbide depressions were not observed on the surfaces of the Wright F1537 low carbon implants. Micropits about 1 to 3 μm in diameter and less than 1 μm deep were occasionally present in the highly polished worn areas in all of the simulator-tested implants.

The transition zone around the main wear zone was visible to the naked eye as a 1 to 5 mm wide whitish and light brown, roughly circular band. The brownish area was covered with tenacious, thin deposits containing calcium phosphate (Figure 7). Thicker deposits were initially observed in the outer periphery of the transition zone, but these were substantially removed during the cleaning process. In some cases, areas in the transition zone had been polished smooth covered with fine third-body scratches. Under the SEM, the whitish area was seen to contain clusters of micropits, depressions without presence of third-body scratches (Figures 8 and 9). Numerous large third-body scratches were typically located between the polished area and the non contact zone.

The micropits were observed in the main wear zone and/or the transition on all of the simulator-tested implants except two out of seven of the Wright implants tested in the MMED machine at the Jo Miller Laboratory. One of these was an F1537 alloy tested without EDTA and the second was an F75 alloy tested with EDTA. In both cases, the components were covered with a dense pattern of third-body scratches in the main wear and transition zones.

Wear Morphology of Clinically Retrieved Implants

Although the distribution of the main wear zone on the clinically retrieved Metasul™ implants was not as obvious as on the simulator-tested components, it appeared

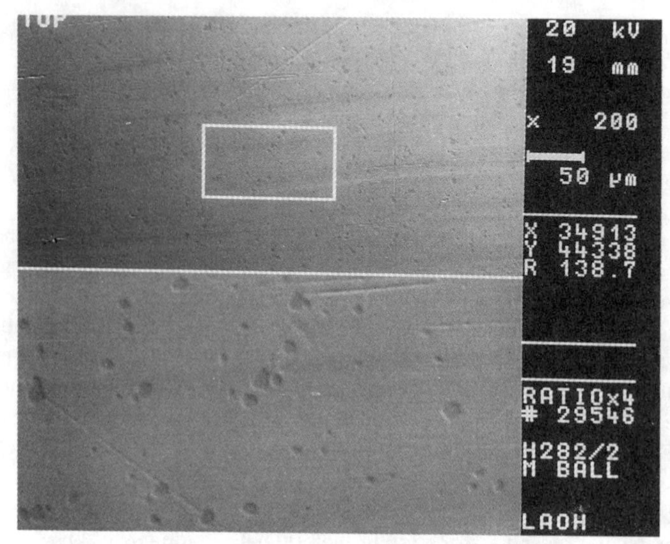

Figure 3: *Main wear area of a Metasul™ ball tested in the Stanmore MK III simulator (top: X200, bottom: X800). The original rough surface was worn away, and fine scratches and carbide craters were present.*

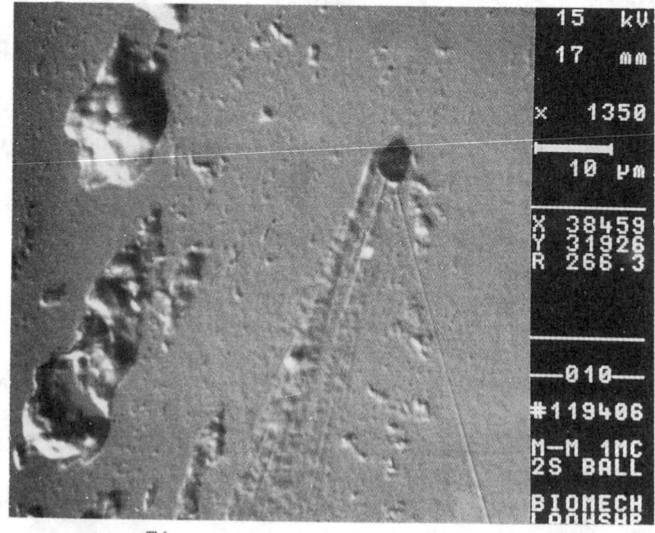

Figure 4: *Metasul™ ball tested in the JVL Laboratory simulator (one million cycles, inverted position, X1350). Left side shows two large "ghost" carbides holes and the right side shows scratches produced by a recently fragmented carbide (carbide "comet").*

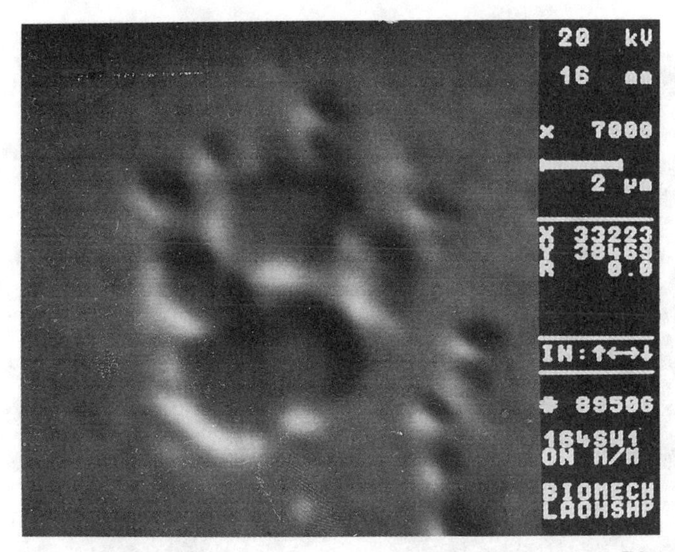

Figure 5: *Carbide depressions in the main wear area of Metasul™ ball tested in the Intermedics Orthopaedics Laboratory simulator (X7000). The carbide was below the level of the worn surface, possibly due to dissolution.*

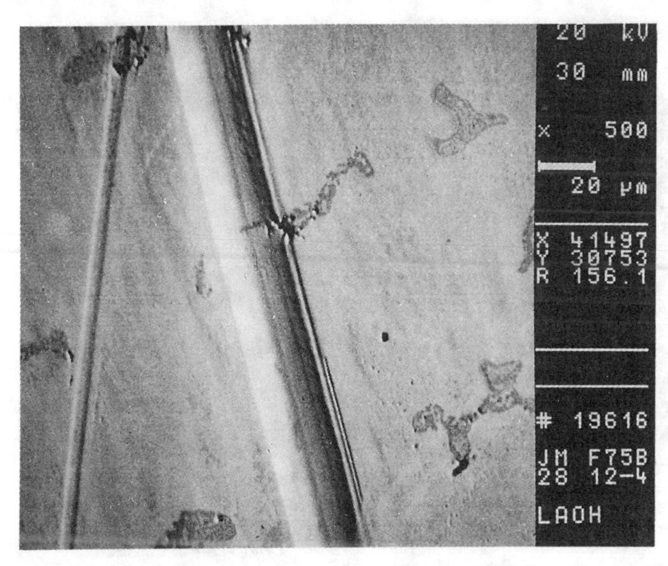

Figure 6: *The main wear zone of a Wright Medical high carbon ball tested in the Jo Miller Laboratory simulator (X500). Micropits were present at the boundary of the irregular shaped carbides.*

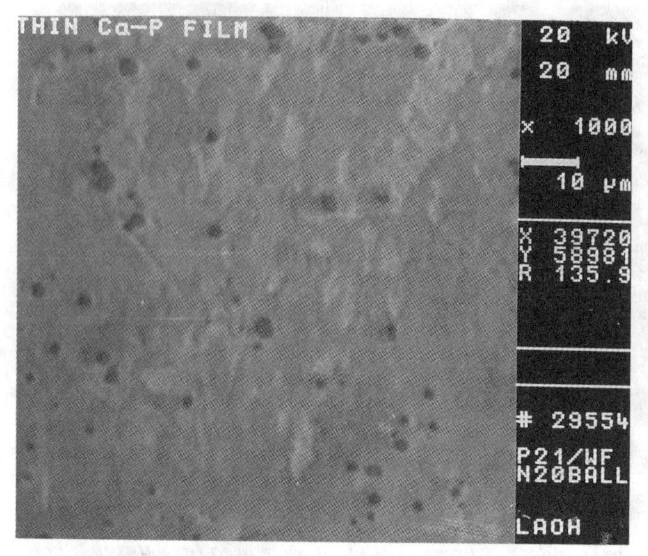

Figure 7: *Transition zone of a Metasul™ implant tested in the AMTI simulator (X1000). The surface was covered with a tenacious thin film deposit containing calcium and phosphorous.*

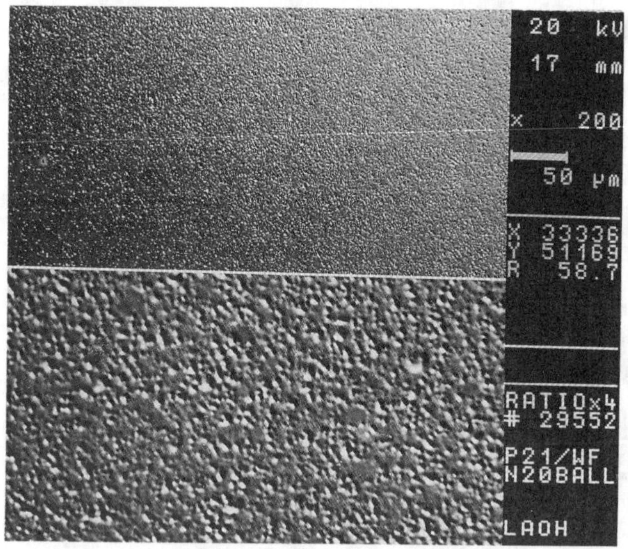

Figure 8: *Transition zone of a Metasul™ ball tested in the AMTI simulator (top:X200, bottom: X800). A narrow band of the surface was covered with numerous micropits and round carbide craters.*

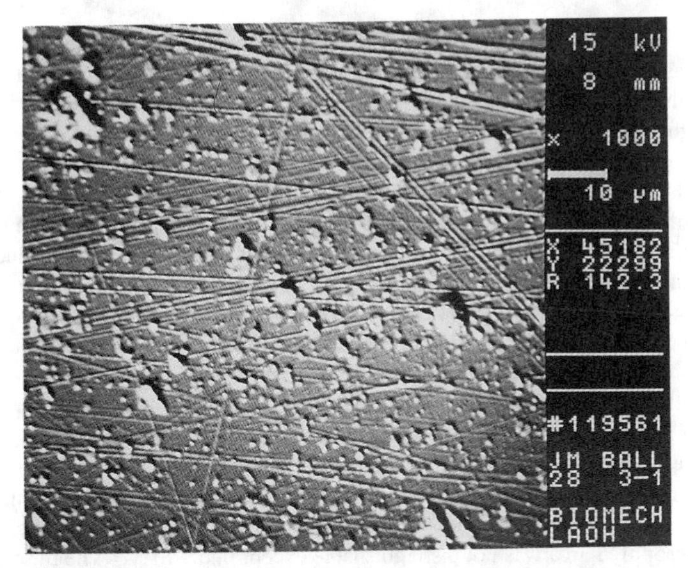

Figure 9: *Transition zone of a Wright Medical low carbon ball (X1000). A narrow band of the surface was covered with numerous micropits and fine third-body scratches.*

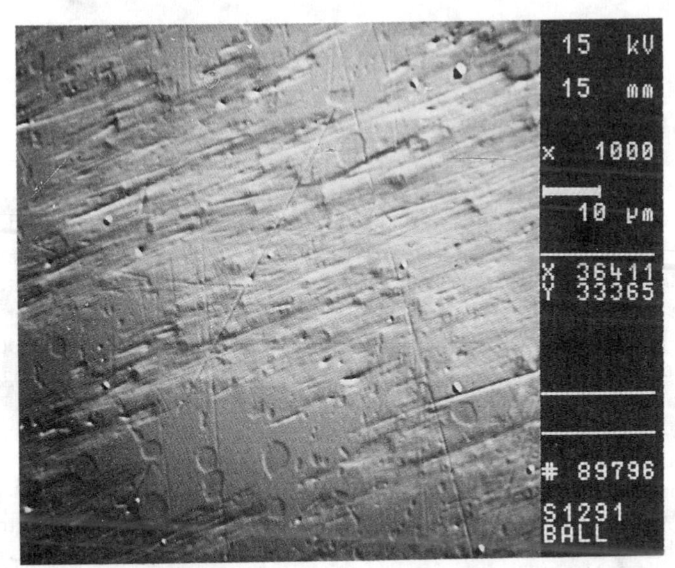

Figure 10: *Transition zone of a retrieved Metasul™ ball. The mound containing carbides was polished smooth, and carbides bumps were transformed into shallow craters in the polished areas (X1000).*

to be relatively concentrated on the balls and distributed on the cups, and the wear morphology was very comparable to the simulator-tested. In the transition area of the clinical retrievals, the protruding and bumpy surface was worn smooth without carbide dislodging (Figure 10). Even though evidence of dislodged carbides was not observed in the transition zone, most of the components had sustained considerable third-body abrasive scratching in the transition and main bearing zones. Most of the main bearing zone was smoothly polished, leaving fine, third-body scratches and shallow-bottomed carbide craters, comparable to the simulator-tested implants (Figure 11). One component that was revised for recurrent dislocation exhibited a large abrasive track across the center of the ball (apparently due to dragging across the rim of the metal acetabular socket). However, the edge of the track had been polished flat during subsequent use, and the extent of third-body damage in the implant was comparable to the other implants.

Two retrieved components exhibited a pattern of numerous micropits, from 1 to 3 μm in diameter and about 1 μm deep, covering much of the main bearing zones on the ball and cup (Figure 12). The micropits were located mostly in the matrix (i.e., between the large carbides) and at the edge of the carbide depressions, but not within the carbides. On one component, the area covered with micropits appeared whitish to the eye while, on the second, the micropitted area was not distinguishable except under SEM. The third-body scratches were less dense and shallower in the pitted area compared with the non-pitted, polished areas. As on the simulator-tested implants, thin, tenacious deposits of calcium phosphate-based precipitate were found in the transition areas of the retrieved implants, while the thicker deposits had been removed during the cleaning process.

Discussion

The similarity of the appearance of the bearing surfaces suggested that the wear mechanisms generated in the simulators were the same as those occurring in vivo with the metal-metal hip prostheses, both for first-generation [6,11,12] and second-generation implants. Both in vitro and in vivo, it was apparent that many of the surface carbides were dislodged from the surface of the contact zones during the wear-in phase and acted as third-body particles, generating extensive abrasive scratching and, probably, elevated early wear rates. The metal-metal bearings exhibited the ability to "self-polishing," i.e., to polish out these third-body scratches, as well as the residual scratches from the original polishing. Even the severe damage that occurred during subluxation (i.e., as the ball was dragged across the metal rim of the acetabular shell) was substantially polished out during subsequent use. In contrast, such surface damage was not repaired outside of the contact zones.

Particularly in the high-carbon alloys, the surface carbides that were not dislodged were eventually worn to the level of the surrounding matrix. The shallow, flat-bottomed depressions, which also exhibited the typical composition of carbides on EDAX, were found only in the main wear zones of the simulator-tested specimens and the clinically retrieved implants, and only for the high carbon alloys. Muratoglu et al. [7] observed similar flat-bottomed carbide depressions on clinically retrieved cobalt-chrome balls, both from metal-polyethylene and first generation metal-metal hip prostheses. The texture of the floor of the depressions, measured using an atomic force microscope, suggested that they had been formed in part by corrosion. The fact that the carbide depressions observed in the present study were below the level of the surrounding matrix, and only formed in the area where the surface was polished smooth without dense scratches, was consistent with their being formed by dissolution of chrome carbides, rather than by mechanical wear (Figures 3 and 5). That is, an initially protruding carbide may have been worn by abrasion to the level of the surrounding matrix, and then reduced below this level by dissolution (Figure 10).

Micropits have also been observed previously on first and second generation metal-metal implants, however, a common denominator for their formation is not yet apparent. Walker [12] described "smoky" regions on the main contact zones of some early retrieved McKee-Farrar metal-metal hips, which were found to contain extensive fine pits. He suggested that the micropits resulted from a fatigue-pitting mechanism. More recently, Rieker et al. [8] observed micropits on some first generation Muller type implant and second generation Metasul™ implants, and attributed their formation to adhesive wear, rather than corrosion. Rieker further reported that the wear rates of those Metasul™ implants with micropits were within the range of those without micropits.

In the present study, micropits were found on most of the simulator tested implants and on two out of eight second generation Metasul™ retrievals The distribution of the micropits on the bearing surface was comparable to that of the matrix carbides in a cobalt-chrome alloy [10]. Metallographs of the Metasul™ implants showed large, rounded grain boundary carbides and fine dispersed carbides in the matrix (Figure 13), indicating that micropit formation was associated with fine matrix carbides, and was sensitive to the local contact conditions. That is, on clinically retrieved implants, the micropits were found primarily in the main contact zone and the transition zone, where the surface had been polished smooth and was almost free of third-body scratches. In contrast, on the simulator-tested specimens, micropits were observed primarily in a narrow band of well-polished surface in the transition zone. The fact that, in some cases, the micropits were observed clustered at the edge of large carbides suggested that the high energy state of the boundary, both for large grain boundary carbides and for fine matrix carbides, may have facilitated local chemical attack which, in turn, allowed the matrix carbides to be dissolved below the level of the surface and/or to be broken out by the repeated adhesive/abrasive wear processes. In fact, due to the lack of third-body scratches in the areas with micropits, dissolution of matrix carbides is a more reasonable explanation than dislodging.

The formation of micropits was independent of the lubrication conditions used in the various simulators, which included variations in concentration of the serum, the presence of EDTA, or the particular antibiotic used. Originally, EDTA was added to the serum lubricant in hip simulator tests of metal-polyethylene and metal-ceramic implants to minimize precipitation of calcium phosphate onto the surface of the balls [5]. Since heavy layers of calcium phosphate were not typically observed on retrieved metal-polyethylene or ceramic-polyethylene implants, they were considered to be an artifact, possibly due to the elevated temperatures that are reached after several hours of uninterrupted running in the simulator [3]. However, since deposits containing calcium phosphate are typically present on retrieved metal-metal implants [6,9,11,12], it has been suggested that EDTA should not be used in simulator tests of metal-metal implants. On the other hand, Chan et

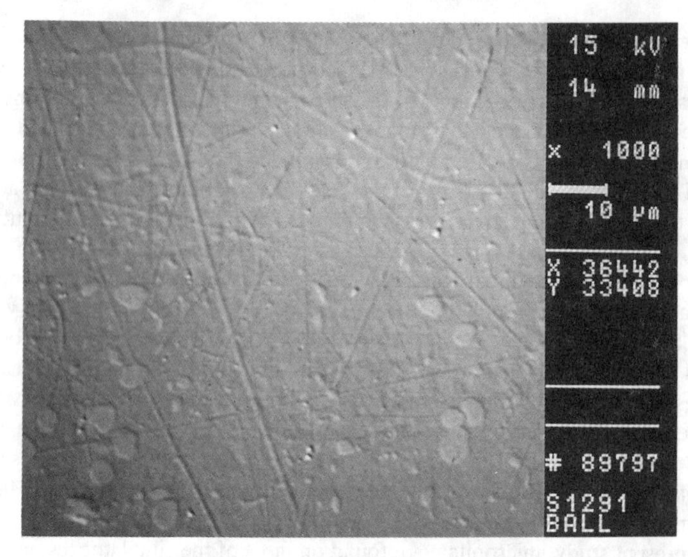

Figure 11: *Main wear area of a retrieved Metasul™ ball. The surface was polished smooth and covered with fine third-body scratches and round carbide craters (X1000).*

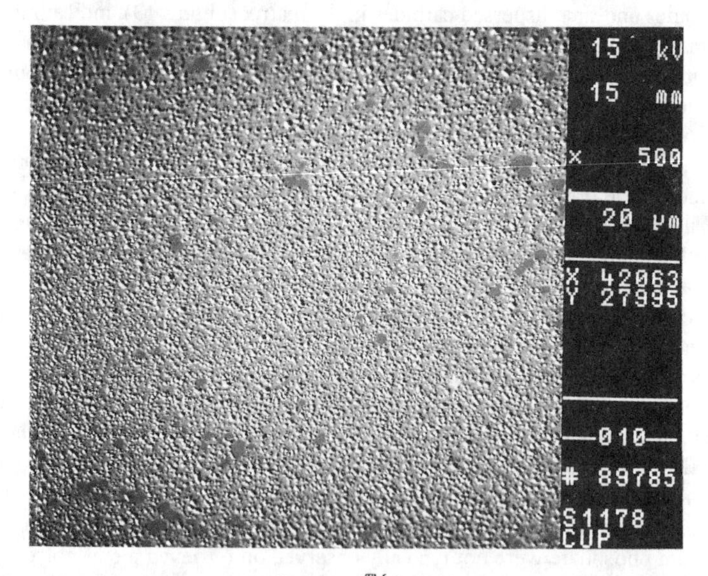

Figure 12: *Area of a retrieved Metasul™ ball that appeared whitish to the eye. The surface was covered with numerous micropits and rounded carbide craters. Third-body scratches were rare in the micropitted area (X1000).*

al. [2] have reported that the amount of wear in simulator tests was comparable whether or not EDTA was added to the serum and, since the formation of these interferes with the weighing and/or dimensional techniques used to determine the amount of wear, it might be preferable to use EDTA in order to maximize the accuracy of the wear measurements. -This issue should be given careful consideration by investigators performing laboratory wear tests of the second-generation metal-metal implants.

Conclusion

Although the location and distribution of the worn zones on the implants differed somewhat among the various simulators, depending on the particular load-motion patterns applied, the type of wear induced in each of them appeared very comparable to that occurring with metal-metal implants in vivo. Thus, provided that the magnitude of the contact stresses applied and the sliding distance per cycle are reasonably comparable to those in vivo, it can be expected that these hip simulators would also generate relative amounts of wear for two candidate materials comparable to that in vivo [8]. Nevertheless, additional studies should be directed toward identifying the mechanisms of formation of the shallow depressions and the micropits and their effect on the wear rates of the metal-metal implants.

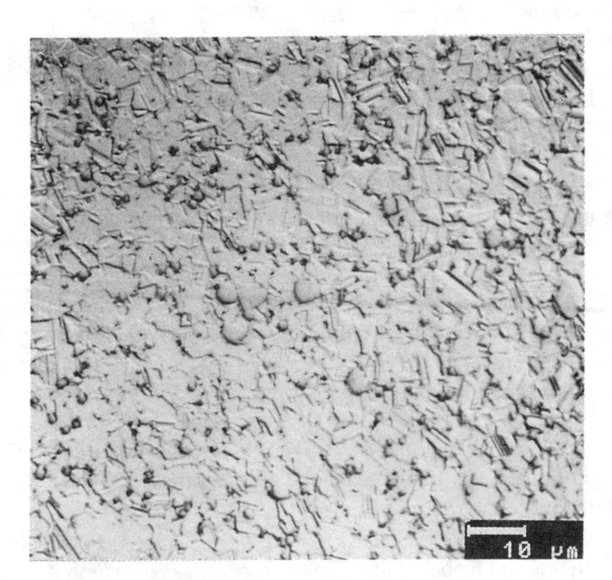

Figure 13: *Metallograph of a Metasul™ ball showing large round carbides and fine dispersed carbides.*

References

[1] August, A. C. , Aldam., C. H., and Pynsent, P.B., "The Mckee-Farrar Hip Arthroplasty. A Long-Term Study," *J. Bone Joint Surg.*, Vol. 68B, 1986, pp. 520-527.

[2] Chan, F.W., Bobyn. J.D., Medley, J.B., Krygier, J.J., Podgorsak, G.F., and Tanzer, M., "Design Factors That Control Wear of Metal-Metal Total Hip Implants," *Transactions, Society for Biomaterials*, New Orleans, 1997, p. 77.

[3] Lu, Z., and McKellop, H., "Frictional Heating of Bearing Materials Tested in a Hip Joint Wear Simulator," *Proc. Instn. Mech. Engrs.,* Part H, Vol. 211, 1997, pp.101-108.

[4] McCalden, R.W., Howie, D. W., Ward, L., Surbramanian, C., Nawana, N., and Pearcy, M.J., "Observation on the Long-Term Wear Behavior of Retrieved McKee-Farrar total Hip Replacement Implants," *Transactions, Orthopaedic Research Society,* Vol. 20, 1995, p. 242.

[5] McKellop, H., Lu, B., and Benya, P., "Friction, Lubrication and Wear of Cobalt-Chromium, Alumina and Zirconia Hip Prostheses Compared on a Joint Simulator," *Transactions, Orthopaedic Research Society,* Vol. 17, 1992, p. 402.

[6] McKellop, H., Park, S. H., Chisa, R., Door, P., Lu, B., Norman P., Grigoris, P., and Amstutz, H., "In-Vivo Wear of 3 Types of Metal on Metal Hip Prostheses During 2 Decades of Use," *Clinical Orthopaedics*, Vol. S129, 1996, pp. 128-140.

[7] Muratoglu, O. K., Jasty, M., and Harris, W. H., "In Vivo Corrosive Wear of the Carbide Phase in Cast CoCr Femoral heads. Metal on Polymer and Metal on Metal," *Transactions, Orthopaedic Research Society*, Vol. 22, 1997, p. 765.

[8] Rieker, C.B., Koettig, P., Schoen, R., Windler, M., and Wyss U.P., "Clinical Wear Performance of Metal-on-Metal Hip Arthroplasties," *Alternative Bearing Surfaces in Total Joint Replacement, ASTM STP* 1346, J. J. Jacobs and T.L. Craig, Eds., American Society for Testing Materials, 1998, pp **??-??**

[9] Semlitsch, M., Streicher, R.M., and Weber, H., "Wear Behavior of Cast CoCrMo Cups and Balls in Long-Term Implanted Total Hip Prostheses," *Orthopaede,* Vol. 18, 1989, pp. 377-381.

[10] Smith, W. F., "Nickel and Cobalt Alloys," *Structure and Properties of Engineering Alloys*, McGraw-Hill, New York, 1981, pp. 458-502.

[11] Walker, P. S., Salvati, E., and Hotzler, R. K., "The Wear on Removed McKee-Farrar Total Hip Prostheses," *J. Bone Joint Surg.*, Vol. 56A, 1974, pp. 92-100.

[12] Walker, P. S., "Friction and Wear of Artificial Joint," *Human Joint and Their Artificial Replacements*, Charles C Thomas, Publisher, Springfield, 1977, pp. 368-422.

Claude B. Rieker[1], Petra Köttig[1], Rolf Schön[1], Markus Windler[1] and Urs P. Wyss[2]

CLINICAL WEAR PERFORMANCE OF METAL-ON-METAL HIP ARTHROPLASTIES

REFERENCE: Rieker, C. B., Köttig, P., Schön, R., Windler, M., and Wyss, U. P., "**Clinical Wear Performance of Metal-on-Metal Hip Arthroplasties,**" *Alternative Bearing Surfaces in Total Joint Replacement, ASTM STP 1346*, J. J. Jacobs and T. L. Craig, Eds., American Society for Testing and Materials, 1998.

ABSTRACT: Thirty old (1st generation) Cobalt-Chromium metal-on-metal (Müller design) hip components and 83 new (2nd generation) Cobalt-Chromium metal-on-metal (METASUL™ design) hip components were examined for their in-vivo wear behaviour. The in-vivo wear behaviour of these retrievals was compared with their in-vitro wear behaviour. A running-in period of about one year is observed where the in-vivo wear rate for the whole bearing is approximately 25 μm/year. After this running-in period, the measured in-vivo wear rate of the whole bearing decreases to about 5 μm/year. A very good consistency is found between the in-vitro and in-vivo wear rate. The examination of the wear pattern shows abrasive wear for all the prostheses and some adhesive-fatigue wear areas for 10 per cent of the prostheses. The observed wear rate is independent of the wear mechanisms.
The metal-on-metal bearing can be considered as a very low wear articulation system.

KEYWORDS: hip prosthesis, metal-on-metal, wear mechanisms, wear rate

---

[1]Research scientists, Sulzer Orthopedics, PO Box 65, CH-8404 Winterthur, Switzerland.
[2]Research manager, Sulzer Orthopedics, PO Box 65, CH-8404 Winterthur, Switzerland.
METASUL™ is a trademark of Sulzer Orthopedics Ltd., PO Box 65, CH-8404 Winterthur, Switzerland.

Introduction

A healthy human hip joint has minimum friction and almost no wear due to optimal lubrication [1] which, under normal conditions, completely separates the two articulation surfaces. In the case of osteoarthritis or rheumatoid arthritis, the lubricating capacity decreases, leading to wear of the hip joint surfaces, which in turn leads to increased friction and also intense pain [2]. Under such circumstances the natural joint has to be replaced by artificial hip prosthesis.

As all the materials actually used to manufacture hip prostheses are unable to produce a permanent lubricating film, the prosthesis's surfaces are always subject to wear. The amount of wear particles released control the longevity of the implant fixation [3]. Polyethylene liners wear at an average linear wear rate of 0.1 - 0.2 mm per year depending on the material combination (metal-on-polyethylene or ceramic-on-polyethylene) [4]. This linear wear rate produces a very large number of polyethylene particles overloading the elimination's capacities of the lymphatic tissues, leading to the late loosening of the hip joints [5]. Excellent results of some of the old metal-on-metal prostheses [6] lead to a reassessment of metal-on-metal hip bearing by Sulzer Orthopedics in 1983. The first implantation of the second generation metal-on-metal METASUL™ bearing (Sulzer Orthopedics Ltd.- Switzerland) was made in 1988. To date, more than 60 000 second generation metal-on-metal hip joints (120 000 single components) have been produced.

The wear behaviour of 30 single metal-on-metal retrievals of the first generation (Müller design) and 83 single metal-on-metal retrievals of the modern second generation is examined. The in-vivo wear behaviour is compared with in-vitro experiments (hip simulator).

Experimental method

Materials

The 30 single metal-on-metal retrievals of the first generation (Müller design) manufactured between 1966 and 1970 were made of cast Co-28Cr-6Mo-0.2C alloy (ASTM F-75 / ISO 5832-4). The diameters of the heads were either 37 mm or 42 mm. The implantation time varies between 36 and 337 months (mean follow-up: 187 months). Most revisions were due to a late loosening. Due to an incomplete documentation, a precise statistic for the reasons of these revisions can not be given.

The 83 single metal-on-metal retrievals (head or cup) of the second modern generation manufactured after 1987 were made of a wrought high Carbon Co-28Cr-6Mo-0.2C alloy (ASTM F-1537 / ISO 5832-12). The initial roughness R_a (Mahr-Perthometer stylus surface analyser) of these components is about 0.020 - 0.025 μm. Eighty retrievals have a 28 mm diameter and 3 retrievals have a 32 mm diameter. The implantation time varies between 2 and 72 months (mean follow-up: 18 months). Due the different causes of revision, most of the retrieved components were single component (head or cup). The reasons for revision are given in Table 1.

TABLE 1 – *Reason for retrievals*

Reasons for retrievals	-
Dislocations	35%
Stem loosening	17%
Cup loosening	17%
Others (infection, ossification)	31%

Hip simulator

The hip simulators used (Stanmore Mk-III manufactured by Anderman and Ryder Ltd. - Kingston upon Thames - UK) are mechanically operated with fixed characteristics given in Table 2.

TABLE 2 – *Mechanical characteristic of the hip simulator*

Properties	Value
Flexion - Extension	21° - 21°
Abduction - Adduction	5° - 11°
Internal / External rotation	9° - 9°
Maximum load (double peak)	1 550 N
Temperature	20 °C
Frequency	0.5 Hz

The femoral head is self-aligned into the acetabular component having an inclination angle of 45°, corresponding approximately to an in-vivo situation. The wear tests are lubricated with a stabilised mixture of Ringer's solution with 33 per cent of calf serum, buffered to a pH of 7.2. This lubricant has almost the some amount of proteins and the same content of salts than the healthy human synovial fluid. The lubricant is filtered with a 0.2 μm filter to remove all the possible sources of contamination. A comparison between the healthy synovial fluid and the used lubricant is given in Table 3.

TABLE 3 – *Characteristics of the lubricant*

Constituent (g/l)	Healthy synovial fluid	Lubricant
Water	970.00	973.00
Sodium	3.30	4.76
Potassium	0.16	0.19
Calcium	0.06	0.05
Chloride	3.80	4.77
Protein	17.00	20.33
Hyaluronic acid	3.20	-

Wear measurements

The wear of the components is measured by a co-ordinate measuring machine (CMM5 manufactured by SIP - Geneva - Switzerland) having a spatial resolution lower than 1 μm in the area of measurement. A measurement is made every 7.5 degree on 12 concentric circles as well as on the pole of the component (577 measurements for each component).

For the retrieved components (1st and 2nd generation of the metal-on-metal bearings), the wear is simply defined by the maximum deviation from the ideal sphericity.

For the hip simulator components, the surface dimensions of the head and cup were measured by the co-ordinate measuring machine prior each experiment. These measurements were used as reference values and afterwards compared with the measurements made every 500 000 cycles. The wear is defined by the maximum deviation obtained by comparing the measurements made after a given number of cycles with the reference values.

These two methods (retrieved components and hip simulator) give the local deepest wear (worst case) and are not comparable with the wear value measured by the gravimetric method used by some other laboratories [7] for hip simulator experiments. The gravimetric method gives the mean wear value and not the local deepest wear.

Due to the imprecision of repositioning the components on the co-ordinate measuring machine and due to a permanent organic deposited film found on the components, the precision of the wear measurements is estimated to be around ± 2 μm (scatter bar in the hip simulator results).

Results

Hip simulator

Figure 1 shows the in-vitro wear behaviour (maximum wear for the two components [head and cup] in function of the number of cycles) of three modern metal-on-metal bearings. The first and the second bearings have been already published [8]. For the first bearing where the clearance was too large (more than 200 μm), the wear increases steadily and reaches about 90 μm after 2.5 millions cycles. For the second and third bearings with an optimised clearance (about 100 μm), the total wear after one million cycles approaches about 25 μm. This wear rate corresponds to a running-in period. After this running-in period, the wear rate for the two bearings with an optimised clearance varies between 4 and 10 μm per million cycles. The negative wear rate found with the third bearing between 1 and 2 millions cycles is due to a permanent organic deposited film found on the components. No explanation has been found to explain the differences observed in the wear rates between the second and third bearings.

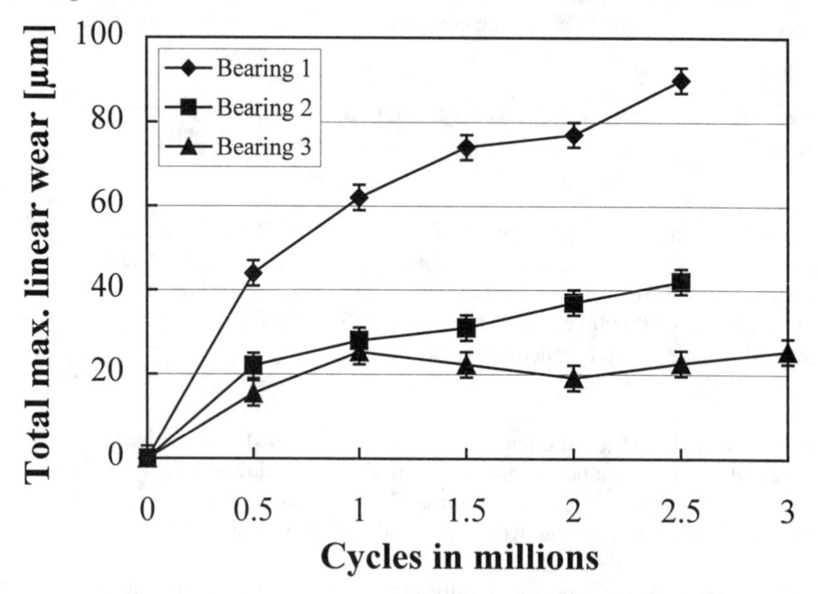

Figure 1: *Wear of three modern metal-on-metal bearings (hip simulator)*

Retrieved Müller metal-on-metal prostheses (1st generation)

Figure 2 shows the in-vivo wear rate (maximum wear rate for the components [head or cup] in function of in-vivo implantation time) for the 30 Müller metal-on-metal prostheses. The wear rate of 24 Müller metal-on-metal prostheses has been already published [9]. The maximum wear rate (6.2 μm/year) was found for a head having an implantation time of 120 months. The wear amount of the heads and of the cups is identical. The mean wear rate for all the retrieved Müller metal-on-metal components (cup or head) is 2.2 μm/year.

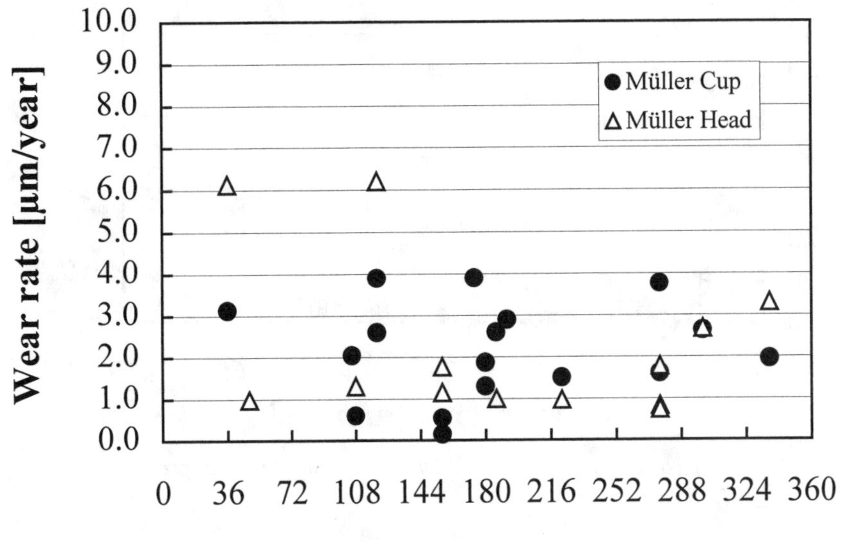

Figure 2: *In-vivo wear rate of retrieved Müller metal-on-metal prostheses (1st generation)*

Retrieved modern metal-on-metal prostheses

Figure 3 shows the in-vivo wear rate (maximum wear rate for the components [head or cup] in function of in-vivo implantation time) for the 83 modern metal-on-metal components. The wear rate of 44 modern metal-on-metal components has been already published [9]. Two wear behaviours can be observed: a moderate wear rate (between 20 and 80 μm/year) and a low wear rate (below 20 μm/year). All 4 retrievals with the moderate wear rate were revised for mechanical problems: 2 for recurrent dislocations, one for cup tilting and one for a "squeaking hip". Figure 3 shows some cups have virtually zero wear. Unfortunately, most of these cups were revised without the corresponding head and therefore it is not possible to investigate this very low wear phenomenon.

Figure 4 shows the mean in-vivo annual wear rate and its standard deviation of the 83 modern metal-on-metal prostheses calculated for every year spent in-vivo. This representation of the annual wear rate shows that the wear rate lowers with the implantation time (wear rate for the 1st in-vivo year: about 25 μm/year for the whole bearing, wear rate after the 2nd year in-vivo: about 5 μm/year for the whole bearing). This Figure 4 shows also that the wear rate of the heads is higher than the cups' wear rate.

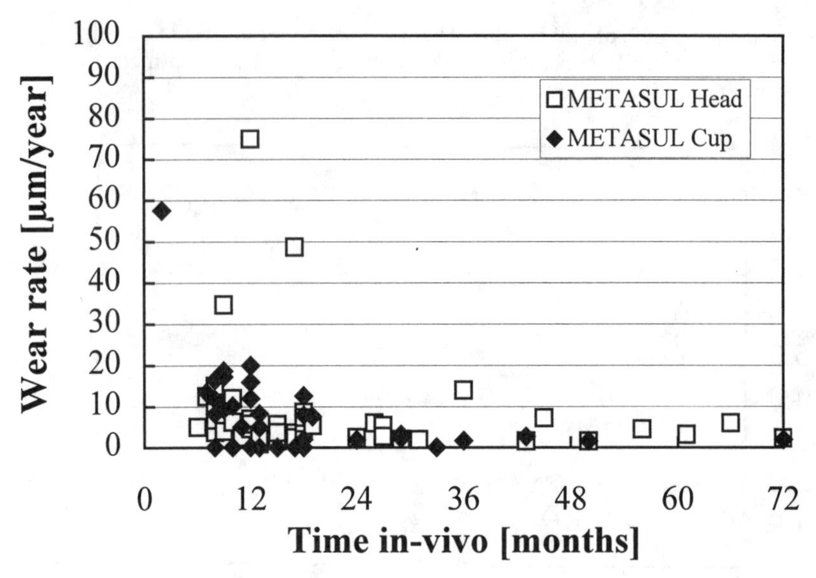

Figure 3: *In-vivo wear rate of retrieved modern metal-on-metal prostheses (2nd generation)*

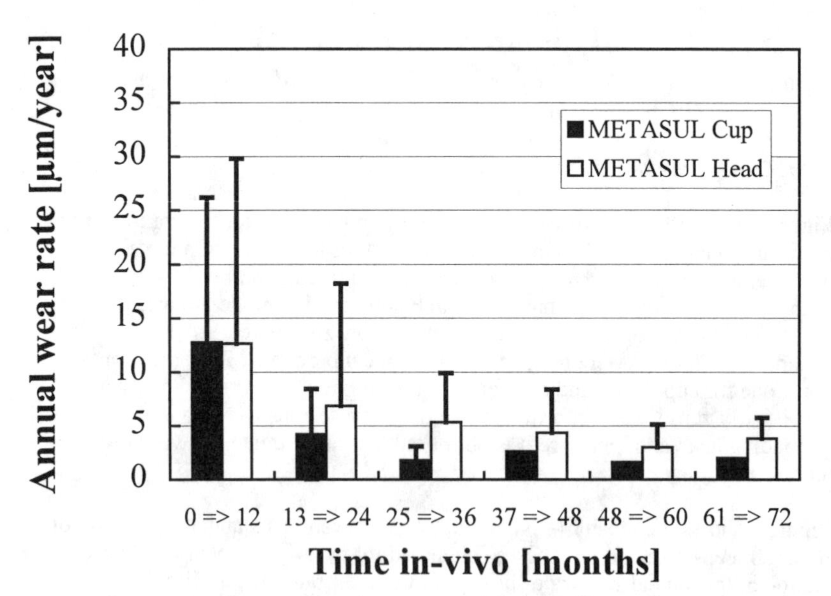

Figure 4: *In-vivo annual wear rate of retrieved modern metal-on-metal prostheses (2nd generation)*

Retrieved metal-on-metal prostheses (1st and 2nd generation)

Figure 5 shows the wear rate for the two generations of metal-on-metal prostheses. The ordinate of Figure 5 shows only the low wear rate of the modern metal-on-metal retrievals to increase the readability of the figure. It can be observed that the two generations of metal-on-metal prostheses seem consistent in describing the same general phenomenon.

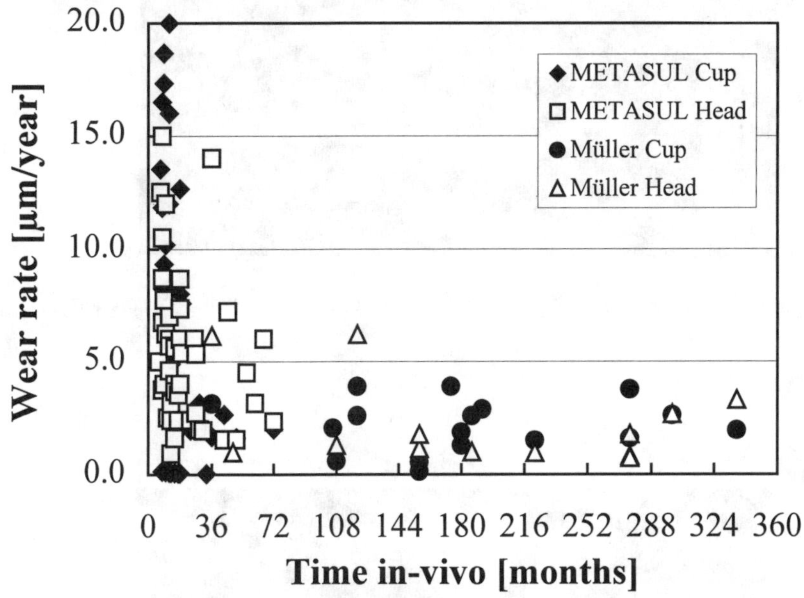

Figure 5: *In-vivo wear rate of retrieved metal-on-metal prostheses (1st and 2nd generation)*

Wear mechanisms of retrieved modern metal-on-metal prostheses (2nd generation)

Figures 6 and 7 show two SEM micrographs of typical worn surfaces of modern metal-on-metal retrievals. The wear pattern on Figure 6 is seen on all the specimens and can be characterised by two types of scratches. The first type is relatively large scratches (width: about 5 µm, depth: about 5 µm, and some millimetres in length). The second type of scratches is described as minor scratches and they can be described as polished large scratches. The arrow on Figure 6 shows this polishing procedure.

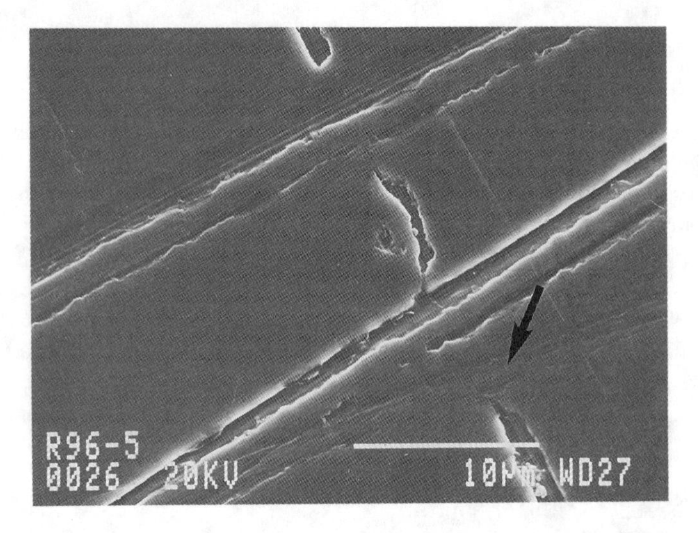

Figure 6: *Worn surface of modern metal-on-metal retrievals - Scratched areas*

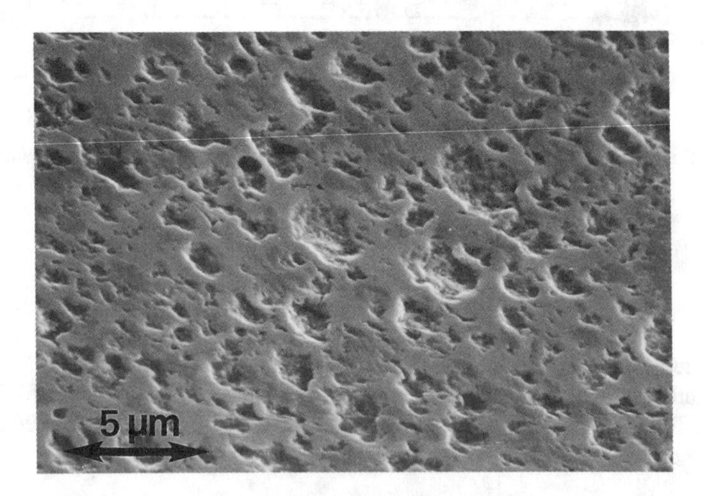

Figure 7: *Worn surface of modern metal-on-metal retrievals - Micro-pits areas*

The wear pattern on Figure 7 is seen on loaded areas on about 10 per cent of the specimens. Without optical magnification, these micro-pits areas are seen as "smoky" areas. The SEM investigation allows to characterise these "smoky" areas as micro-pits areas having a size of about 1 µm - 2 µm in diameter. The depth of these micro-pits was measured by two methods: by SEM micrograph in the transversal plane and by a laser profilometre. These two methods give a 0.3 µm - 0.5 µm depth for these micro-pits. Components with micro-pits areas have the same wear rate than components without any "smoky" areas.

Discussion

The in-vitro results (hip simulator) show that the clearance between the head and the cup is a very important parameter to control the amount of wear for metal-on-metal bearings. This importance of the clearance has been confirmed by the examination of old metal-on-metal retrievals (1st generation) [6], by theoretical calculation of lubricant film thickness [10], and by other in-vitro hip simulator experiments [11, 12]. The running-in period observed in the hip simulator is a typical tribological behaviour for mechanical bearings and has also be confirmed [11] by other laboratories.

The in-vitro results (for the bearings with the correct clearance) are consistent with the in-vivo results (under the supposition that a patient walks one million steps per year). The mean wear rate for the modern metal-on-metal components retrieved in the first year in-vivo (global wear rate: about 25 µm/year for the whole bearing [cup and head]) is higher than the wear rate for the modern metal-on-metal components revised after more than two years (global wear rate: about 5 µm/year). The same global behaviour is observed with the hip simulator experiments.

The linear wear rate for the metal-on-metal bearings is as least 15 times lower than the linear wear rate observed for the bearings metal-on-polyethylene or ceramic-on-polyethylene, and this low wear rate is a very plausible explanation for the excellent preliminary clinical results of metal-on-metal bearings observed in Europe [13], [14].

The 3 implants (on 4) with a wear rate above 20 µm/year had a mechanical instability (recurrent dislocations or cup tilting). These mechanical instabilities modify the geometry of the bearings, resulting in a moderate wear rate (between 20 and 80 µm/year). Even if this wear rate is about 10 - 15 times higher than the normal wear rate for metal-on-metal bearings, this wear rate is much smaller than the polyethylene wear rate observed in similar cases in metal-on-polyethylene bearings or ceramic-on-polyethylene bearings. A possible explanation for the "squeaking" head (the fourth retrieval with a wear rate higher than 20 µm/year) may be a deficiency of lubrication allowing some resonance or slip-stick mechanisms to take place between the head and the cup.

As shown on Figure 5, the wear rate of the two types of retrievals (Müller metal-on-metal prostheses of the 1st generation [ball diameter 37 / 42 mm and Co-Cr-Mo cast alloy] and modern metal-on-metal prostheses of the 2nd generation [ball diameter 28 / 32 mm and Co-Cr-Mo wrought alloy]) is consistent with wear rate of about 5 μm/year, even if the type of alloys (cast versus wrought) is different.

As shown on Figure 6, the abrasive wear is the typical wear mechanism for the metal-on-metal bearings. Due to the remarkable ductility of the Cobalt alloy, the abrasive scratches are closed by the normal relative movements between the two components of the bearing. This polishing procedure improves the surface finish over time, allowing a reduction of the wear rate. This mechanism was already observed for the 1st and for the 2nd generation of metal-on-metal bearings [15, 16].

As shown on Figure 7, the micro-pits are always situated in the load bearing area of the surface. The corrosion resistance of these retrievals was measured according the ASTM standard G5 (solution: 0.9% NaCl for pH 4.0 and 0.15 mol HCl for pH 1.0, temperature: 40°C). The result of these measurements (E_{Break} = 575 mV_{SCE} for a pH 4.0 and E_{Break} = 800 mV_{SCE} for a pH 1.0) allow us to exclude any types of pitting corrosion. Due to the typical morphology of these micro-pits, the wear mechanism forming these micro-pits can be characterised as adhesive wear. The adhesive wear is a typical wear phenomenon for the bearings made in the same metal for the two components [17]. This type of wear was already observed in retrieved metal-on-metal prostheses of the 1st generation [18] and in hip simulator experiment with modern metal-on-metal bearings made by another manufacturer [19]. Walker [18] presented this wear pattern as fatigue wear, which is another way of describing the same wear mechanism. This adhesive-fatigue wear cannot be seen as a catastrophic wear mechanism, as the wear rate for the components with this adhesive-fatigue wear is exactly the same as the one measured for the components having the more conventional abrasive wear pattern.

Conclusions

This study of more than 100 metal-on-metal retrievals shows that the wear rate for this type of bearing is significantly lower (at least 15 times lower) than the wear rate for metal-on-polyethylene or for ceramic-on-polyethylene bearings. As this wear rate shows no tendency to increase with the implantation time, the metal-on-metal bearing can be a possible solution to improve the life's expectation of hip joint prostheses.

References

[1] Ungethüm, M., "Tribologie der Gelenke und Endoprothesen", *Osteosynthese und Endoprothese*, edited by Perren S.M., Birkhäusen Verlag, 1984, p. 91 - 100.

[2] Schurz, J., "Biorheologie: Probleme und Ergebnisse in der Medizin", *Naturwissenschaften*, Vol. 70, 1983, p. 602 - 608.

[3] Campbell, P.A. et al., "Cytokine Production in Human Macrophages Containing Wear Debris", *Fifth World Biomaterials Congress*, Toronto, 1996, p. 547.

[4] Zichner L., and Lindenfeld T., "In-vivo-Verschleiss der Gleitpaarungen Keramik-Polyethylen gegen Metall-Polyethylen", *Orthopäde*, Vol. 26, 1997, p. 129 - 134.

[5] Harris W.H., " The Problem is Osteolysis", *Clinical Orthopaedics and Related Research*, Vol. 311, 1995, p. 46 - 53.

[6] Semlitsch M., Streicher R.M., and Weber H., "Verschleissverhalten von Pfannen und Kugel aus CoCrMo-Gusslegierung bei Langzeitig implantierten Ganzmetall-Hüftprothesen", *Orthopäde*, Vol. 18, 1989, p. 377 - 381.

[7] Saikko V., and Pfaff H.-G., "Wear of Alumina-on-Alumina Total Replacement Hip Joints Studied with a Hip Joint Simulator", *Performance of the Wear Couple BIOLOX forte in Hip Arthroplasty,* edited by W. Puhl, Enke, 1997, p. 117 - 122.

[8] Streicher R.M. et al., "Metal-on-Metal Articulation for Artificial Hip Joints: Laboratory Study and Clinical Results", Proc. Instn. Mech. Engrs., Vol. 210, part H, 1996, p. 223 - 232.

[9] Schmidt M., Weber H., and Schön R., "Cobalt Chromium Molybdenum Metal Combination for Modular Hip Prostheses", *Clinical Orthopaedics and Related Research*, Vol. 329S, 1996, p. S35 - S47.

[10] Jin Z.M., Dowson D., and Fisher J, "Analysis of Lubrication Mechanisms in Hard Bearing Surfaces for Artificial Hip Joint Replacements", Proceedings of the Institution of Mechanical Engineers, Proc. Instn. Mech. Engrs, Vol. 211, part H, 1997, p. 247 - 256.

[11] Chan F.W. et al., "Design Factors that Control Wear of Metal-Metal Total Hip Implants", *23rd Annual Meeting of the Society for Biometarials*, New Orleans, 1997, p 77.

[12] Farrar R., and Schmidt M.B., "The Effect of Diametral Clearance on Wear between Head and Cup for Metal on Metal Articulations", *43rd Orthopaedic Research Society* , San Francisco, 1997, p. 71.

[13] Weber B.G., "Experience with the METASUL™ Total Hip Bearing System", *Clinical Orthopaedics and Related Research*, Vol. 329S, 1996, p. S69 - S77.

[14] Wagner M., and Wagner H., "Preliminary Results of Uncemented Metal-on-Metal Stemmed and Resurfacing Hip Replacement Arthroplasty", *Clinical Orthopaedics and Related Research*, Vol. 329S, 1996, p. S78 - S88.

[15] McKellop H. et al., "Twenty-year Wear Analysis of Retrieved Metal-Metal Prostheses", *Fifth World Biomaterials Congress*, Toronto, 1996, p. 854.

[16] McKellop H. et al., "Clinical Wear Performance of Modern Metal-on-Metal Hip Arthroplasties", *43rd Orthopaedic Research Society* , San Francisco, 1997, p. 766.

[17] Ludema K.C., "Sliding and Adhesive Wear", *ASM Handbook*, Vol. 18, 1992, p. 236 - 241.

[18] Walker P.S., "Friction and Wear of Artificial Joints", *Human joints and their artificial replacements*, edited by C.C. Thomas, Springfield, 1977, p. 368 - 409.

[19] Park S.-H. and al., "Wear Morphology of Metal-Metal Implants: Hip Simulator Tests Compared to Clinical Retrievals", *Alternative Bearing Surfaces in Total Joint Replacement, ASTM, STP 1346*, J.J. Jacobs and T.L. Craig, Eds., American Society for Testing and Materials, 1998.

Ceramic–on–Ceramic Bearings

Marcus L. Scott[1] and Jack E. Lemons[2]

THE WEAR CHARACTERISTICS OF SIVASH®/SRN® CO-CR-MO THA ARTICULATING SURFACES

REFERENCE: Scott, M. L. and Lemons, J. E., "**The Wear Characteristics of Sivash®/SRN® Co-Cr-Mo THA Articulating Surfaces,**" *Alternative Bearing Surfaces in Total Joint Replacement, ASTM STP 1346*, J. J. Jacobs and T. L. Craig, Eds., American Society for Testing and Materials, 1998.

ABSTRACT: The objectives of this study were to characterize and quantify the wear for fourteen explanted Sivash/SRN total hip articulating components. A stereoscope and MicroVu optical measuring system were used to microscopically characterize the wear patterns on the bearing components, while a Checkmaster coordinate measuring machine (CMM) was used to estimate both the linear and volumetric wear of the components. Three distinct zones on the component surfaces were revealed: noncontact, transition, and wear (load-bearing). Maximum wear occurred most often on the superolateral aspect of the femoral head components. The combined linear and volumetric wear rates of the bearing couples averaged 17 μm/year and 5.2 mm^3/year, respectively. The combined linear wear rates decreased significantly ($p= 0.03$) with a longer time in situ. The service life of the implants was found to increase significantly with decreasing radial clearance ($p= 0.03$), but no significant correlation was found between radial clearance and either linear or volumetric wear rates.

KEYWORDS: total hip replacement, wear, metal-on-metal, tribology, osteolysis

---

One of the most important and significantly frequent long-term complications of all total hip arthroplasties (THA) is loosening of prosthetic components. The generation of particulate debris from cement and wear of prosthetic surfaces incites a biological response, characterized by the formation of a reactive soft tissue membrane between the prosthesis or cement and the host bone. The constituents of this membrane are believed to mediate the resorption of bone and other connective tissue, resulting in implant

---

[1] Graduate Assistant, Department of Biomedical Engineering, University of Alabama at Birmingham, 1075 13th St. South, Hoehn Room 370, Birmingham, AL 35294-4440.
[2] Professor, Department of Biomaterials, University of Alabama at Birmingham, 1919 7th Ave. South, SDB Box 29, Birmingham, AL 35294-0007.

loosening [*1,2*]. In particular, polyethylene wear has been found to elicit adverse tissue responses which contribute to periprosthetic bone resorption and subsequent osteolysis and late component loosening [*3-6*]. The need to reduce or eliminate polyethylene debris has led to renewed interest in metal-on-metal joints as an alternative to conventional total hips.

Previous experiences with metal-on-metal THA have yielded mixed results. The McKee-Farrar metal-on-metal hip prosthesis exhibited a high incidence of early failure [*7-9*]. The main cause of failure was found to be loosening of the stems at the bone/cement interface [*10,11*]. The bearing surfaces of retrieved McKee-Farrar implant often demonstrated irregular sizing, geometry, and poor finish, contributing to the generation of high frictional torques from equatorial contact of the bearing surfaces [*12,13*]. Suboptimal femoral neck and stem designs have also been proposed to have played a role in loosening of McKee-Farrar THA components [*14,15*]. Despite these shortcomings, numerous cases of McKee-Farrar replacements demonstrating outstanding long-term performance and remarkably low wear rates have been reported [*16-19*]. From these long-term studies, volumetric wear rates of metal-on-metal components have been estimated to be 10-25 times smaller than that of metal-on-polyethylene components. New evidence suggesting that an increased volume of polyethylene wear particles may contribute more to component loosening than increased frictional torque has sparked further interest in the reexamination of metal-on-metal bearing surfaces [*20*].

In addition to the McKee-Farrar THA, other metal-on-metal total hip endoprostheses were implanted in the United States. The Sivash/SRN design utilized a femoral head that was constrained within the acetabular cup to prevent dislocation. Like the McKee-Farrar endoprosthesis, the articulating surfaces were nominally made of a Co-28Cr-6Mo as-cast alloy (ASTM F75- Specification for Cast Co-Cr-Mo Alloy for Surgical Implant Applications) which was known to have resistance to wear. Originally developed in Moscow, the Sivash prosthesis never gained wide popularity outside the U.S.S.R., but was used by several surgeons in the southeastern part of the United States [*21*]. In light of the renewed interest in metal-on-metal THA articulations, numerous new designs of metal-on-metal prosthesis will be introduced in the coming years. The purpose of the present study was to characterize and quantify the wear for an available series of explanted Sivash/SRN THA articulating components in order to better understand the wear processes that occurred in an earlier generation metal-on-metal design.

Materials and Methods

Fourteen retrieved Sivash/SRN THA devices were evaluated in this study (Table 1). The retrieved implants had been implanted for periods ranging from 1.8 to 22 years, with an average in vivo duration 9.1 years. Nine were revised for aseptic loosening, one each for femoral nonunion, infection, and implant fracture, and two for unknown reasons. Three non-implanted prostheses served as controls. The original surface and any areas of wear or removal damage on articulating component were identified and mapped using stereomicroscopy. The components were then ultrasonically cleaned in both an acetone bath and an enzymatic detergent bath to remove any proteinacious deposits, and the articulating surfaces were reexamined using stereomicroscopy. The surfaces of the cups and heads were further examined with the MicroVu® optical measuring system (MicroVu Corp.). Either an indirect or coaxial light source was used to illuminate the viewing field, and the images were digitally captured and stored in a bitmap file.

TABLE 1--*Clinical information and wear data on retrieved implants.*

No.	Years *In Situ*	Reason For Removal	Clearance (μm)	Linear Cup Wear (μm)	Linear Head Wear (μm)	Volumetric Cup Wear (mm^3)	Volumetric Head Wear (mm^3)
1	1.8	femoral nonunion	74	61	11	14.07	0.55
2	2.0	N/A	69	63	3	4.05	0.01
3	4.5	loosening	91	123	70	102.31	20.36
4	5.2	loosening	103	67	18	37.65	3.70
5	5.8	loosening	115	51	20	21.27	2.75
6	7.0	infection	115	74	89	29.65	30.50
7	7.3	loosening	85	30	3	2.35	0.02
8	8.0	loosening	73	25	15	0.63	1.25
9	8.5	N/A	56	56	16	13.80	1.27
10	11.0	loosening	90	50	20	5.23	2.03
11	12.2	loosening	74	59	6	26.97	0.06
12	12.3	loosening	81	309	61	73.13	20.47
13	20.0	loosening	60	53	37	5.49	7.54
14	22.0	implant fracture	61	64	56	9.97	14.68

Each femoral head component was then secured in a Checkmaster® (Helmel Engineering Products, Inc.) coordinate measuring machine (CMM). The surface of each head was probed at 24 evenly spaced locations every 5° latitudinally from the apex (0°) to 110° for a total of 529 points per head. A sphere-fitting technique was used to quantitate wear on the articulating components using a C++ program called SPHRFIT which simultaneously translates the center of a sphere (x_0, y_0, z_0) and varies its radius (ρ) in order to minimize the sum of the squared errors between the measured surface dimensions and the sphere. Initially, points which had been microscopically identified as lying in areas of wear or areas of surgical removal damage were removed from the surface data array, and a sphere was fit to the remaining data points. The deviations of the remaining data points from the best-fit sphere were then inspected. If a deviation was negative and nonsymmetric about the polar axis, then it was assumed that the head had been worn or had been manufactured substantially out of round. Data points from such cases were removed from the array and another sphere was fit to the remaining points. Once an optimum fit had been attained to the non-worn regions of the head, the radial distance, r_i, from sphere center of each remaining surface data points was determined. The point demonstrating the smallest r_i value was then identified, and its value of r_i was taken as the critical sphere radius, ρ_c. Any of the original 529 surface points with a r_i value below ρ_c were considered the result of in vivo wear. The linear wear depth of worn regions was taken as the difference between ρ_c and r_i.

For each cup component, manufacturing drawings were used to align the origin of the CMM with the origin of the original non-worn spherical surface of each cup. Then, the surface of each cup was probed at 22 evenly spaced locations every 5° latitudinally from the apex (0°) to 105° for a total of 463 points per cup. The r_i of each point from sphere center was then determined, and the magnitude and location of wear were determined by comparing the r_i values of the retrieved cups with the r_i values of corresponding points on the non-implanted cups.

A previously described numerical program was used to calculate the volume of wear over the surface of each component [*17*]. The average wear rate for each component was calculated by dividing the final wear (maximum depth or total volume) by the duration of implantation. The average combined wear rate of each retrieved prosthesis was calculated by summing its cup and head wear rates. The original, as-manufactured clearance for each bearing couple was calculated as the difference between the radii of the final best fit spheres for the nonworn surface data on the femoral head and the acetabular cup components. A correlation analysis (Pearson's coefficient) was used to assess relationships between wear rates and either clearance or time in situ.

Results

There was minimal surface damage apparent to the naked eye. The load bearing regions of the articulating surfaces appeared polished and mirrorlike, while the noncontact zones appeared dull and to be covered with randomly oriented light scratches. Proteinacious deposits were often seen adhering to the unworn areas of the retrieved components.

Stereomicroscopic and MicroVu examination generally revealed three distinct zones on the articulating surfaces of the retrieved implants— noncontact, transition, and load bearing (wear). The noncontact zones exhibited the original surface as produced by the manufacturer. The surface of the noncontact zones on the heads contained residual polishing scratches and a network of raised and rounded-off metallic-carbides, some of which were greater than 30 μm in length (Fig. 1*a*). Noncontact zones with little or no surface carbides present were more subject to light abrasion when compared to regions with surface carbides (Fig. 1*b*). The noncontact zones along the unpolished surface of the acetabular cups showed pronounced machining marks as well as what appeared to be torn-out carbides (Fig. 2*a*). On all control cup bearing surfaces, regions of randomly-oriented, light scratches were located at the apex and also in a thin band running just below the rim of the cup (Fig. 2*b*).

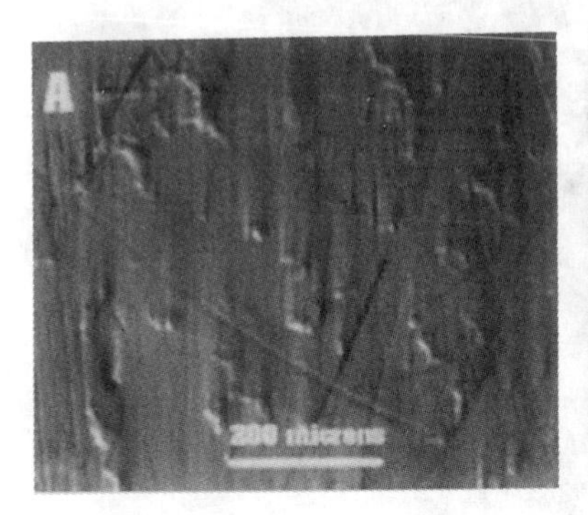

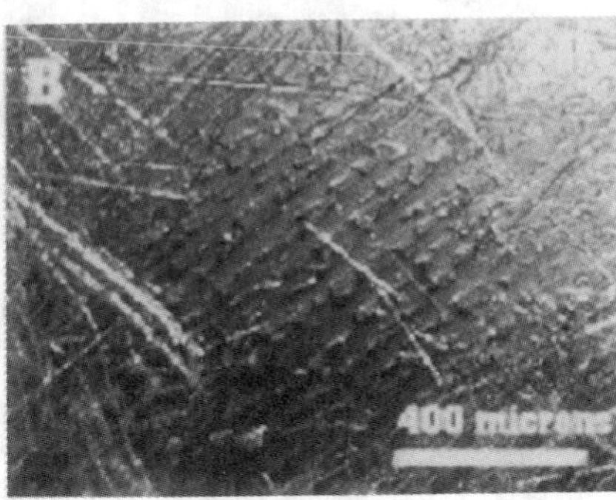

FIG. 1--*Microvu digital images showing nonworn (original) surfaces of Sivash femoral head components: (a) a non-implanted head with residual polishing scratches and raised, rounded carbides; (b) carbide network imparts scratch resistance to surface of a retrieved head.*

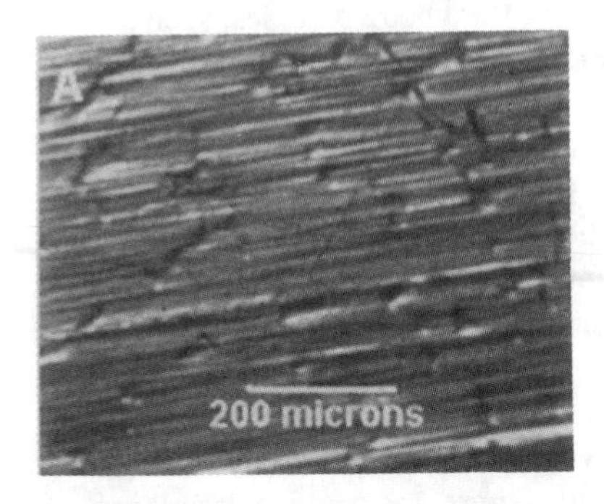

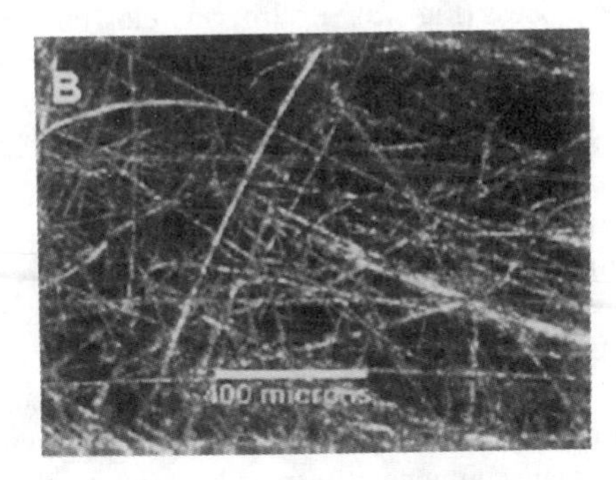

FIG. 2--*Microvu digital images showing nonworn (original) surfaces of Sivash cups: (a) a control cup with residual machining marks and carbide pullout; (b) typical dull, scratch-filled region located at apex and just below rim of the control cups.*

Typically, a dense pattern of third body scratches was located between the load bearing surfaces and the noncontact surfaces of both the cups and heads (Fig. 3*a*). The transition zone was sharply set off from the load bearing regions, and often times a criss-cross pattern of abrasion was present (Fig. 3*b*).

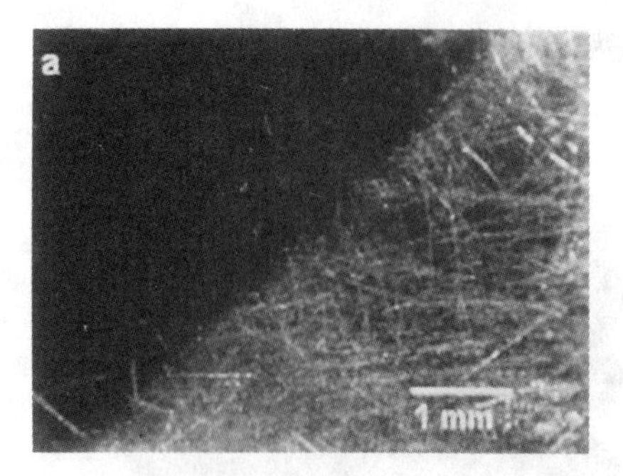

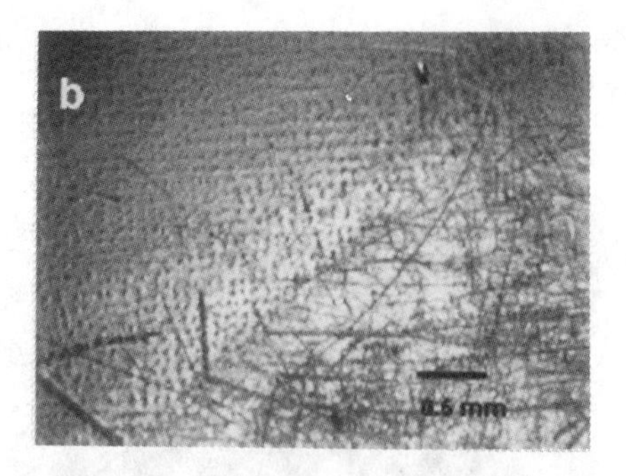

FIG. 3--*Microvu digital images showing transition zones typically seen along the Sivash bearing surfaces: (a) indirect light source shows a head with a smoothly polished wear zone that is sharply set off from the highly scratched transition zone; (b) coaxial light source shows criss-cross pattern of scratches bordering wear zone.*

The load bearing zones had a similar appearance on both the heads and cups. Generally, these wear zones were more polished than the surfaces of the nonimplanted prostheses. In many areas, scratches, both those from residual polishing and third body abrasion, had been worn away and replaced with fine surface scratches (Fig. 4*a*). In the wear zones, raised carbide features were found only bordering the transition zones where both lower contact stresses and linear wear would be expected (Fig. 4*b*). Often times what appeared to be casting microporosities and/or carbide pullout had been revealed by the wear process (Fig. 4*c*). Rolling and plowing effects of third body particles, such as bone cement components, bone, or dislodged carbides, were evident on portions of the load bearing surfaces (Fig. 4*d*).

Six of the retrieved femoral head components showed wear zones in which maximum wear occurred in the superior lateral region (Fig. 5). Two additional heads (prostheses 4 and 6) also showed a superolateral location of maximum wear, but in addition, a smaller inferomedial wear band was present (Fig. 6). Zones of maximum wear were located inferiorly and medially on the surface (Fig. 7) of two heads (prostheses 1 and 5), while prosthesis 10 showed an equatorial band of wear (Fig. 8). The wear zone locations of three of the heads (prostheses 2, 7, and 11) were not described due to the low number of worn surface points on each head. The in vivo orientations of the retrieved acetabular cup components were unknown, therefore no attempt was made at describing the in vivo locations of wear zones. However, maximum wear of the mating cups was found to occur near the cup rim for all but one of the heads showing superolateral maximum wear. For the heads showing superolateral wear and a band of inferomedial wear, the mating cups showed wear zones near both the pole and the rim. The mating cups of the inferiorly worn heads showed regions of maximum wear near the equator, while the equatorially worn head was mated with a cup worn at its pole.

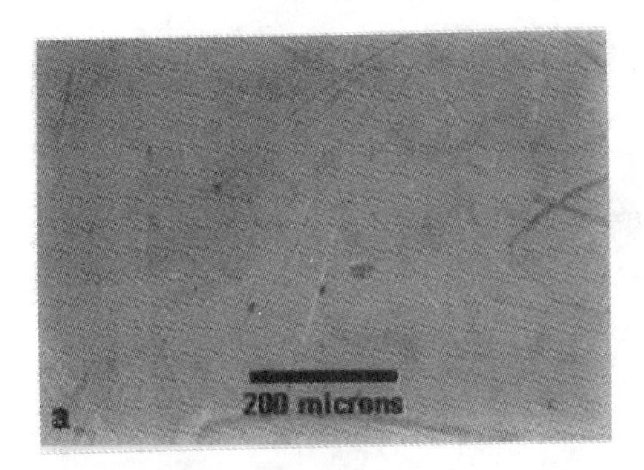

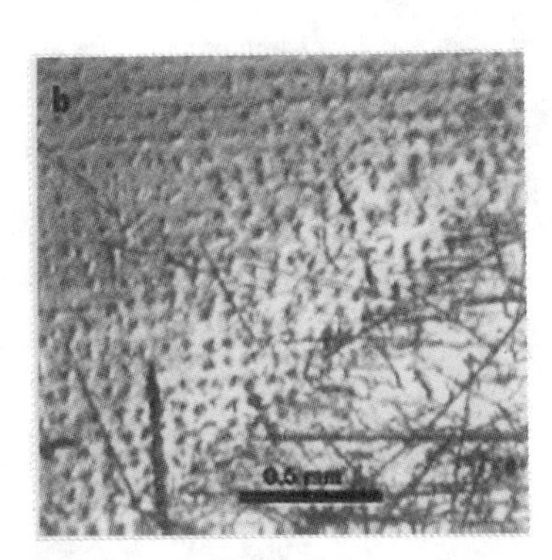

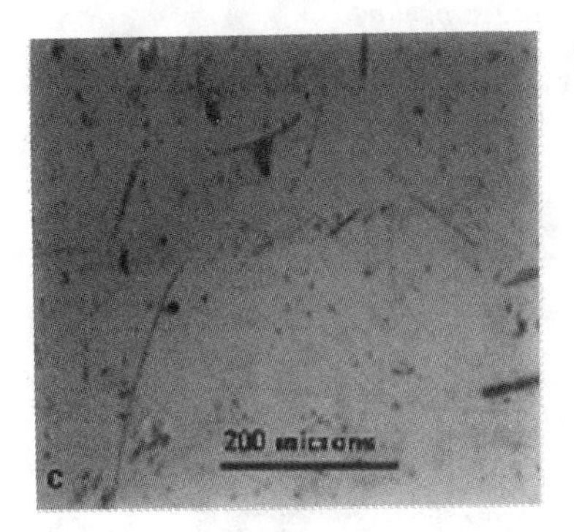

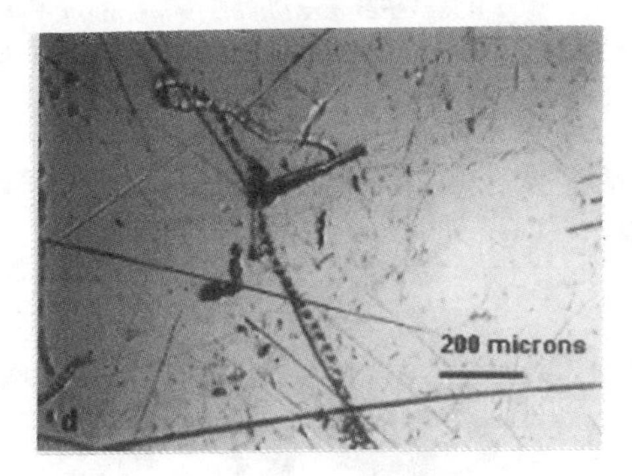

FIG. 4--*Microvu digital images showing load bearing (wear) zones typically seen along the Sivash bearing surfaces: (a) a retrieved cup with a smoothly polished wear zone; (b) raised carbide precipitates found bordering the transition zone; (c) casting microporosities on a retrieved head; (d) rolling and plowing tracks caused by third body abrasion.*

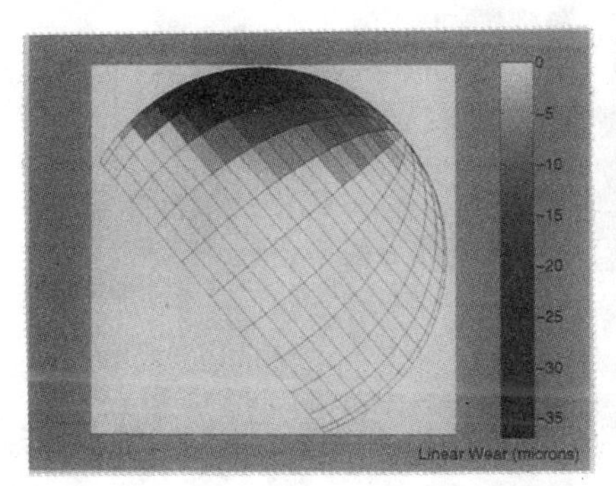

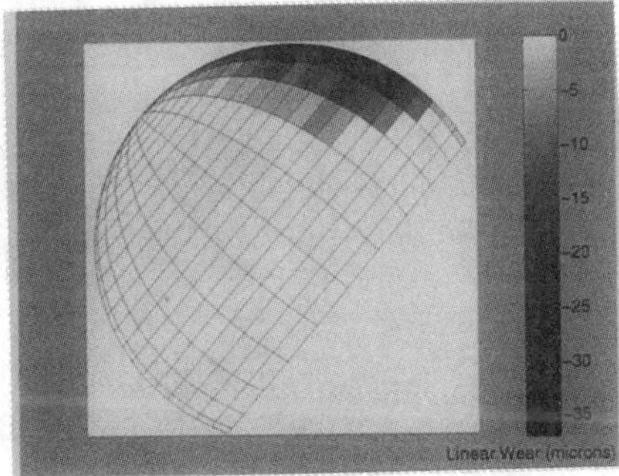

FIG. 5--*Femoral head component 13 showing wear centered superiorly and laterally.*

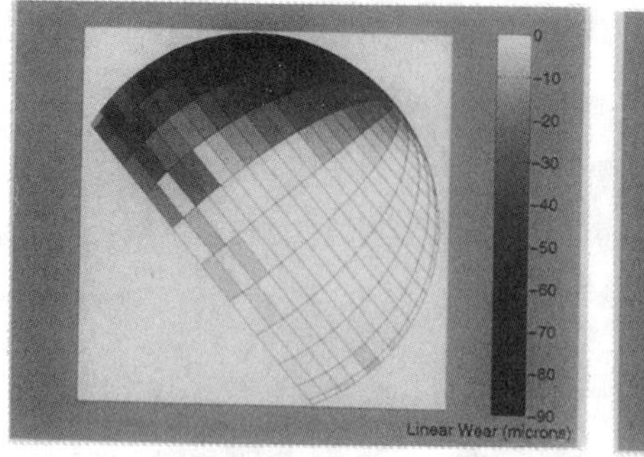

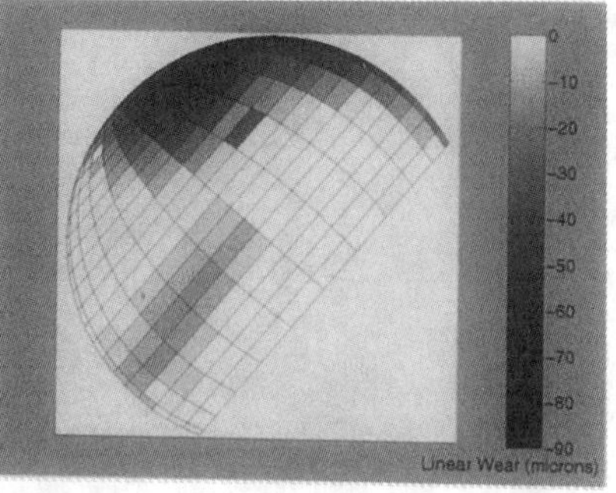

FIG. 6--*Femoral head component 6 showing superiorly centered wear and an inferomedial band of wear.*

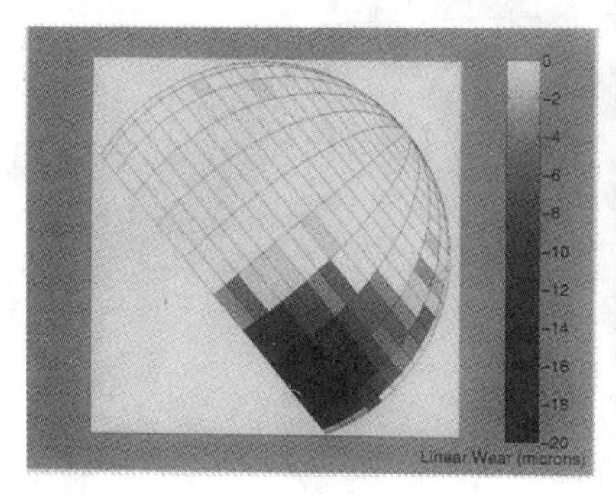

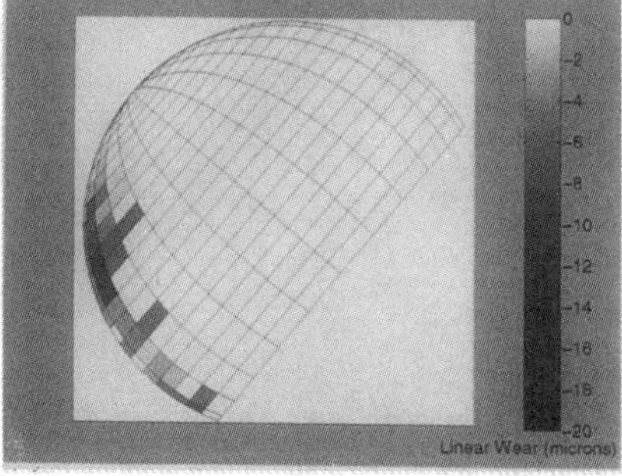

FIG. 7--*Femoral head component 5 showing wear centered inferiorly and medially.*

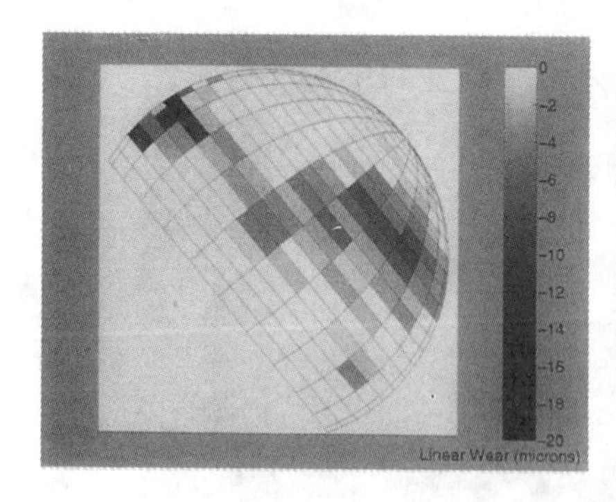

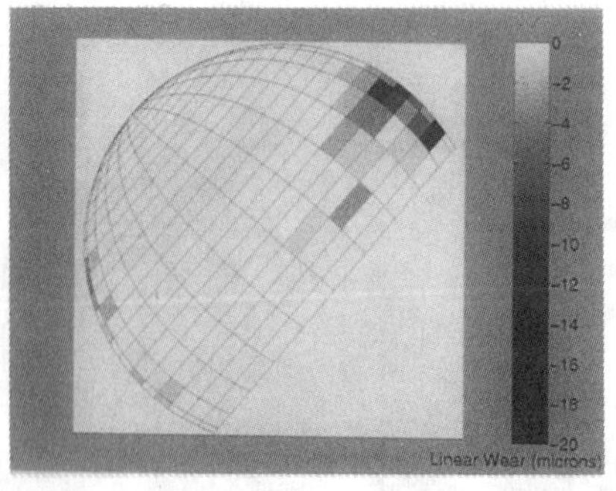

FIG. 8--*Femoral head 10 showing equatorial band of wear.*

The three nonimplanted femoral heads were found to have an average radius of 13.997±0.003 mm and an average sphericity (R_{MAX} minus R_{MIN}) of 0.037±0.020 mm. The three nonimplanted acetabular cups were found to have an average radius of 14.073±0.003 mm and an average sphericity of 0.077±0.003 mm. The large values of cup sphericity may be explained in part by a machined-in deviation (polar relief) found at the apex of each nonimplanted cup. Nevertheless, the average sum of control head and cup sphericity was found to be 0.114±0.023 mm.

The average linear wear rates were found to be 13 μm/yr and 4 μm/yr and the average volumetric wear rates were found to be 4.2 mm^3/yr and 1.0 mm^3/yr for the retrieved cups and heads, respectively. Both the cup ($R = -0.61$, $p = 0.02$) and combined ($R = -0.59$, $p = 0.03$) average linear wear rates were found to decrease with longer time in situ (Fig. 9). There was also slight trend of decreasing volumetric wear with longer time in situ for both the cups ($p = 0.14$) and combined wear ($p = 0.18$), but these trends had lower statistical reliability than the linear wear trends (Fig. 10). Excluding the implants which failed for non-mechanical reasons, i.e., infection or unknown reasons, the time in situ was found to increase with decreasing radial clearance between articulating components ($R = -0.65$, $p = 0.03$) (Fig. 11). However, no statistically significant correlation was found between radial clearance and either average linear and volumetric wear rates.

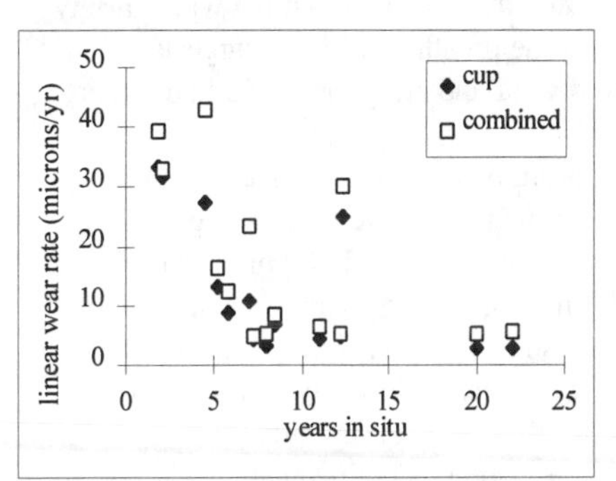

FIG. 9--*Linear wear rates vs. time in situ for both cup and combined wear.*

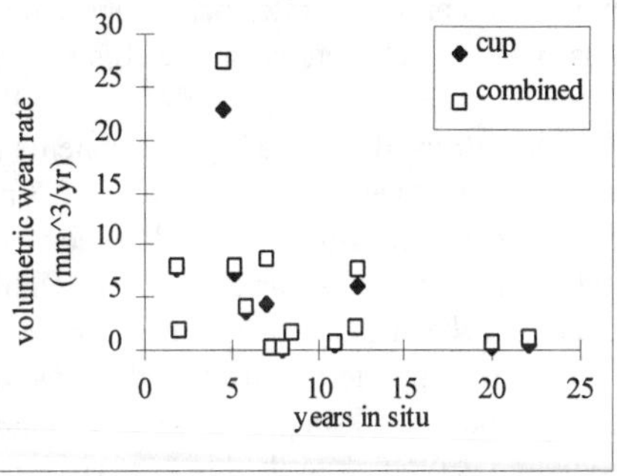

FIG. 10--*Volumetric wear rates vs. time in situ for both cup and combined wear.*

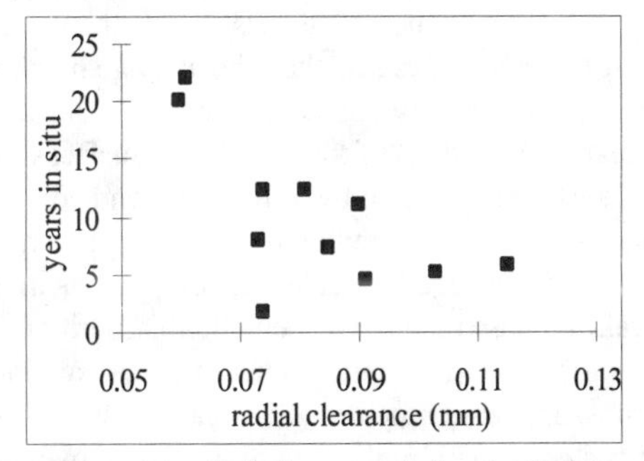

FIG. 11--*Time in situ vs. radial clearance of articulating components.*

Discussion

The appearances of the articulating components were in general agreement with the results of previous metal on metal hip implant studies [*17,18*]. The worn surfaces appeared smoother than the noncontact surface, and although surface profilometry was not performed, it was assumed that the surface roughness values of the worn-in surfaces were less than those of the original, as manufactured surfaces. Typically, polishing of bearing surfaces involves the production of very small abrasive particulates [*22*], thus submicron sized metallic wear particles, such as those found in retrieved periprosthetic tissue [*23,24*], may have been involved in the polishing of the contact surfaces. However, closer examination of the bearing surfaces and characterization of wear particulate produced from periprosthetic tissue are needed to draw any conclusions about the in vivo wear mechanisms of the devices in this study.

Walker and Gold stressed the importance of avoiding equatorial contact on the femoral head in order to reduce the frictional torque and wear generated during metal-on-metal articulation [*25*]. Specifically, Walker suggested that contact between the femoral head and acetabular cup be kept within 50° of the pole of the head. Interestingly, none of the retrieved Sivash femoral heads in this study achieved Walker's criterion of keeping contact (wear) zones within 50° of the pole of the femoral head. The areas of maximal wear depth were typically located between 60° and 80° from the pole, with a wide variety of times in situ and wear rates being reported among the prostheses. This suggests no clear association between the surface distribution of wear and either time in situ or wear rate.

The retrieved articulating components in this study showed combined average linear (5-43 μm/yr) and volumetric (0.3-27.3 mm^3/yr) wear rates well below those typically seen in metal-on-polyethylene components (100 μm/yr and 100 mm^3/yr). An initial break-in phase was observed in which high linear and volumetric wear rates were calculated for the articulation couples retrieved after short in vivo service (Figs. 9,10). Typically, the longer term retrievals demonstrated dramatically lower wear rates, thus indicating a post-break-in phase of steady state wear. In tribology, the break-in phenomenon is often described in terms of the ratio, λ, which is defined as:

$$\lambda = h/\sigma \qquad (1)$$

where h is the fluid film thickness and σ is the composite surface roughness of the two articulating surfaces [*26*]. When the value of λ is less than 1, the thickness of the fluid film between the sliding surfaces becomes less than the average height of the asperities on the sliding surface, resulting in asperity contact and possibly adhesive wear (in the absence of effective boundary lubrication) of the contacting surfaces. Higher values of λ result in higher degrees of surface separation by a fluid film and correspondingly lower levels of wear, and this has been demonstrated experimentally for a metal-on-metal THA articulating couple [*27*]. For the retrieved articulating components in this study , the high wear rates seen in the break-in phase may have been due to asperity contact due to an initially low λ ratio. The surfaces of the nonimplanted bearing components, especially those of the unpolished cups, appeared much rougher than the worn surfaces of the retrieved components, thus a correspondingly low initial λ ratio may have contributed to the initially high wear rates of the retrieved components. This initial wearing process led to changes in the microtopography, i.e., wearing down of surface asperities, of the contact zones that resulted in a subsequent increase in the λ ratio of the articulating system. Thus, break-in produced a "self-healing" of the contact zones on the articulating surfaces, resulting in the lower average wear rates for the long-term retrieved implants in this study. This same phenomenon has previously been reported for McKee-Farrar and Metusal retrieved metal-on-metal THA articulating couples [*19*].

The prosthesis service life was found to increase with decreasing radial clearance between articulating components (Fig. 11). Large clearances may lead to a reduced contact area, loss of squeeze film action, and rapid wear, thus resulting in early failure of the implant [*28*]. However, no correlation was found between radial clearance and either linear or volumetric wear rates, thus the reason for the extended life of the bearing couples with smaller radial clearances seems unclear.

While conclusions from a small sample size must be drawn with caution, this study indicates that the majority of lifetime articular wear (and debris) was generated early in the service life of a first generation metal-on-metal hip prosthesis. The incidence of high early wear was due to the breaking-in of the articulating components. However, while the running-in of mating surfaces such as the rough, relatively aspherical bearing components of three decades ago seems inevitable, designers and manufacturers must ask if this breaking-in phase is avoidable in a modern metal-on-metal THA bearing couple. Certainly, a manufacturing process that decreased the early burden of wear debris on surrounding tissue caused by the breaking-in period of metal-on-metal bearing components could increase the life expectancy of the implants. However, while a manufacturing process such as the running-in of mated bearing couples prior to implantation could produce favorable changes in the microtopography of the articulating system, e.g., decreased surface roughness, unfavorable changes in the macrogeometry of the bearing couple, e.g., increased clearance, could also result. Thus, design parameters and manufacturing techniques must be optimized in order to avoid the breaking-in phenomenon associated with metal-on-metal THA bearing couples.

Conclusions

(1) Due to the unfavorable original surface microtopography, i.e., high composite surface roughness, and macrogeometry, i.e., large deviations from sphericity, the Sivash/SRN metal-on-metal THA articulating surfaces experienced an initial breaking-in phase which resulted in initially high linear and volumetric wear rates of up to 43 μm/year and 27 mm^3/year, respectively.

(2) The breaking-in of the rough, relatively aspherical bearing surfaces produced contact zones with surface characteristics (lower composite surface roughness) that better promoted fluid film lubrication and decreased asperity contact, thus reducing long-term wear rates of the articulating surfaces. The bearing couples with the longest service life in the present study demonstrated linear and volumetric wear rates of approximately 5 μm/year and 1 mm^3/year, respectively.

(3) Time in situ was found to increase with decreasing radial clearance between articulating components. However, radial clearance was not related and either linear or volumetric wear rates.

(4) Polar contact, as defined by Walker [*25*], was not achieved by any of the retrieved femoral head components in this study. The areas of maximal wear depth were typically located between 60° and 80° from the pole, with a wide variety of times in situ and wear rates being reported among the prostheses. Thus, no clear association between the surface distribution of wear and either time in situ or wear rate was found.

Acknowledgments

The support of Crystal Medical, Inc. for equipment is gratefully acknowledged.

References

[1] Amstutz H. C., Campbell P., Kossovsky N., and Clarke I. C., "Mechanism and Clinical Significance of Wear Debris-Induced Osteolysis," *Clinical Orthopaedics and Related Research*, Vol. 276, 1992, pp. 7-18.

[2] Goldring S. R., Schiller A. L., and Roelke M., "The Synovial Like Membrane at the Bone-Cement Interface in Loose Total Hip Replacements and Its Proposed Role in Bone Lysis," *Journal of Bone and Joint Surgery*, Vol. 65A, 1983, pp. 575-574.

[3] Cates H. E., Faris P. M., Keating E. M., and Ritter M. A., "Polyethylene Wear in Cemented Metal-Backed Acetabular Cups," *Journal of Bone and Joint Surgery*, Vol. 75B, 1993, pp. 249-253.

[4] Ritter M. A., Keating E. M., Faris P. M., and Brugmo G., "Metal-Backed Acetabular Cups in Total Hip Arthroplasty," *Journal of Bone and Joint Surgery*, Vol. 72A, 1990, pp. 672-677.

[5] Schmalzried T. P., Jasty M., and Harris W. H., "Periprosthetic Bone Loss in Total Hip Arthroplasty: The Role of Polyethylene Wear Debris and The Concept of the Effective Joint Space," *Journal of Bone and Joint Surgery*, Vol. 74A, 1992, pp. 849-863.

[6] Schmalzried T. P., Kwong L. M., Jasty M. et al., "The Mechanism of Loosening of Cemented Acetabular Components in Total Hip Arthroplasty: Analysis of Specimens Retrieved at Autopsy," *Clinical Orthopaedics and Related Research*, Vol. 274, 1992, pp. 60-78.

[7] Bentley G. and Duthie R. B., "A Comparative Review of the McKee-Farrar and Charnley Total Hip Prostheses," *Clinical Orthopaedics and Related Research*,

Vol. 95, 1973, pp. 127-142.

[8] Dobbs H. S., "Survivorship of Total Hip Replacements," *Journal of Bone and Joint Surgery*, Vol. 62B, 1980, pp. 168-173.

[9] McKee G. K., "Total Hip Replacement- Past, Present and Future," *Biomaterials*, Vol. 3, 1982, pp. 130-135.

[10] August A. C., Aldam C. H., and Pynsent P. B., "The McKee-Farrar Hip Arthroplasty- A Long-Term Study," *Journal of Bone and Joint Surgery*, Vol. 68B, 1986, pp. 520-527.

[11] Jantsch S., Schwagerl W., Zenz P., Semlitsch M., and Fertschal W., "Long-Term Results After Implantation of McKee-Farrar Total Hip Prostheses," *Archives of Orthopaedic Trauma Surgery*, Vol. 110, 1991, pp. 230-237.

[12] Walker P., Ed., *Human Joints and Their Artificial Replacements*. Charles C. Thomas, Springield, IL, 1977.

[13] Wilson J. N., Scales J. T., "Loosening of Total Hip Replacements with Cement Fixation. Clinical Findings and Laboratory Studies," *Clinical Orthopaedics and Related Research*, Vol. 72, 1970, pp. 145-160.

[14] Walker P., "Metal-on-Metal Lubrication in Artificial Human Joints," *Wear*, Vol. 21, 1972, pp. 377-392.

[15] Crowninshield R. D., Brand R. A., Johnston R. C., and Milroy J. C., "The Effect of Femoral Stem Cross-Sectional Geometry on Cement Stresses in Total Hip Reconstruction," *Clinical Orthopaedics and Related Research*, Vol. 146, 1980, pp. 71-77.

[16] Kothari M., Bartel D. L., and Booker J. F., "Surface Geometry of Retrieved McKee-Farrar Total Hip Replacements," *Clinical Orthopaedics and Related Research*, Vol. 329S, 1996, pp. 141-147.

[17] McKellop H., Park S-H., Chiesa R., Doorn P., Lu B., Normand P., Grigoris P., and Amstutz H., "In Vivo Wear of 3 Types of Metal on Metal Hip Prostheses During 2 Decades of Use," *Clinical Orthopaedics and Related Research*, Vol. 329S, 1996, pp. 128-140.

[18] Semlitsch M., Streicher R. M., and Weber H., "Long-Term Results with Metal/Metal Pairing in Artificial Hip Joints," In *Technical Principles, Design and Safety of Joint Implants*, Buchhorn G. H. and Willert H. G., Eds., Hogrefe & Huber, Seattle, 1994, pp. 62-67.

[19] Schmidt M., Weber H., and Schon R., "Cobalt-Chromium Molybdenum Metal Combination for Modular Hip Prostheses," *Clinical Orthopaedics and Related Research*, Vol. 329S, 1996, pp. 35-47.

[20] Mai M. T., Schmalzried T. P., Dorey F. J., Campbell P. A., and Amstutz H. C., "The Contribution of Frictional Torque to Loosening at the Cement-Bone Interface in Tharies Hip Replacements," *Journal of Bone and Joint Surgery*, Vol. 78A, 1996, pp. 505-511.

[21] Amstutz H. C. and Grigoris P., "Metal on Metal Bearings in Total Hip Arthroplasty," *Clinical Orthopaedics and Related Research*, Vol. 329S, 1996, pp. 11-34.

[22] Rabinowicz E., *Friction and Wear of Materials*, Wiley, New York, 1995, pp. 209-211.

[23] Maloney W. J., Smith R. L., Schmalzried T. P. et al., "Isolation and Characterization of Wear Particles Generated in Patients Who Have Had Failure of a Hip Artrhoplasty Without Cement," *Journal of Bone and Joint Surgery*, Vol. 77A, 1995, pp. 1301-1310.

[24] Maloney W. J., Smith R. L., Huene D., and Rubash H., "Characterization of In Vivo Wear Particles Isolated from Membranes Around Failed Cementless Total Hip Replacements," *Transactions of the Society for Biomaterials*, Vol. 15, 1992, p. 28.

[25] Walker P. S. and Gold B. L., "The Tribology (Friction, Lubrication, and Wear) of All Metal Artificial Hip Joints," *Wear* , Vol. 17, 1971, pp. 285-299.

[26] Ludema K. C., *Friction, Wear, Lubrication. A Textbook in Tribology*, CRC Press, Boca Raton, FL, 1996, pp. 165-166.

[27] Chan F. W., Bobyn J. D., and Medley J. B., "Engineering Issues and Wear Performance of Metal-Metal Hip Implants," *Transactions of the Orthopaedic Research Society*, 1997, p. 763.

[28] Schey J. A. "Systems View of Optimizing Metal on Metal Bearings," *Clinical Orthopaedics and Related Research*, Vol. 329S, 1996, pp. 115-127.

Herbert G. Richter[1], Gerd Willmann[2], and Katrin Weick[3]

IMPROVING THE RELIABILITY OF THE CERAMIC-ON-CERAMIC WEAR COUPLE IN THR

REFERENCE: Richter, H. G., Willmann, G., and Weick, K., **"Improving the Reliability of the Ceramic-on-Ceramic Wear Couple in THR,"** *Alternative Bearing Surfaces in Total Joint Replacement, ASTM STP 1346*, J. J. Jacobs and T. L. Craig, Eds., American Society for Testing and Materials, 1998.

Abstract

The alumina-on-alumina wear couple which was introduced about 20 years ago has received new attention because of its superior wear behavior. Improved material properties and new design concepts provide solutions which overcome the restrictions of the older cup design. The new design makes use of the beneficial properties of both ceramic and metal materials in a modular cup assembly. In this paper the material aspects are briefly reviewed first: the mechanical strength of medical grade alumina has been improved by about 40 % between 1978 and 1996. Results of finite element analysis of the stresses found in the ceramic cup insert are presented: it was found that the metal back cone angle has to be larger than the insert cone angle in order to minimize tensile stresses in the cup insert. In addition, stresses in the cup insert are minimized if the radial gap between cup insert and ball head is around 40 μm. The finite element results are confirmed by experimental findings on the resistance to static load and on fracture patterns. Also reported are results of cyclic fatigue experiments at up to 10^7 cycles which result in a fatigue limit of at least 19 kN. Preliminary results on the stability of the cup assembly under directionally oscillating loads show that there is no detectable motion between the cup insert and the metal back after a few load cycles.

Keywords: total hip replacement, ceramic cup insert, ceramic liner, stress distribution, resistance to static load, cyclic fatigue, fracture pattern, mechanical stability

---

[1]Manager, Engineering Test Group, Research and Development Division, CeramTec AG, Plochingen, Germany
[2]Director R&D, Medical Products Division, CeramTec AG, Plochingen, Germany
[3] Student, University of Stuttgart, Stuttgart, Germany

Introduction

Avoiding wear debris is one of the most vital goals in the design of total hip replacement components. Among the different approaches to this goal the alumina-on-alumina wear couple already has received particular attention. It is known that the alumina-on-alumina wear couple produces minimal particulate debris. This material combination using a monobloc alumina cup has been in use for more than 20 years.

Aluminum oxide has been used for components for hip joint prostheses for more than 20 years. In this time period the material properties have been improved continuously by several means. These include improved raw material processing, powder preparation under clean room conditions and advanced sintering technology [1-2]. The results of these continuous and on-going improvements can be illustrated by a diagram showing the increase in strength of BIOLOX® achieved over the time period from 1978 to 1996 (Figure 1). It can be seen that the material strength has been improved by about 40 %. The strength data were obtained in 3-point-bending testing on tapered specimens.

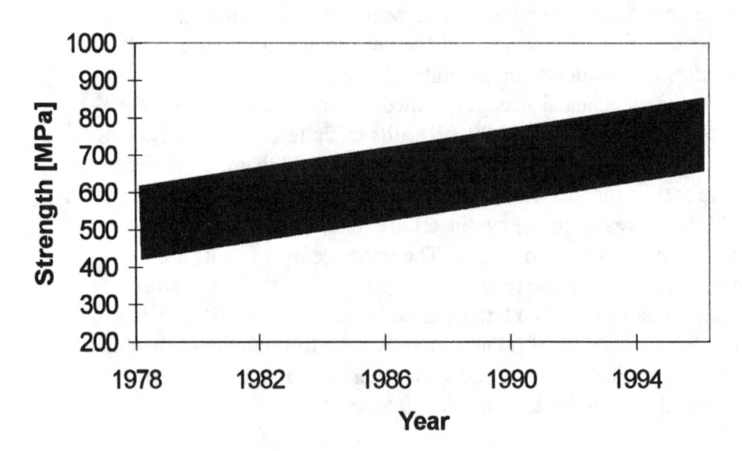

FIG. 1--Increase of the strength of alumina by continuous material improvement over the time period 1978-1994

The original design of alumina-on-alumina wear couples with a monobloc ceramic cup turned out not to make the best use of the properties of the ceramic material. Alumina has a low potential of osseointegration [3]. In an improved design the beneficial properties of both metals and ceramics were combined. The alumina liner or alumina insert provides optimum wear characteristics when used together with an alumina femoral head, whereas the metal back provides both the appropriate backing of the ceramic inserts and the flexibility in the implantation together with good osseointegration potential. These design aspects have been described elsewhere [4, 5] in detail.

BIOLOX®: Trademark of CeramTec (former Feldmühle), Plochingen, Germany

In this paper results on the load bearing capability and the performance of ceramic cup inserts of the new design are presented with particular regard to material and design issues.

Material

The investigations were performed on specimens and on components for total hip joint replacement, i.e. on ceramic cup inserts together with ceramic ball heads, made of BIOLOX alumina ceramics. This material meets all requirements of ISO 6474 2nd edition (Implants for surgery – Ceramic materials based on high purity alumina). In addition to these requirements the material is hot isostatically pressed. Typical properties of this material are a grain size of 2 µm , a density of >3.98 g/cm^3, a bending strength of >500 MPa, a Young's modulus of 380 GPa and a Poisson's ratio of 0.23.

The tests were run on components for total hip joint replacement of a nominal diameter of 28 mm; the outer diameter of the cup insert was 37 mm; the cone angle of the cup inserts corresponds to a rate of taper C = 1:3 according to ISO 1119 (Series of conical tapers and taper angles).

Wear couples of other ceramic materials are not covered in this study.

Experimental Methods

The Finite Element Analysis software Pro/MECHANICA STRUCTURE® was used for determining stress distributions in the ceramic cup insert. For the Finite Element Analysis a model was set up which comprises a ceramic insert, a metal back and a simulated bone (see Figure 2). Table 1 gives the elastic constants that were used in the Finite Element Analysis.

Table 1 - *Elastic constants used in the Finite Element Analysis*

Material	Young's Modulus, GPa	Poisson's ratio
Alumina ceramics	380	0,23
Metal back	115	0,35
Bone	0,5	0,33

Pro/MECHANICA STRUCTURE®: Trademark of Parametric Technology, Waltham, Mass

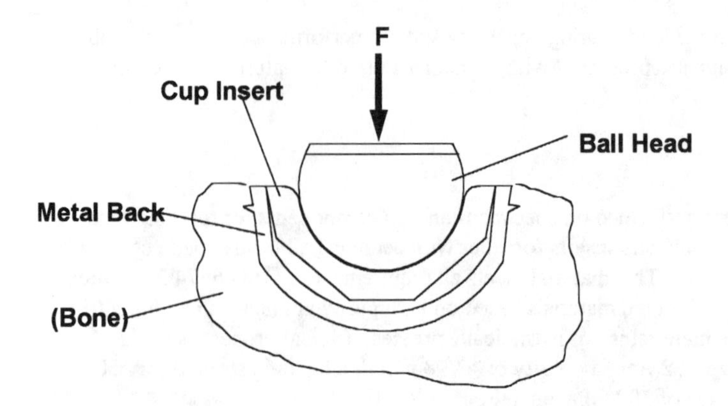

FIG. 2--Finite Element Analysis model comprising a ceramic cup insert in a model metal back

The resistance of the ceramic cup inserts to static load was measured following the principles given in ISO 7206 (Implants for surgery – Partial and total hip joint prostheses - Part 5: Determination of resistance to static load of head and neck region of stemmed femoral components). The experimental set-up is shown in Figure 3. The ceramic cup insert is fixed in a metal back which is embedded in a container using an epoxy as the embedding materials. The load is applied through a ceramic ball head. Guided by the results of the Finite Element Analysis, our standard test used ball heads whose diameters are in the center of the tolerance field. Additionally, to investigate the dependence on the diameter mismatch, ball heads with various diameters were also used in some tests. The resistance to static load was measured in an universal testing machine at a cross head speed of 2 mm/min. At least 10 specimens were used for each test series.

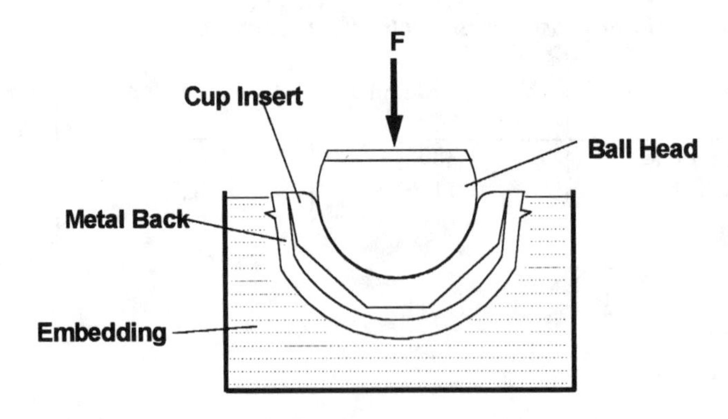

FIG. 3—Set-up for measuring the resistance of cup inserts to static load.

The same experimental set-up was used to determine the fatigue limit. The fatigue experiments were run with a lower load of 0,5 kN and upper loads of 31 kN, 28 kN, 25 kN, 22 kN and 19 kN. These experiments were performed with Ringer solution as the surrounding medium and with a load cycle frequency of 5 Hz.. Ceramic cup inserts which reach 10 million load cycles are regarded as "survivors".

Experiments have been initiated to study the stability of the press fit connection between ceramic cup insert and metal back. The main purpose is to investigate whether the conical press fit at an angle of ca. 18° can be regarded as safe and stable under loading conditions that vary in magnitude and in direction.

The experimental set-up is shown in Figure 4. The ceramic cup insert can be loaded at varying directions and with varying load levels. The relative movement of a ceramic cup insert and a metal back is measured by strain-gage based miniature displacement transducers having a resolution of around 0.5 µm. The relative movement is continuously recorded. Two displacement transducers are located 180 ° apart from each other in the plane of the oscillating loads at positions adjacent to the insert and the metal back (see Figure 3).

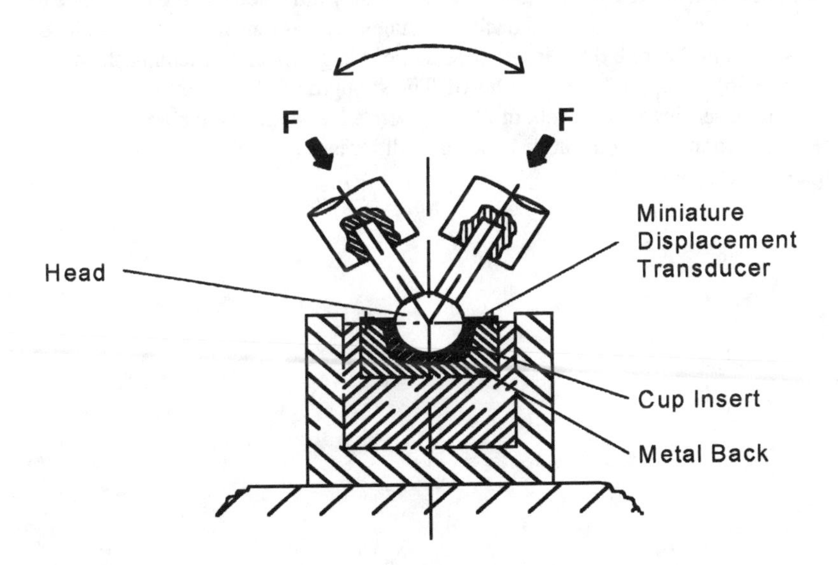

FIG. 4--Set-up for loading the ceramic cup insert/metal back system under loads which varies with regard to load level and direction

Results and Discussion

Finite element analysis

The stress distribution within the ceramic insert and consequently its predicted load bearing capability is strongly influenced by three parameters: the difference of insert cone angle and metal back cone angle, the difference of ball head and insert diameter and the surface structure of the conical surface of the metal back.

The general stress distribution in the ceramic insert which is loaded by a ceramic ball head is shown in Figure 5: A certain amount of stress concentration is found on the conical surface and at the outer bottom surface.

The calculated stress on the conical surface of the cup insert is almost independent of the diameter of the ball head, whereas the stress at the bottom surface increases with decreasing ball head diameter (see Figure 7). Figure 7 illustrates the dependence of the stress at the bottom surface on the ball head diameter.

The stress distribution in the ceramic insert is also strongly influenced by the difference in the cup insert cone angle and the metal back cone angle. This is illustrated in Figure 8: In the case illustrated in Figure 8a) the insert cone angle is larger than the metal back cone angle, in Figure 8b) the opposite case is shown. The strength of the system of metal back and ceramic cup insert increases by about 25 % dependence when positive cone angle differences are used instead of negative cone angle differences. Details of the dependence are still under investigation.

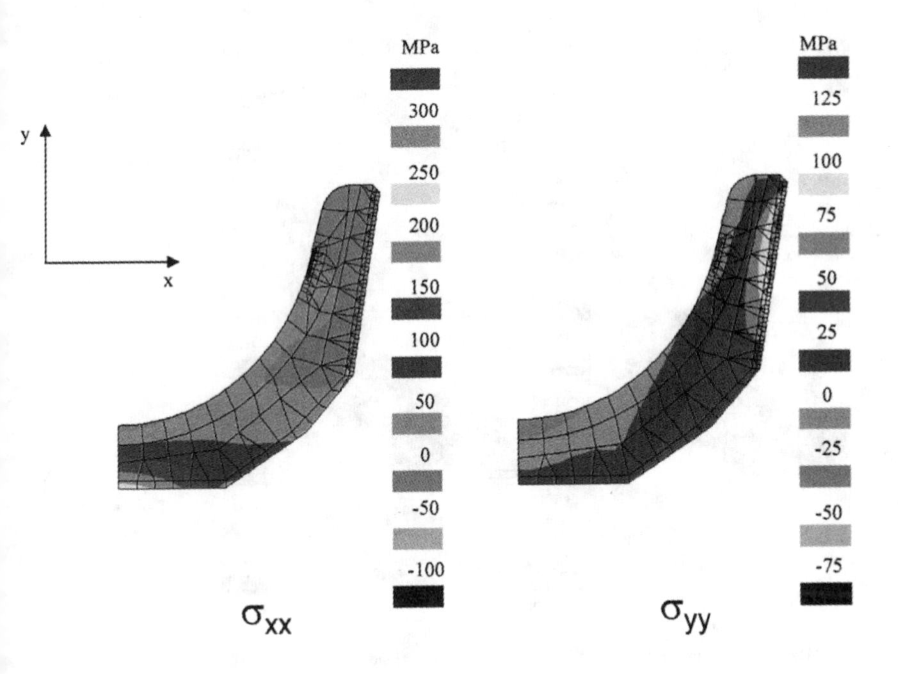

FIG. 5--General stress distribution in a ceramic cup insert fixed in a metal back which is embedded in bone

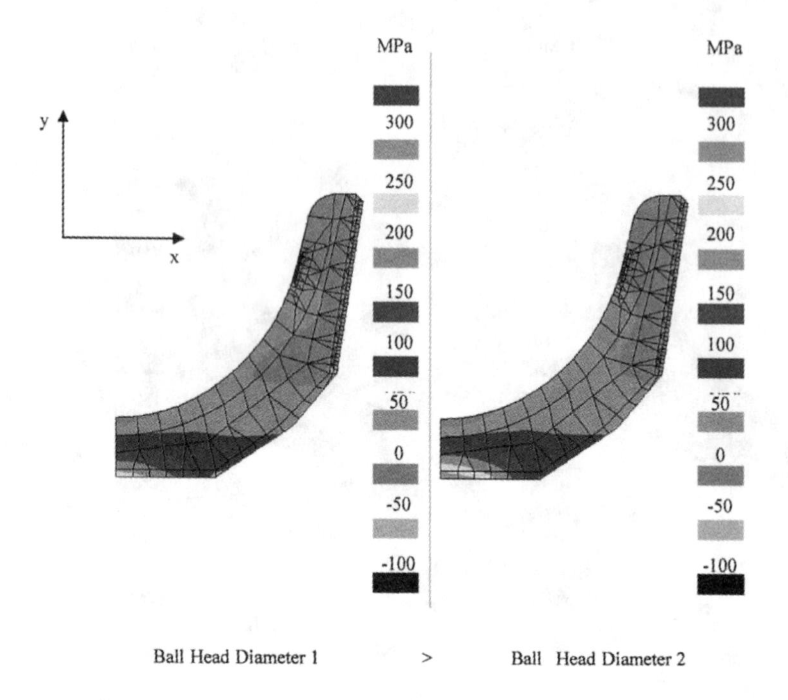

FIG. 6--Increasing stress concentration at the bottom surface of the ceramic insert with decreasing head diameter

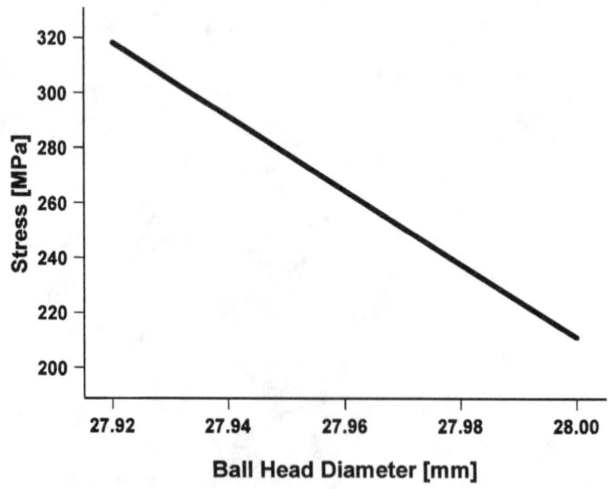

FIG. 7--Dependence of the stress at the bottom surface on the ball head diameter.

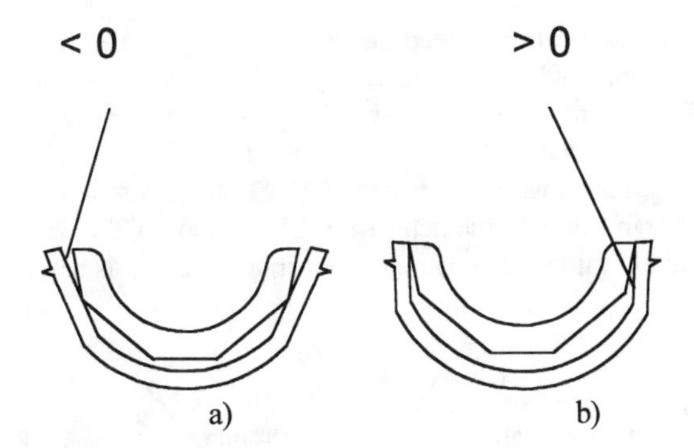

FIG. 8--Cone angle difference
a) Difference of "insert cone angle - metal back cone angle" is negative
b) Difference of "insert cone angle - metal back cone angle" is positive

Experimental results with axial load

Figure 9 shows the Weibull distribution of the strength of ceramic cup inserts evaluated according to ASTM Standard Practice for Reporting Uniaxial Strength Data and Estimating Weibull Distribution Parameters for Advanced Ceramics (C 1239). The breakage forces cover a range from 50 to 90 kN. They are similar to the strength of corresponding alumina ball heads.

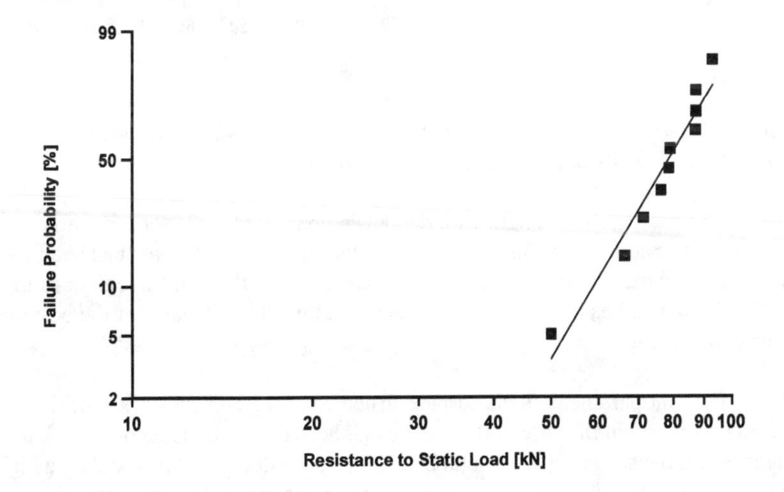

FIG. 9—Weibull distribution of the strength, i.e. resistance to static load of alumina cup inserts.

The results of strength variation with ball head diameter are in agreement with the Finite Element Analysis results mentioned above. The strength distributions measured with ball head diameters of 27.994 mm and 27.92 mm respectively are shown in Figure 9. The average strength is 78 kN when the cup is loaded by a head of a diameter 27.994 mm, and 35 kN when it is loaded by a head with a diameter of 27.92 mm. There is a 50 % decrease in strength with a decrease in ball head diameter from 27.994 mm to 27.92 mm. Here 27.994 mm is the most likely value in the diameter distribution; 27.92 is below the lower tolerance limit.

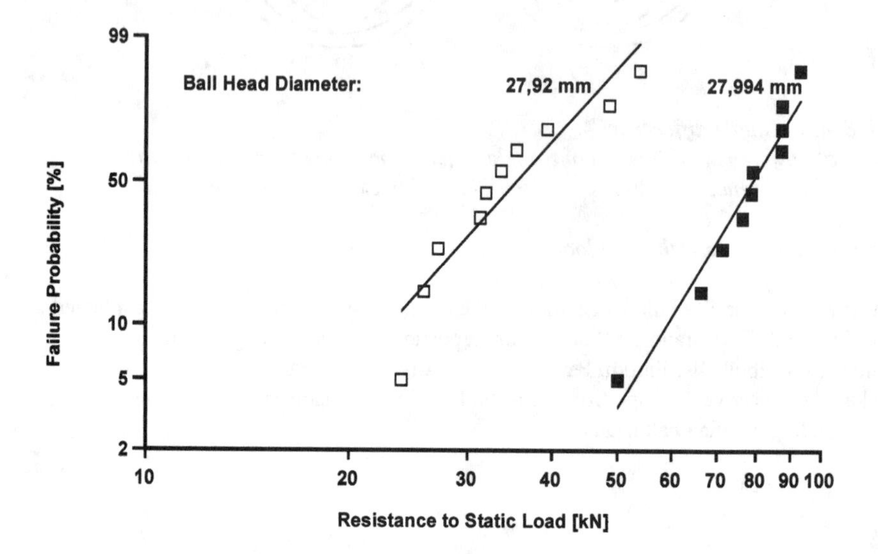

FIG. 10--Strength distributions measured on ceramic cup insert with heads with diameters of 27.994 mm and 27.92 mm respectively

Associated with the decrease in strength with decreasing ball head diameter is a marked change in the fracture pattern (see Figure 11). In the case of the 27.994 mm ball head the predominant fracture pattern is one of a circumferential crack in the conical region: In the case of the 27.92 mm ball head, the fracture origin is predominantly located at the bottom surface of the ceramic cup insert.

An additional important parameter is the surface structure of the conical surface of the metal back. As was found in the case with ceramic ball heads and metal spigots [6, 7], a certain roughness on the surface of the metal back cone is needed in order to obtain a high load bearing capability. This is because, without surface roughness, there is a low friction situation leading to a low load bearing capability.

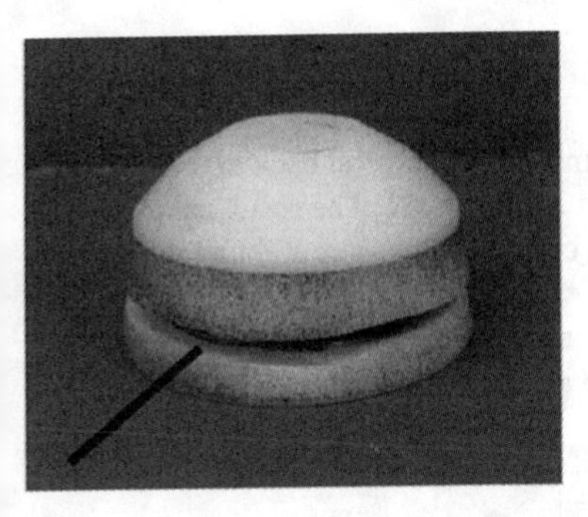

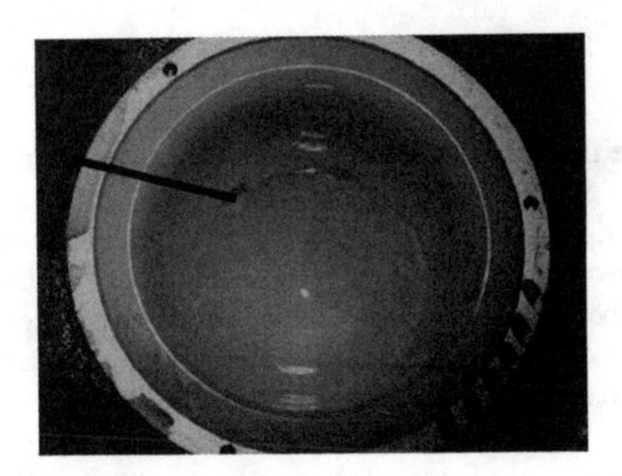

FIG. 11--Fracture patterns on ceramic cup insert
Test ball diameter: (a) 27.994 mm head, (b) 27.92 mm head

Axial cyclic load

In addition to experiments which were run with quasistatic, i.e. slowly increasing load, experiments with oscillating loads were run in order to determine the fatigue behavior of ceramic cup inserts. Figure 12 shows the SN diagram. As expected, the number of survivors increases with decreasing upper load. A threshold level seems to be reached at around 19 kN. This trend is in agreement with common fatigue behavior of ceramic

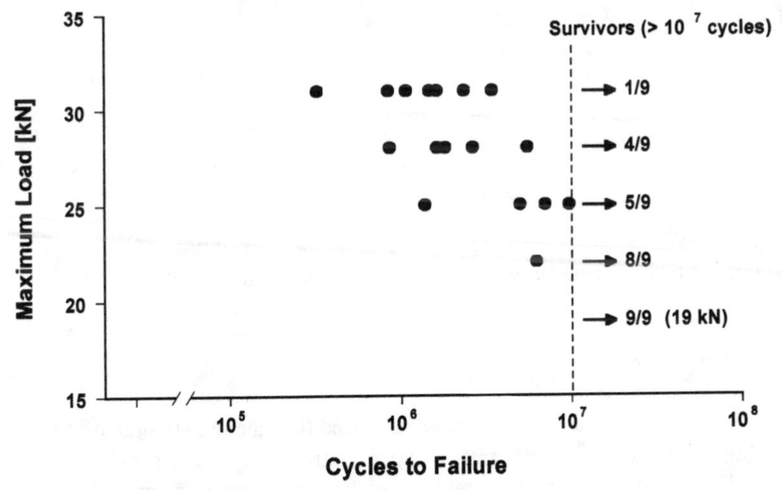

FIG. 12--SN diagram for BIOLOX forte cup inserts

materials. The fatigue limit lies at around 30 % of the short term strength, i.e. the resistance to static load. Most oxide materials used for technical applications have their fatigue limit at around 25 % of their short term strength.

Directionally oscillating loading

Before the start of the test the ceramic cup insert is assembled in the metal back at a fixed load of 500 N. So far the tests were run with a maximum load of 5 kN. The results show that a significant irreversible relative movement between ceramic cup insert and metal back only takes place over the first few loading cycles. Later on no significant relative movement could be found. Figure 13 shows a typical experimental finding. Additional experiments are currently under way which will take into account variations of the angle of oblique loading, load level and metal back design.

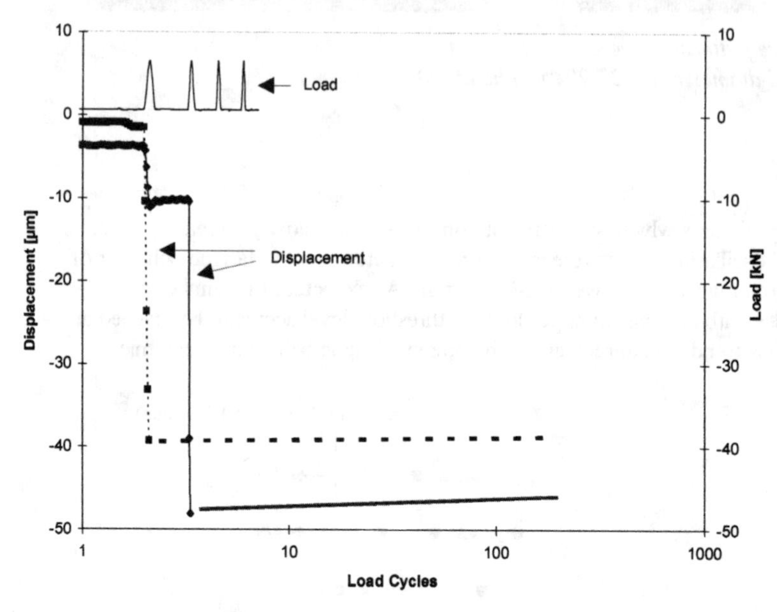

FIG. 13--Relative displacement between cup insert and metal back at two points 180° apart from each other in the plane of directionally oscillating loading.

Conclusion

Continuous material improvement processes have increased the inherent strength of the medical grade alumina BIOLOX® significantly. Proper control of parameters such as cone angle difference, diameter difference and metal back surface structure is critical for achieving optimum load bearing capability in the cup insert assembly with ceramic inserts. The ceramic insert/metal back system has a fatigue strength 19 kN for 100 % survival at 10 million cycles. A significant relative movement between the ceramic insert and the metal back occurs only in the very early stage of the directionally cyclic loading history.

References

[1] Richter, H.G.; Willmann, G., "Reliability of Ceramic Components for Total Hip Endoprostheses," *Die Keramikpaarung BIOLOX in der Hüftendoprothetik (The Wear Couple BIOLOX for Hip Prostheses),* W. Puhl, Ed., Enke Vlg., Stuttgart, 1997, pp77-83

[2] Willmann, G., "Ceramic Components for Total Hip Arthroplasty", *Orthopedic Int.* 5 (1997) 269-277

[3] Willmann, G., "Ceramic cups for total hip replacement, part 3: Osseointegration of monolithic ceramic sockets",. *Biomedizinische Technik* 42 (1997) 256.263

[4] Blömer, W., Design Aspects of Modular Inlay Fixation, *"Performance of the Wear Couple BIOLOX forte in hip arthroplasty.* Proceedings of the 2nd Symposium on Ceramic Wear Couple, W. Puhl, Ed. Enke, Stuttgart, 1997

[5] Dalla Pria, P., "Recent Innovations Relating to the Use of Ceramic-Ceramic Hip Joint Prostheses", W. Puhl, Ed. *"Die Keramikpaarung BIOLOX in der Hüftendoprothetik*, Enke, Stuttgart, 1996

[6] Richter, H.G., Willmann, G., Wimmer, M. and Osthues, F.G., "Influence of the Ball/Stem-Interface on the load bearing capability of modular total hip endoprostheses", *Modularity of Orthopedic Implants, ASTM STP 1301*, Jack E. Parr, Michael B. Mayor, and Donald E. Marlowe, Eds., American Society for Testing and Materials, Philadelphia, 1996

[7] Bachnik, M., Hasenpusch, M., et al, "The Effect of Hardness and Surface Quality of Metal Tapers on the Fracture Load of Ceramic Ball Heads in Hip Endoprostheses", *Biomedizinische Technik* Vol 39, No. 12, 1994, pp 302-306.

Bernard Cales and Jérôme Chevalier[1]

WEAR BEHAVIOR OF CERAMIC PAIRS COMPARED ON DIFFERENT TESTING CONFIGURATIONS

REFERENCE: Cales, B. and Chevalier, J., "**Wear Behavior of Ceramic Pairs Compared on Different Testing Configurations,**" *Alternative Bearing Surfaces in Total Joint Replacement, ASTM STP 1346*, J. J. Jacobs and T. L. Craig, Eds., American Society for Testing and Materials, 1998.

ABSTRACT: The wear properties of ceramic pairs including a biomedical grade zirconia ceramic (PROZYR®) were studied. In a simple disk-on-disk wear test in synthetic serum, the best wear behavior was observed with alumina-zirconia pairing. These tests also showed that the zirconia-zirconia combination can be considered for hip joint applications because it demonstrates wear behavior close to the classic alumina-alumina pairing. Hip simulator tests up to 10 million cycles for zirconia-alumina combinations confirm the previous experiments. It is clearly shown, if zirconia ceramic material and convenient wear test procedures are used, that the wear behavior of zirconia ceramic in ceramic-ceramic pairing is outstanding. The wear performance of zirconia was similar to, if not better than, that of alumina. Furthermore, tensile stresses in heads and cups, determined using finite element analysis, were found to be significantly higher in ceramic-on-ceramic bearings than in conventional ceramic-on-polyethylene couplings. This may influence the incidence of ceramic component fractures in ceramic-on ceramic bearings and may have implications concerning ceramic material selection for this application.

KEYWORDS: zirconia ceramic, ceramic-on-ceramic, wear test, hip joint simulator, finite element analysis, total hip prosthesis

---

Ultra High Molecular Weight Polyethylene (UHMWPE) has been widely used since the beginning of the 60's as a material to manufacture acetabular cups. However, the wear of polyethylene is today one of the major concerns in the total hip arthroplasty community. It is the production of small submicron polymer debris that is believed to be responsible for adverse tissue response and subsequent osteolysis and implant loosening[1-4]. Therefore, there is a growing interest in alternative "hard-on-hard" combinations such as metal-on-metal or ceramic-on-ceramic.

The concept of the Total Hip Prosthesis (THP) bringing into play hard materials for both the femoral head and the acetabular cup is not recent. It was introduced in the 60's

---

1 Manager and research engineer, respectively, Biomedical Activity, Norton Desmarquest, Z.I. n°1, rue de l'Industrie, 27025 Evreux Cedex, France.

with implants such as the Ring [5], McKee-Farrar [6] or Müller [7] metallic prostheses. Metal-metal hip implants have shown mixed clinical results. On the one hand, a number of the earlier McKee-Farrar implants were retained in the body even after more than 20 years with no evidence of surface degradation or tissue response [8]. On the other hand discouraging results were sometimes mentioned [9,10]. The issue of the metallic corrosion and ion release has also been often questioned in the literature [9,10]. Some recent papers deal with the so-called "second generation of metal-metal hip implants" exhibiting low in-vitro wear rates [11]. Recent papers also deal with cobalt (Co) and chromium (Cr) release in patients implanted with metal-metal THP [9,10].

Ceramics were introduced in orthopaedy by Boutin at the beginning of the 70's. Biomedical grade ceramics, alumina and zirconia, are highly wettable, hard and inert. They therefore lead to low frictional torques, low wear rates and they are extremely scratch resistant. So, they appear very appropriate for the production of hip joint components. Alumina-alumina hip prostheses have exhibited excellent clinical results, with very low wear rates, typically less than 5 mm per year as compared with the 100 mm classically obtained for the polyethylene cups associated with metallic heads [12-14]. However, alumina is brittle and some fracture cases were reported for the head in the literature. not only for the alumina-UHMWPE combination, but also for the alumina-alumina THPs [15,16] . Furthermore, the fracture rate seems to be significantly higher for the alumina-alumina combination than for alumina-polyethylene, probably because of increased stresses in the head for a "hard-on-hard" system [16]. For instance, Fritsch and Gleitz [16] made a review of different case reports of THP using different ceramic sources. They found 12 fractures for a total of 5170 alumina-UHMWPE THPs, leading to a fracture rate between 0 and 1.6% with a mean at 0.2%, while for 5530 alumina-alumina THPs they indicate 40 fractures with a fracture rate between 0 and 13.4% with a mean at 0.7%.

Biomedical grade zirconia ceramic was introduced in the mid-1980's as an alternative to alumina ceramic because it presented much higher mechanical performances, i.e., at least double strength and toughness [17,18]. Zirconia allows, for example, the production of small 22 mm heads, which are not reliable, mechanically, with alumina. There have been about 300,000 zirconia hip joint heads implanted throughout the world. They were all combined with UHMWPE acetabular cups. The use of a zirconia head bearing against a ceramic acetabular cup is therefore attractive in the sense that it should decrease the in-vivo fracture probability of ceramic-ceramic THPs. However, little is known about the wear performance of a zirconia bearing against another ceramic for a hip joint prosthesis application. Some papers showed disastrous wear properties of so-called "biomedical grade" zirconia ceramics, but little was known about physico-chemical parameters of the studied materials (processing, grain size, purity, density, etc.) [19]. Moreover, a recent publication has shown that the wear behavior of zirconia ceramic is highly dependent not only on microstructure parameters, but also on test conditions (load, speed and lubrication) [20]. A preliminary study with a pin-on-disk device has shown zirconia-zirconia or zirconia-alumina combinations could work as well as alumina-alumina [24]. Therefore, the aim of the present work was to study the wear properties of a biomedical grade zirconia ceramic: PROZYR® (Norton Desmarquest, Evreux, France) bearing against itself or a biomedical grade alumina and to compare with the well documented alumina-alumina systems. An attempt has also been made to determine the tensile stresses in hard-hard bearing systems using finite element analysis (FEA), in order to understand the reported higher fracture rate for ceramic-ceramic systems.

Experimental Method

Materials

Zirconia and alumina were tested as bearing materials. The zirconia ceramic was a 3Y-TZP, i.e., a tetragonal zirconia stabilized with 3% mol. yttria, commercially available under the name PROZYR®. The material was processed by cold isostatic pressing, pressureless sintering and further hot isostatic pressing (HIP) to obtain a density of 6.1 for a mean grain size of 0.4 ± 0.05 μm. The biomedical grade alumina ceramic was very pure and processed according to the same procedure to obtain a density of 3.98 for a mean grain size of 2 ± 0.5 μm. The other physical and chemical properties of the studied materials are in agreement with the standards (ISO 6474 and ISO 13356).

Experimental Tests

Disk-on-Disk -- The reciprocating disk-on-disk test is presented in Figure 1. It is similar to the standard VAMAS test used to examine tribological properties of water faucet ceramic parts. This test was considered by the authors as more severe and more representative than the conventional pin-on-disk tests because, in addition to tensile stresses, shear stresses are induced by the rotation of one disk on the other one. Four grooves are machined on disk 1 to provide a good lubrication of the two bearing surfaces. The flat surfaces of the disks are oscillating against each other at an angle of ±120°. at a frequency of 0.16 Hz and under a constant load F = 500 N. This gives a mean contact stress of 1.5 MPa and a total sliding distance of 25 km for a testing time of 30 days (1.5 million cycles).

The disks were machined and polished with diamond tools, with the same care as used for femoral heads. The roughness parameters were measured by means of an optical interferometer (MicroXAM, Phase Shift Technology, Tucson, AZ). Surface of typically 150 μm x 150 μm were scanned using a monochromatic light and the surface texture was obtained by optical interferometry. The following parameters were routinely controled : Ra, Rv (lowest valley), Rp (highest pic) and PV = Rp+ Rv.

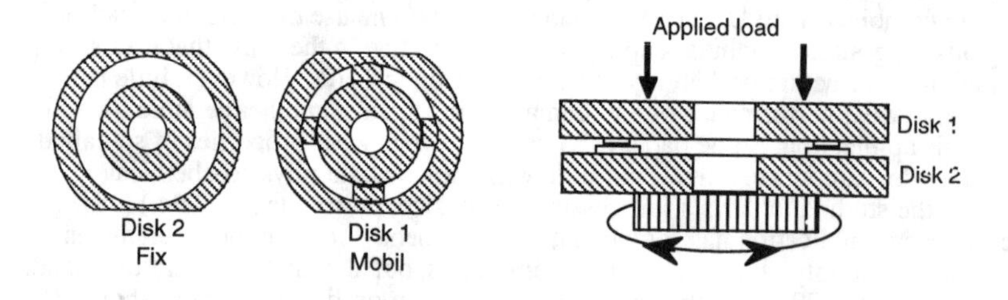

FIG. 1--*Schematic of the disk-on-disk wear test.*

The initial roughness of the disks ranged from Ra= 2 to 4 nm and from Ra= 2 to 5 nm for the zirconia or alumina disks, respectively. The flatness was controlled to be less than 1 mm for each disk. The choice of the lubricant is fundamental because it has a direct influence on the tribological properties of a given material combination. Water should be avoided because it does not give wear results representative of the in-vivo situation. Polineni has shown that a lubricant should present a protein content of about 25 to 35 g/L to approach the physiological fluid [25]. In this study, a synthetic serum (Plasmion®, Rhône Poulenc Roger Bellon) was used because it contains 30 g/L of proteins and is less sensitive to bacterial degradation than bovine serum. The temperature of the lubriquant was room temperature.

Quantitative measurements consisted of in-situ friction coefficient measurements and wear rate. The wear track profile was determined on disk 2 after the test using a profilometer along 4 radial directions, at 0°, 90°, 180° and 270°, with a sufficiently sensitive scale. The wear track cross-sectional area was then determined by an average of the 4 measurements. The wear volume was calculated from the equation:

$$V = \pi(r_0 + r_i) \quad (1)$$

where A is the mean wear track cross-sectional area and ro and ri the outer and inner radius of the wear track respectively.

Additionally, monoclinic content measurements were conducted for the zirconia disks before and after the test to investigate the wear-induced tetragonal to monoclinic transformation. Monoclinic content was determined from an X-Ray Diffraction analysis [21]. Scanning Electron Microscopy (SEM) was used to visualize the topography of the disks after the test.

Two tests were performed for each bearing combination in order to avoid statistical errors on a single specimen.

Hip Simulator -- Simple pin-on-disk or ring-on-disk tests cannot determine the potential use of a bearing combination without the support of more sophisticated hip simulator wear tests. Thus, a series of 8 head-cup pairs was tested on a 4-channel hip simulator (MTS, Eden Prairie, MN). Tests were conducted with commercially available Co-Cr and zirconia (PROZYR®) 28mm femoral heads and UHMWPE cups and on alumina or zirconia prototype acetabular cups. The same synthetic serum as for disk-on-disk tests was used as lubricant, at a temperature of about 37°C. Two zirconia head/alumina cup combinations were tested first up to 10 million cycles and two zirconia head/zirconia cup systems are currently under testing (2 million cycles). The cups were glued with a cup fixture and the head mounted on a taper. The simulator permits one rotation (flexion-extension) with a physiological angle of ±25°. The load is applied hydraulically in the vertical direction through the head and follows the J. Paul curve (maximum load : 2600 N, frequency : 1 Hz) [27].

The roughness, the diameter and the mass of the bearing components were measured before each test. The roughness was measured by means of the optical interferometer and the diameter with a micrometer. The mass was measured with a balance with a precision of ± 0.5 mg. The mass loss was recorded during the ongoing test only for the head because the cup was hardly removable from the cup fixture. This was not considered as an issue because wear was expected to occur mostly on the head, zirconia being less hard than alumina. However, it was decided to measure the weight of the cup at the end of the test. The other "on line" measurements were the roughness of both the head and the cup. Finally, the monoclinic fraction was also measured before and after the wear tests for all zirconia components. Visual inspection and scanning electron microscopy were conducted at the end of the tests to conclude the analysis.

Finite Element Analysis-- The stress map in total hip prostheses was made by finite element analysis (FEA) using Ansys 5.3 software (Ansys Inc. Houston, PA) in non-linear conditions. The metallic taper, the ceramic head, the ceramic or the polyethylene cup and the metal back were all simulated in the FEA with appropriate contact elements at the interfaces. According to previous studies, a friction coefficient of 0.15 was introduced at the ceramic/metal interfaces [24]. The stress distribution in the ceramic head and cup was analyzed, but the analysis was focused on the tensile stresses in the head to understand the reported head fractures in ceramic-ceramic bearing systems. Young's modulus and

Poisson's ratio were respectively 115 GPa and 0.31 for the taper and metal back, 220 GPa and 0.29 for the zirconia ceramic, 330 GPa and 0.29 for the alumina ceramic and 340 MPa and 0.42 for the polyethylene. A 2D axisymetric model was used with axial loading. The external surface of the metal back was blocked and the bottom of the taper was displacement constrained.

Results and Discussion

Results for the Disk-on-Disk Wear Test

Figure 2 represents the variation of the torque measured for alumina-alumina, zirconia-zirconia, alumina-zirconia and zirconia-alumina pairings up to 1.5 million cycles. For all combinations, a decrease of the torque is observed during the first thousand cycles, followed by a plateau value. This phenomenon is generally explained by the accommodation of the two surfaces at the beginning of the experiment and is commonly observed in ceramic disk-ceramic disk tests. It probably corresponds to an improvement of the flatness of the contact area. As a consequence the torque during the first 250,000 cycles cannot be properly analyzed.

The value of the torque in the stationary regime appears to be lower for the symmetric combinations (alumina-alumina or zirconia-zirconia) than for the "composite" combination zirconia against alumina.

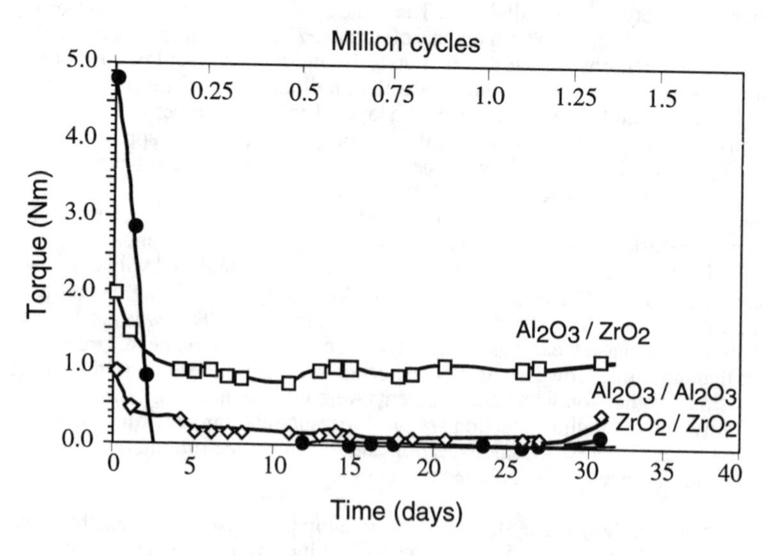

FIG. 2--*Variation of the torque for different ceramic-ceramic pairs.*

Table I summarizes the wear rates in mm3/km calculated from the wear track measurements. A wear factor is also reported. It is 1 for the lowest wear rate and equal to the ratio of the wear rate to the lowest wear rate for the other combinations. It appears the lowest wear factors are obtained with the composite zirconia against alumina combinations. The difference between alumina-zirconia and zirconia-alumina is due to the scatter observed for wear measurements. The difference between the composite and the monolithic combinations is large and this result indicates that zirconia against alumina pairing represents the best combination. The zirconia-zirconia pairing exhibits a wear factor of the same order compared with alumina against alumina.

Table 1 --Wear parameters of the disk-on-disk experiments.

Disc 1/ Disc 2	ZrO_2 / ZrO_2	Al_2O_3 / Al_2O_3	Al_2O_3 / ZrO_2	ZrO_2 / Al_2O_3
Friction coeff.	0.005	0.006	0.09	0.016
Wear (mm^3 / km)	2.7 10^{-3}	1.5 10^{-3}	1.6 10^{-4}	4 10^{-4}
Wear factor	17	10	1	2
Initial roughness (µm Ra)	2-4 nm	2-5 nm	2-5 nm	2-5 nm
Final roughness (µm Ra)	1-5 nm	3-6 nm	2-5 nm	2-5 nm

SEM observations show no evidence of surface degradation for any ceramic disks. This was confirmed by the optical interferometer measurements showing the roughness of the ceramic components did not appear to be changed by the wear tests; wear tracks consisted of a slight "polishing" of the surface.

This simple test indicates the best wear behavior was the alumina-zirconia pairing. This is in agreement with previous work conducted with the pin-on-disk method [24]. It also shows that the zirconia-zirconia combination can be considered for hip joint applications because it gives a wear behavior close to the classic alumina-alumina pairing. This result is in disagreement with some previous studies on the wear behavior of biomedical grade zirconia ceramics [19]. This can be explained by a number of factors such as the test configuration, the applied pressure, the lubricant and the zirconia material itself. The good result obtained in this work for the zirconia-zirconia pairing can be related to the lubrication by the proteins contained in the synthetic serum and also to the high resistance to low temperature transformation (aging) of the presently studied zirconia. It was shown in a number of papers that the wear properties of zirconia ceramics are directly related to the propensity of a given zirconia to transform from the tetragonal to the monoclinic phase, but the role of the T->M transformation on the wear properties of zirconia is not obvious [22, 28]. In this work, the monoclinic fraction does not increase significantly after 1.5 million cycles (1 month wear testing). In any event, this work confirms the obvious fact that wear testing can give fundamentally different conclusions, depending on a great number of parameters. Thus, for a hip prosthesis application, it should be necessary to test any bearing system on a hip simulator, under physiological conditions, before determining its potential use in-vivo.

Hip Simulator Results

A first series of hip simulator results is shown in Figure 3, which shows also the mass loss of the cup for a zirconia head-alumina cup combination, compared with Co-

Cr/UHMWPE and zirconia/UHMWPE systems. As previously reported, the zirconia/UHMWPE system exhibits a significantly lower polyethylene weight loss than the classical Co-Cr/UHMWPE [3,23]. The observed wear rate of the Co-Cr/UHMWPE system, which is about 5 mg per million cycles, is much more lower than the observed in vivo UHMWPE wear rate for the same system. Polyethylene wear rates between 50 and 100 mg per year (equivalent to per million cycles) have been reproted in the litterature [29-31]. Significantly lowest wear rates are generally observed for in-vitro tests. In the present case, the used lubricant, which is made of denatured collagen, charaterized by longer chemical chains than albumine and globuline present in the human fluid, could be at the origin of the low polyethylene wear rate observed for the Co-Cr/UHMWPE system.

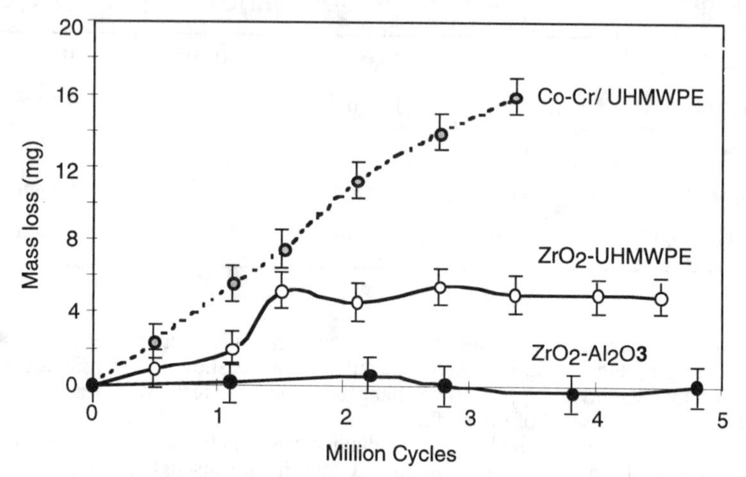

FIG. 3--*Mass loss of the cup for different bearing systems tested on the hip simulator.*

The polyethylene weight loss for the zirconia/UHMWPE system exhibits two rates, the first one up to about 1.5 million cycles corresponding to the plastic deformation/wear of the small grooves resulting from the machining of the polyethylene cup. After 1.5 million cycles, the polyethylene surface bearing against the zirconia head is very smooth and the polyethylene wear seems to be very low with the weight loss being negligible.

In the case of the zirconia head/alumina cup combination, no significant weight loss was measured and the weight of the zirconia head after 5 million cycles remains unchanged. This result is in fair agreement with the disk-on-disk wear test, showing, contrary to what was reported in the literature [19], zirconia-alumina systems could be used for hip joint prostheses, provided the ceramics exhibit the appropriate characteristics.

Hip simulator tests of up to 10 million cycles are reported in Table 2 for two zirconia-alumina combinations. They both confirm the previous experiments, with no significant weight loss of the zirconia head after 10 million cycles. Weight loss measurements on the alumina cup were hindered by remaining glue and metal transfer from the fixture on the external surface. The roundness and the diameter of both the head and the cup were found unchanged, the variation being under the detection limit. Also, there was no significant change in the surface roughness of the two ceramic parts. The roughness (Ra) of the head was slightly lower after the test because of a slight "polishing" of the surface. The roughness of the cup was slightly increased because of the presence of some scratches on the alumina surface.

In the two tests, after 10 million cycles, no monoclinic content was detectable on the zirconia head. This is in complete disagreement with previously reported results which attributed a poor wear behavior of zirconia ceramics to a rapid transformation of tetragonal phase into monoclinic phase [19]. In the present study, the zirconia ceramic is a commercial product which is characterized by a density equal to theoretical density, a very low grain size and a precisely controlled yttrium oxide content (5.15 ± 0.20 wt%), which are the main physical parameters to control phase stability of 3Y-TZP ceramics [26]. Therefore, this study shown that, if proper zirconia ceramic material is used, the wear behavior of zirconia ceramic in ceramic-ceramic pairing for THPs is outstanding, similar if not better than that of alumina.

Table 2 --Surface characteristics of heads and cups after 10 million cycles on hip simulator

	Weight Loss (g) [± 0.0005]	Initial Surface Roughness	Final Surface Roughness	Initial Monoclinic Content (%)	Final Monoclinic Content (%)
Zirconia Head 1	+ 0.0004	Ra=1.8 nm PV= 108 nm	Ra=1.1 nm PV=67nm	< 2% (no detect.)	< 2% (no detect.)
Alumina Cup 1	+ 0.0085 (glue & metal transfer)	Ra=5.5 nm PV=103 nm	Ra=7.2 nm PV=168 nm		
Zirconia Head 2	+ 0.0008	Ra=2.8 nm PV=116 nm	Ra=1.9 nm PV=221 nm	< 2% (no detect.)	< 2% (no detect.)
Alumina Cup 2	non measurable (glue & metal transfer)	Ra=4.9 nm PV=71 nm	Ra=5.0 nm PV=300 nm		

Stress Analysis in Ceramic-Ceramic Pairings

As indicated before, despite the advantage of an outstanding wear behavior, alumina-alumina bearing systems were reported to be characterized by a higher fracture ratio than the alumina-UHMWPE systems, because of higher stresses in hard-on-hard systems [16]. This behavior is of prime importance from a liability point of view.

Table 3 summarizes the maximum tensile stresses in the ceramic head at both the ceramic head/metal taper interface and at the top of the bore. The FEA reveals in both cases, the polyethylene and ceramic cup, that the stress at the ceramic head/metal taper interface is similar and equal to about 130 to 140 MPa for a 10 kN loading. In contrast, the stress at the top of the bore is significantly higher for ceramic-ceramic systems (100 MPa) compared with ceramic-polyethylene systems (60 MPa). This is directly due to the lower contact surface between the head and cup for ceramic-ceramic systems. This difference is very important (+67%) and, even if the stress remains lower than the material fracture strength (no immediate fracture), such a higher tensile stress could be at the origin of increased sub-critical crack growth with short term fracture. The observed higher fracture rate for ceramic-ceramic THPs could thus have an origin in the higher tensile stresses in the ceramic head.

To avoid or reduce such increased sub-critical crack growth and consequent fracture rate, it will be of prime importance to improve the crack resistance of the ceramic material.

Table 3 --Tensile stress in the ceramic head for both ceramic/UHMWPE and ceremic/ceramic combinations

	CERAMIC UHMWPE	CERAMIC CERAMIC
Tensile stress		
at the bore/cone interface	130 MPa	140 MPa
at the top of the bore	60 MPa	100 MPa

In such an analysis, zirconia ceramic appears much more suitable because of its higher fracture strength and toughness compared to alumina and, as previously reported by the authors, by the absence of any sub-critical crack growth in low loading/low stress conditions.

Conclusion

Wear tests in synthetic serum, both disk-on-disk and hip joint simulator, revealed that, contrary to previous reports, zirconia ceramic could be used for ceramic-on-ceramic pairs for THP applications. Zirconia heads on alumina cups appear to be an outstanding bearing system with extremely low wear rate. After 10 million cycles on the hip joint simulator the surface roughness of the head and the cup was unchanged and no phase transformation was detected at the surface of the zirconia head. In addition to the wear behavior, a zirconia head will also offer a higher strength compared to an alumina head, thus contributing to lowering the failure probability. Indeed, finite element analyses confirmed ceramic-on-ceramic bearings generate higher tensile stresses in the head than a conventional ceramic-on-polyethylene couplings.

References

[1] Schmalzried, T.P., Kwong, L.M., Jasty, M., Sedlacek, R.C., Haire, T.C., O'Connor, D.O., Bragdon, C.R., Kabo, J.M., Malcom, A.J. and Harris, W.H., "The mechanism of loosening of cemented acetabular components in total hip arthroplasty. Analysis of specimens retrieved at autopsy," *Clin. Orthop.*, Vol. 274, 1992, pp. 60-78.

[2] Schmalzried, T.P., Guttmann, D., Grecula, M. and Amstutz, H.C., "The relationship between the design, position, and articular wear of acetabular components inserted without cement and the development of pelvic osteolysis," *J. Bone Joint Surg.*, Vol. 76-A, May 1994, pp. 677-688.

[3] Manley, M.T. and Serekian, P., "Wear debris," *Clin. Orthop. and Related Res.*, Vol. 298, 1994, pp. 37-146.

[4] *Implant Wear : The Future of Total Joint Replacement*, T.M. Wright and S.B. Goodman, Ed., American Academy of Orthopaedic Surgeons, 1996.

[5] Ring, P.A., "Complete replacement arthroplasty of the hip by the Ring prosthesis," *J. Bone Joint Surg.,* Vol. 50-B, 1968, pp. 720-731.

[6] McKee, G.K. and Watson-Farrar, J., "Replacement of arthritic hips by the McKee-Farrar prosthesis,"*J. Bone Joint Surg*., Vol. 48-B, 1966, pp. 245-259.

[7] Müller, M.E., "Total hip prosthesis,"*Clin. Orthop.,* Vol. 72, 1970, pp. 46-68.

[8] Schmalzried, T.P., Peters, P.C., Maurer, B.T., Bragdon, C.R. and Harris, W.H., "Long duration metal on metal total hip replacement with low wear of the articulating surfaces,"*J. Arthroplasty*, Vol. 11, 1996, pp. 322-331.

[9] Jacobs, J.J., Skipor, A.K., Doorn, P.F., Campbell, P., Schmalzried, T.P., Black, J. and Amstutz, H.C., "Cobalt and chromium concentrations in patients with metal on metal total hip replacements," *Clin. Orthop. and Related Res*., Vol. 329S, 1996, pp. 256-263.

[10] Black, J., "Metal on metal bearings," *Clin. Orthop. and Related Res*., Vol. 329S, 1996, pp. 244-255.

[11] Chan, F.W., Bobyn, J.D., Medley, J.B., Krygier, J.J., Yue, S. and Tanzer, M., "Engineering issues and wear performance of metal on metal hip implants," *Clin. Orthop. and Related Res*., Vol. 333, 1996, pp. 96-107.

[12] Sedel, L., Nizard, R.S., Kerboul, L. and Witvoet, J., "Alumina-alumina hip replacement in patients younger than 50 years old," *Clin. Orthop. and Related Res*., Vol. 298, 1994, pp. 175-183.

[13] Boutin, P., Christel, P., Dorlot, J.-M., Meunier, A., de Roquancourt, A., Blanquaert, D., Herman, S., Sedel, L. and Witvoet, J., "The use of dense alumina-alumina ceramic combination in total hip replacement," *J. Biomed. Mat. Res*., Vol. 22, 1988, pp. 1203-1232.

[14] Riska, E.B., "Ceramic endoprosthesis in total hip arthroplasty," *Clin. Orthop. and Related Res*., Vol. 297, 1993, pp. 87-94.

[15] Michaud, R.J. and Rashad, S.Y., "Spontaneous fracture of the ceramic ball in a ceramic-polyethylene total hip arthroplasty," *J. Arthroplasty*, Vol. 10, 1995, pp. 863-867.

[16] Fritsch, E. W. and Gleitz, M., "Ceramic femoral head fractures in total hip arthroplasty," *Clin. Orthop. and Related Res*., Vol. 328, 1996, pp. 129-136.

[17] Christel, P., "Zirconia: The second generation of ceramics for total hip replacement," *Bull. Hospital Joint Diseases Orthop. Inst*., Vol. 49, 1989, pp. 170-177.

[18] Calès, B., "Y-TZP zirconia ceramics hip joint heads. Key issues for a high reliability," *Fourth EuroCeramics*, Vol.8, R. Ravaglioli, Ed., Gruppo Editoriale Faenza, Italy, 1995, pp. 45-52.

[19] Willmann, G., Früth, H.J. and Pfaff, H. G., "Wear characteristics of sliding pairs of zirconia (Y-TZP) for hip endoprostheses," *Biomaterials*, Vol. 17, 1996, pp. 2157-2162.

[20] Lee, S.W., Hsu, S.M. and Shen, M.C., "Ceramic wear maps; Zirconia," *J. Am. Ceram. Soc.*, Vol. 76, 1993, pp. 1937-1947.

[21] Garvie, R.G. and Nicholson, P.S., "Phase analysis in zirconia systems," *J. Am. Ceram. Soc.*, Vol. 55, 1972, p. 303.

[22] Birkby, I., Harrison, P. and Stevens, R., "The effect of surface transformation on the wear behaviour of zirconia TZP ceramics," *J. Europ. Ceram. Soc.*, Vol. 5, 1989, pp. 37-45.

[23] McKellop, H., Lu, B., Benya, P. and Park, S.H., *Proceedings of the Orthopaedic Research Society Meeting,* Washington, DC, Feb. 1992.

[24] Chevalier, J., Calès, B., Drouin, J. M. and Stefani, Y., "Ceramic-ceramic bearing systems compared on different testing configurations,"*Bioceramics*, Vol.8, L. Sedel and C. Rey, Ed., Elsevier Science, Cambridge, 1997, pp. 271-274.

[25] Polineli, V. K., Wang, A., Essner, A., Stark, C. and Dumbleton, J. H., "Effect of lubricant protein concentration on the wear of UHMWPE acetabular cups against cobalt- chrome and alumina femoral heads," *23rd Annual Meeting of the Society for Biomaterials,* New Orleans, LA, April 30-May 4, 1992.

[26] Lawson, S., "Environmental degradation of zirconia ceramics," *J. Europ. Ceram. Soc.*, Vol. 15, 1995, pp. 485-502.

[27] Paul, J., "Forces transmitted by joints in the human body," *Proc. Instn. Mech. Engrs.,* Vol. 181, 1966-67, pp. 8-15.

[28] Lee, S. W., Hsu, S. M. and Shen, M. C., "Ceramic wear maps: Zirconia," *J. Am. Ceram. Soc.,* Vol. 76, 1993, pp. 1937-1947.

[29] McKellop, H., Park, S-H., Chiesa, R., Lu, B. and Normand, P., "Twenty-year wear analysis of retrieved metal-metal hip prostheses,"*Fith World Biomaterials Congress,* Toronto, May 29 - June 2, 1996.

[30] Kabo, J. M., Gebhard, J. S., Loren, G. and Amstutz, H. C., "In vivo wear of polyethylene acetabular components," *J. Bone and Joint Surgery*, Vol. 75, 1993, pp. 254-258.

[31] Sychterz, C.J., Moon, K.H., Hashimoto, Y., Terefenko, K.M., Engh, C.A. and Bauer, T.W., "Wear of polyethylene cups in Total Hip Arthroplasty," *J. Bone and Joint Surgery*, Vol. 78-A, 1995, pp. 1311-1314.

Anthony J. Armini[1], Stephen N. Bunker[1], and Darryl M. Huntington[1]

ADHERENT ALUMINA COATINGS BY ION BEAM SYNTHESIS

REFERENCE: Armini, A. J., Bunker, S. N., and Huntington, D. M., "**Adherent Alumina Coatings by Ion Beam Synthesis,**" *Alternative Bearing Surfaces in Total Joint Replacement, ASTM STP 1346*, J. J. Jacobs and T. L. Craig, Eds., American Society for Testing and Materials, 1998.

ABSTRACT: The lower wear rate obtained with bulk alumina femoral hip balls compared to cobalt-chromium alloy balls on ultra-high molecular weight polyethylene is well documented in clinical studies. An alumina coating on a cobalt-chrome component would produce the superior surface properties of the ceramic combined with the desirable bulk properties of the metal. A new technique for forming a blended interface between the alumina coating and cobalt-chrome has been developed. The process uses a high energy ion beam of aluminum impinging on a cobalt-chrome substrate in an oxygen ambient gas to grow the alumina from beneath the metal's surface. Interface thicknesses up to 1200 Angstroms thick have been observed. To date, flat coupons and hip balls, have been coated with coatings 1 micron thick. The coatings were evaluated for polyethylene wear using a laboratory screening tribometer which has been designed to simulate non-linear tracking of the femoral ball on the UHMW polyethylene. The adhesion was measured using a diamond point scratch tester.

KEYWORDS: ion implantation, alumina, ceramic, coating, polyethylene wear, pin-on-disk, cobalt-chrome

---

Polyethylene wear debris is one of the primary causes of loosening resulting in the need for subsequent revision surgery in total joint replacement. Numerous clinical studies [*1-6*] have shown a 38% to 73% reduction in wear when articulating against monolithic/alumina femoral heads. One clinical study, Bragdon et al [*7*] showed no improvement however and one study by Livingston et al [*8*] showed increased wear of Hylamer UHMWPE which the authors did not investigate further. Fig. 1 shows clinical data for both polyethylene wear and total hip replacement (THR) revision rates using CoCr balls vs alumina balls.

---

[1]President, Chief Scientist, and Mechanical Engineer respectively, Implant Sciences Corporation, 107 Audubon Road, #5, Wakefield, MA 01880

Wear rates measured from clinical radiographs of Weber THR designs [*1*] show a 3.7 times reduction in polyethylene wear on average when alumina balls were used instead of CoCr (left side of Figure 1). Revision rates reported for Muller THR designs with CoCr balls were ten times higher than when ceramic balls were used [*8*]. (Right side of Figure 1). These ceramic advantages have not yet been realized on a widespread basis for total knee replacement components.

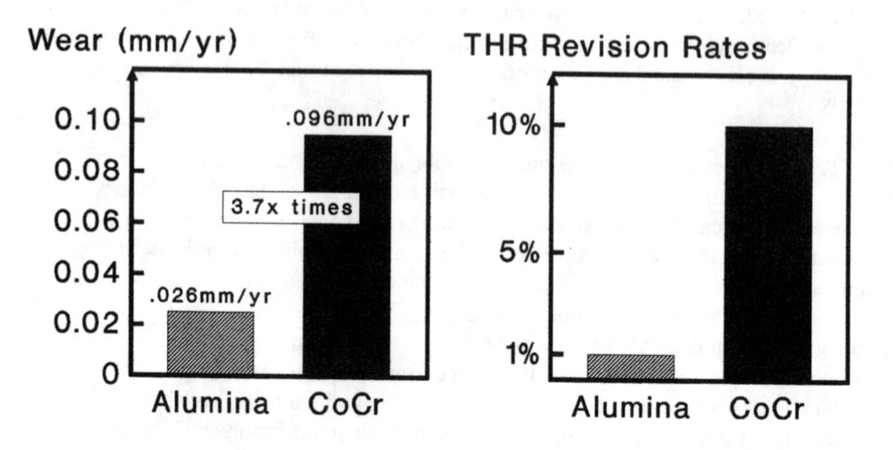

FIG. 1—*Clinical data for UHMWPE wear, CoCr vs monolithic alumina for Weber THR designs (left side) from Ref 1. Revision rates for CoCr vs alumina for Muller THR design (right side) from Ref 8.*

Materials and Methods

Alumina Coating Process

In order to specifically address the femoral knee application, an adherent alumina coating is being developed. However, aluminum oxide is not readily compatible with cobalt chrome alloy with respect to chemical affinity. Samples of CoCr alloy coated by the authors using magnetron sputtering, ion beam assisted deposition, and chemical vapor deposition (CVD) all debonded using a diamond scratch test method [*9*] at loads between 5 and 10 Newtons, while the goal was at least 30 Newtons. Failure occurred at the metal-ceramic interface.

Recently, we have ion implanted aluminum at high energy into CoCr while in an oxygen ambient in order to grow an alumina coating starting from beneath the alloy surface. Through a series of trials at various temperatures and ion beam current densities, it was found that alumina can be grown at a temperature as low as 500°C at an ion beam current density of $25\mu A/cm^2$.

The growth proceeds in three steps as shown in figure 2. In step 1 the aluminum ions are implanted below the surface of the CoCr by virtue of their 90keV kinetic energy.

Subsequently in step 2, oxygen diffuses into the metal and reacts with aluminum atoms diffusing outward toward the surface. In step 3, residual surface CoCr is sputtered away by the ion beam and the alumina coating thickens as additional aluminum and oxygen are reacted. The graded interface between the alumina coating and the CoCr substrate determined by Auger (AES) depth profiling was 660 Angstrom thick, as shown in figure 3.

The alumina coatings thus grown were found to have the same average surface roughness as the uncoated Cobalt-Chrome. Figure 4 shows sample surface roughness profiles for a bare cobalt-chrome control (left) and an alumina coated cobalt-chrome taken with a Sloan Dektak II profilometer located at Implant Sciences Corporation. The alumina coatings also had a straw color typical of oxidized chromium.

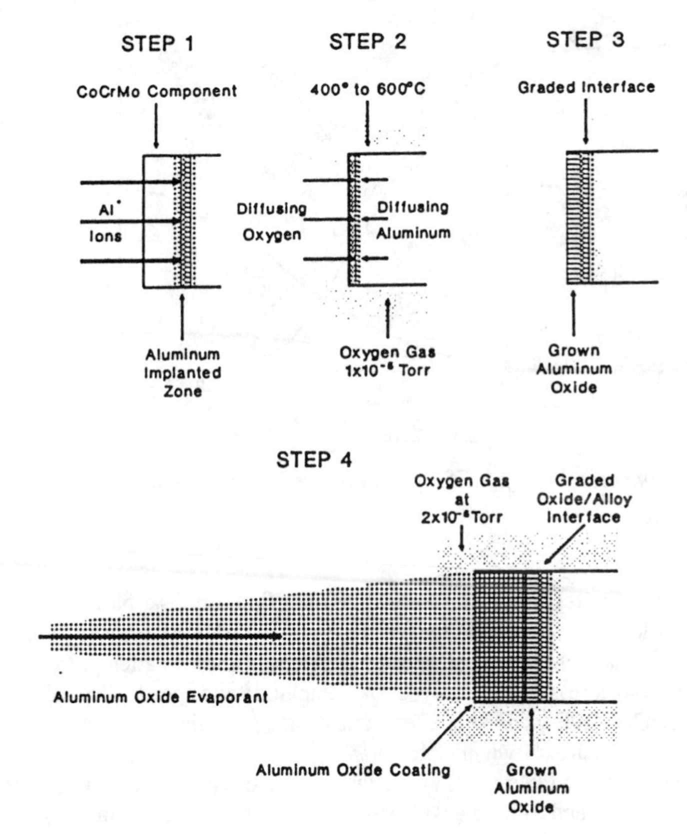

FIG. 2—*Ion beam synthesis of alumina coating on cobalt-chrome*

The smoothness of the coating and the low temperature deposition process used indicate that the alumina is probably amorphous, but x-ray diffraction measurements to determine the crystallinity have not yet been done. Constant load scratch tests using a standard Rockwell-C diamond indentor were performed to measure the adhesion of the alumina coating. Figure 5 shows magnified scratches for the ion beam synthesized alumina (left) and ion beam assisted deposition (IBAD) alumina (right). The left scratch made at 30 Newtons has no delamination at the edges of the scratch whereas the IBAD alumina shows severe delamination at only 10 Newtons.

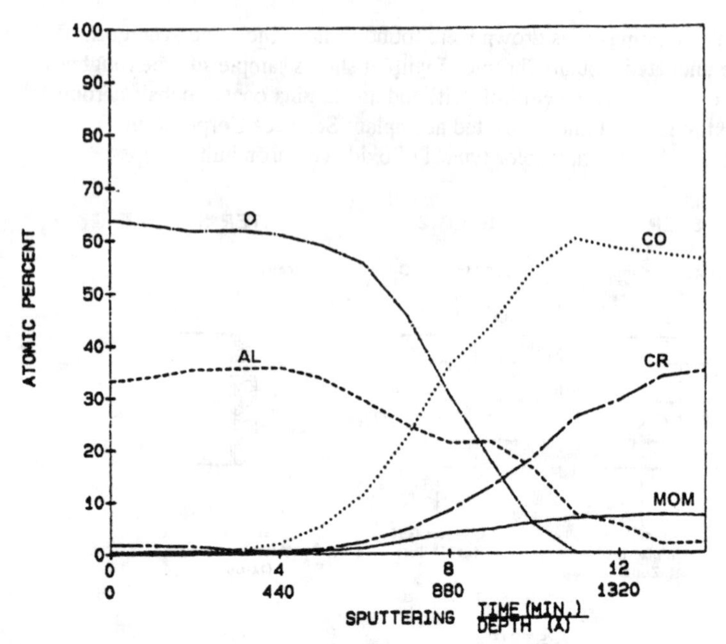

FIG. 3—*Auger election spectroscopy (AES) of alumina-cobalt-chrome interface*

Wear Testing

Laboratory screening tests based on the geometries of pin-on-disk, block-on-journal, and flat-on-disk have been used in the past to evaluate UHMWPE wear. While these devices do not simulate physiological loads or geometries, they do attempt to provide equivalent contact stresses, frequency, stroke amplitude and speed. Typical results from the CoCr/UHMWE wear couple for clinical data, joint simulators, and laboratory screening devices are shown in table 1.

As can be seen from the table a good joint simulator can replicate the low end of the clinical wear data which tend to have a wide variation. Laboratory screening tests typically show wear a factor of 10 or more lower than joint simulators. Recently Bragdon[*13*] and Wang[*14*] have proposed that laboratory screening devices have linear tracking which tends to actually strengthen the UHMWPE and reduces the observed wear. It appears that non-linear tracking, where the track of the metal on the UHMWPE traces out a complex path over an area of the polyethylene, is the key parameter which is responsible for the much higher wear values observed in joint simulators.

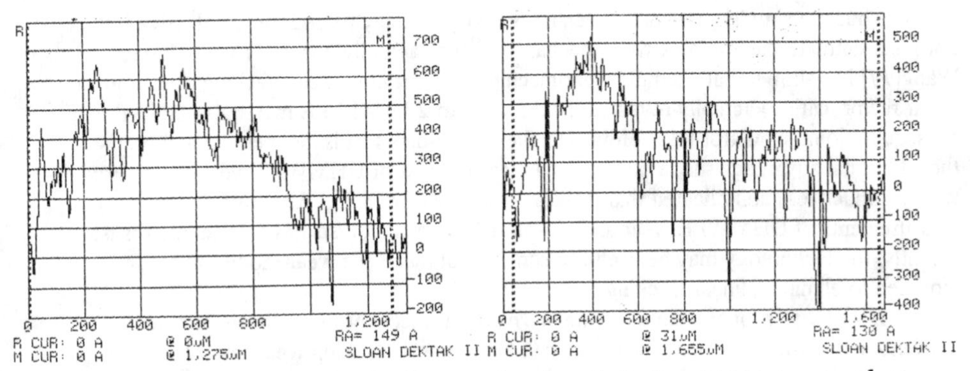

FIG. 4—*Profilometry traces of a Co-Cr control surface (left), Ra=0.015 micron and an alumina coated CoCr (right), Ra=0.013 micron.*

TABLE 1—*Typical average wear for the CoCr/UHMWPE couple*

	Wear Depth ($mm/10^6$ cycle)	Wear Volume ($mm^3/10^6$ cycle)	Methodology
Clinical	0.1 to 0.2/yr.	80-160	Radiographic[*10*]
Joint Simulators	0.10	80	Hip Simulator[*11*]
Screening Devices	~0.01	N/A	Pin-on-Disk[*12*]

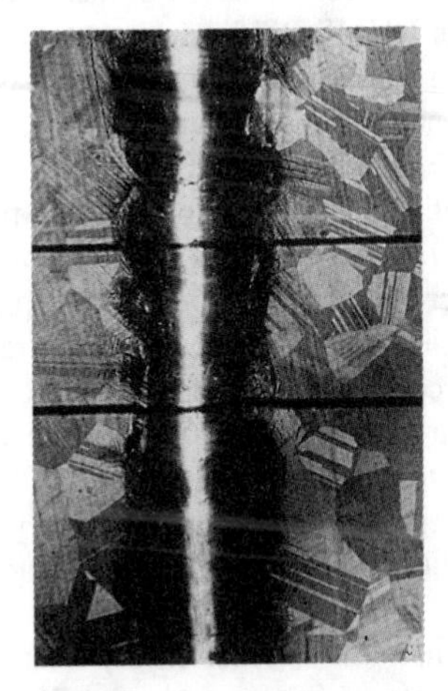
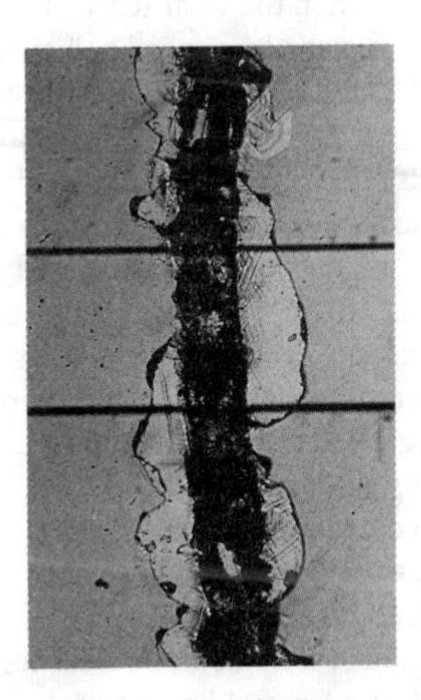

FIG. 5—*Thirty Newton scratch test on ion beam synthesized alumina (left) and a 10 Newton scratch test on IBAD alumina (right).*

Thus the simple, low cost screening test may actually be counter-productive if it does not simulate the complex wear mechanism which actually occurs *in-vivo*. In fact, Wang[*14*] has shown that a simple wear machine without non-linear tracking (line contact linear reciprocating) actually reversed the rankings of 2 UHMWPE materials obtained on a subsequent joint simulator test. However, the pin-on-disk test is inexpensive and offers the additional advantage that a dimensional measurement of UHMWPE wear can be used which is much less complicated than a weight loss measurement. Although dimensional measurements of UHMWPE wear and pin-on-disk screening tests have fallen into disuse recently, the technology may be useful to screen coatings if the wear mode can be modified to eliminate linear tracking.

In order to properly simulate the *in-vivo* wear mechanism, we have modified a conventional pin-on-disk machine to provide a non-linear tracking wear test. This was done by placing the disk and its motor assembly on a translation stage which then allows the radius of the wear track to change continuously during the test. The amount of the radius change was selected using a random number generator in a personal computer to randomly change the radius. The direction of the rotation was also changed at 6 second intervals. Figure 6 shows a photograph of the disk and the linear translation stage. Figure 7 shows a computer simulation of the first 15 rotations of disk. After a few hundred cycles the entire region between the minimum radius and the maximum radius is completely filled with cris-crossing tracks. The ball was also continuously rotated at 1 rpm to eliminate the single wear spot obtained in conventional pin-on-disk tests.

In order to evaluate this new wear tester concept it was necessary to verify two basic concerns:

1. That any creep of the UHMWPE is adequately accounted for
2. That the total wear volume is much higher than in the linear tracking pin-on-disk test.

Static dry and wet creep measurements were made at the same average contact stress (8.2MPa) as used in the wear tests. These measurements consisted of measuring the depth of a dimple made by a metal ball on a plate of UHMWPE for a preset time at a contact stress of 8.2MPa. These measurements yielded conflicting results until it was realized that the static creep amount was greatly influenced by the amount of time used presoaking (in Calf serum). The presoaked UHMWPE gave much less creep than dry disks. Figure 8 shows that the creep for a 1½ hour static contact sharply decreases from the dry conditions and then levels off at slightly above 1/3 of the dry value. We concluded from these tests that after 5 hours of presoak that the creep rate leveled off and therefore these 5 hour presoak creep depths could be used to estimate creep during the wear tests which lasted 230 hours per million cycles. In order to correct for the changes in pressure from the static single point test to the full wear track circumference, the ratio of the areas of a full circle to a single point area was used. This factor was computed to be 187.5 using the Hertzian contact stress model. Thus a 1 hour static creep test with a 220 gram load on a 22mm diameter ball is equivalent to a 187.5 hr linear pin-on-disk test using the same ball at the same load.

A comparison of a single track wear test and a non-linear (cross-shear) wear test were then run on CoCr femoral heads to assess the differences in wear volume. The pin-on-disk wear test parameters are shown in table 2. The creep test results were also used

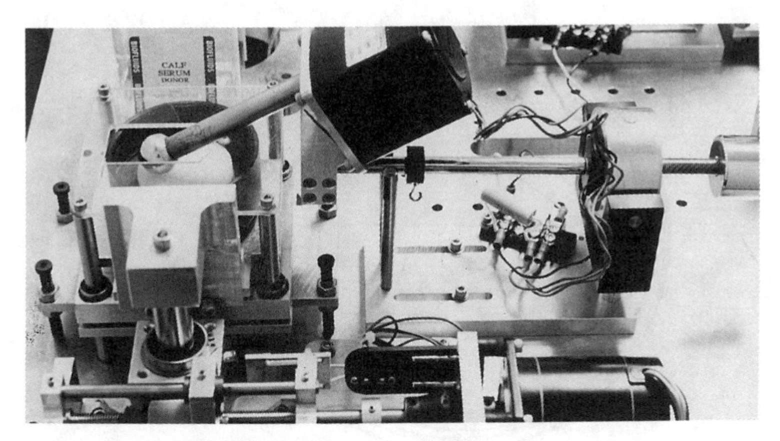

FIG. 6—*Mechanical arrangement of modified pin-on-disk with randomly varied track radius*

to reduce the apparent wear volumes measured in both tests but the magnitude of these corrections was smaller than the data symbols on the graph. Note that the cross-shear tests yielded UHMWPE wear rates which are about 8 times the linear tracking values, which is close to the discrepancy seen between joint simulators and linear tracking screening devices as previously shown in table 1. Figure 9 shows the linear tracking wear vs the cross-shear wear of UHMWPE using CoCr balls in both cases. The reason for this large difference in wear rate can be explained by examining the photographs of the wear track on the two CoCr balls shown in figures 9 and 10. Both CoCr balls themselves also showed some wear. This was manifested as a flat spot on the ring that contacted the UHMWPE. The linear tracking ball (figure 10) was very highly polished in the contact track and showed 3.6 times less wear than the cross-shear ball. The ball used in the cross-shear (figure 11) test was heavily worn and showed numerous scratches which may have been responsible for the heavy UHMWPE wear. Both of these pin-on-disk machines were in a common particle-free clean hood so these scratches could not have been due to particle contamination in only the cross-shear test apparatus. These data give us reasonable confidence to use this cross-shearing test methodology when comparing ceramic coated pins verses CoCr pins.

TABLE 2—*Laboratory wear test parameters*

Parameter		Value
Ball material	-	F799 CoCr (22mm dia.)
Disk material	-	GUR 413 UHMWPE
Load	-	220gram (8.2MPa avg Hertzian Stress)
Speed	-	72 RPM (reversed each 6 sec.)
Track dia.	-	38mm (± 1.5mm random)
Lubrication	-	Bovine serum

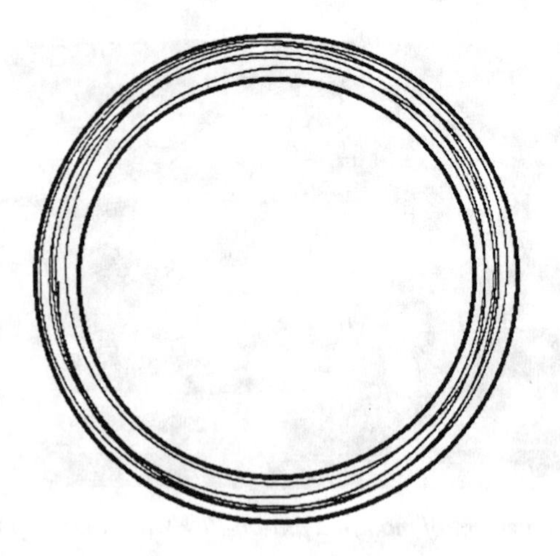

FIG. 7—*Locus of wear track for first 15 turns of disk*

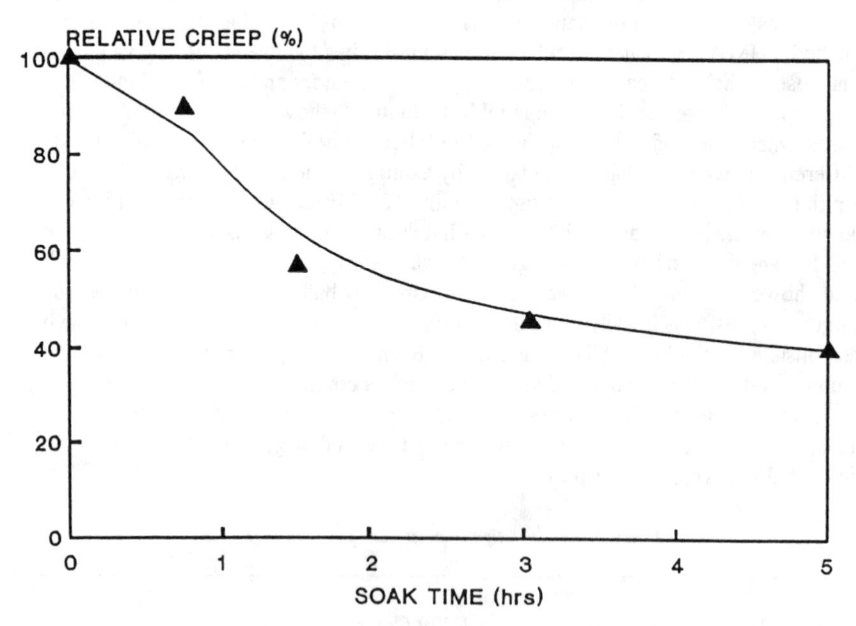

FIG. 8—*Static creep test measurements vs soak time of UHMWPE*

Results

One CoCr control ball and one alumina coated ball were tested to 2 ½ million-cycles using a 2 station wear test machine both in cross-shear mode in order to obtain a preliminary indication of a reduction of wear.

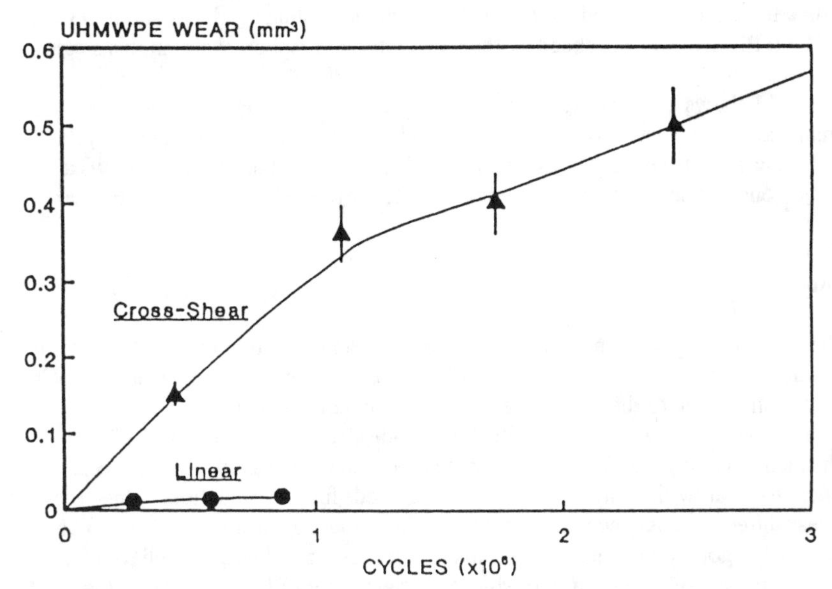

FIG. 9—*Linear tracking wear vs cross-shear wear for CoCr ball on UHMWPE disk*

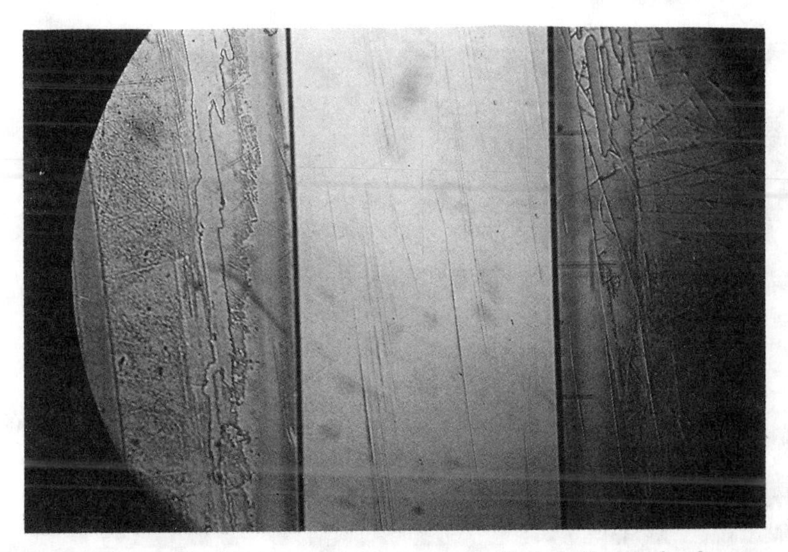

FIG. 10—*Micrograph of Linear tracking groove on CoCr ball. Marker lines are 500 microns apart.*

The wear results of the alumina-coated CoCr ball and the CoCr control are shown in figure 12. The error bars shown are the standard deviations computed from measuring the groove area at four equally spaced points around the UHMWPE wear track. In both cases the data have been corrected for creep. The alumina coating produces about 1/3 the wear of UHMWPE than was produced by the CoCr after 2 ½ million cycles in this single ball test.

Figure 13 shows a comparison of the depth profiles of the UHMWE wear grooves in (a) alumina coated ball and (b) a CoCr control ball at the end of the 2 ½ million cycle test. The photograph of the wear track on the alumina coated ball in figure 13 shows a very polished contact region which may be responsible for the reduced UHMWPE wear observed.

Discussion

These preliminary tests show that the use of an alumina coating on a CoCr femoral head may reduce the wear of UHMWPE to about 1/3 of that caused by an uncoated CoCr head. This is comparable to the wear observed from a monolithic alumina head.

It has also been shown that a modified pin-on-disk test where the radius of the track is changed randomly may be a useful device to screen coatings although the exact amount of cross-shear to simulate in-vivo conditions needs further validation. While the absolute wear differences between ceramic coated CoCr and a control would have to be determined using a good joint simulator and many more test specimens, we believe that this test may properly rank the wear performance in the proper order. In addition the anticipated problems of dimensional UHMWPE creep effects can be surmounted.

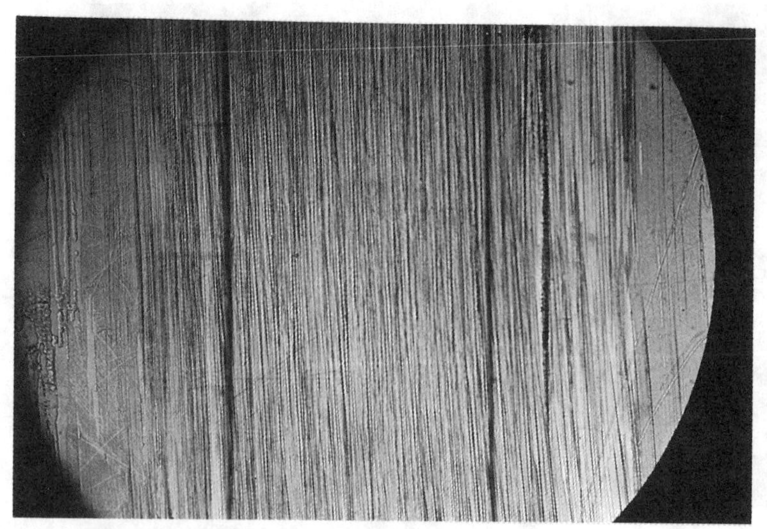

FIG. 11—*Micrograph of cross-shear tracking groove on CoCr ball. Marker lines are 500 microns apart.*

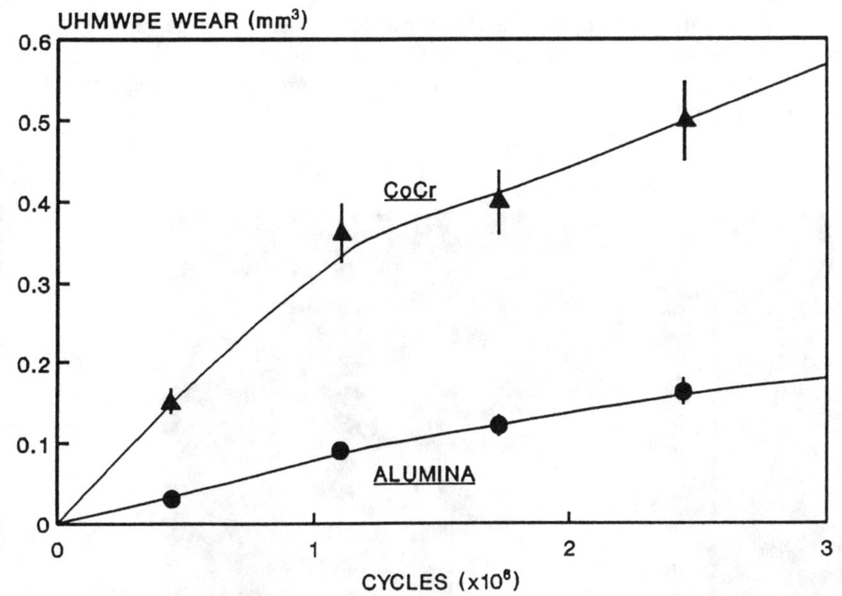

FIG. 12—*Cobalt-chrome cross-shear wear vs. alumina cross-shear wear of UHMWPE*

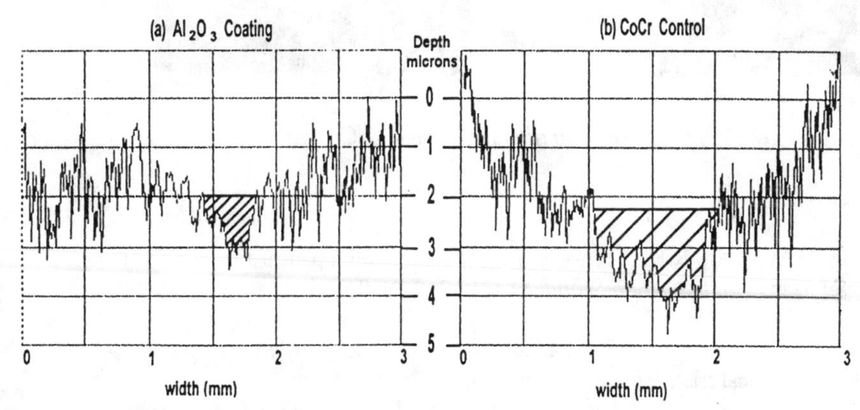

FIG. 13—*Profilometer trace of wear grooves in UHMWPE from (a) alumina coated ball and (b) Cobalt-chrome control ball*

Further tests are planned on variations of the alumina processing to minimize the UHMWPE wear. Zirconia ceramic, made with a similar ion beam technique, will also be evaluated for wear. However, these wear tests did not test for third body wear from bone cement and other hard debris which may become trapped in the joint *in-vivo*. Further tests are planned with thicker alumina coatings to evaluate performance under these conditions.

Progress has also been made in coating complex shapes, such as femoral knee prostheses. These knees coated with 1 micron of alumina show some non-uniformities in the straw color but these are due to optical interference effects rather than large variations in coating thickness. Thus a thin alumina coating on CoCr components may reduce UHMWPE wear to less than 1/3 of present values and therefore, prove to be an important advance in TJR prosthesis design.

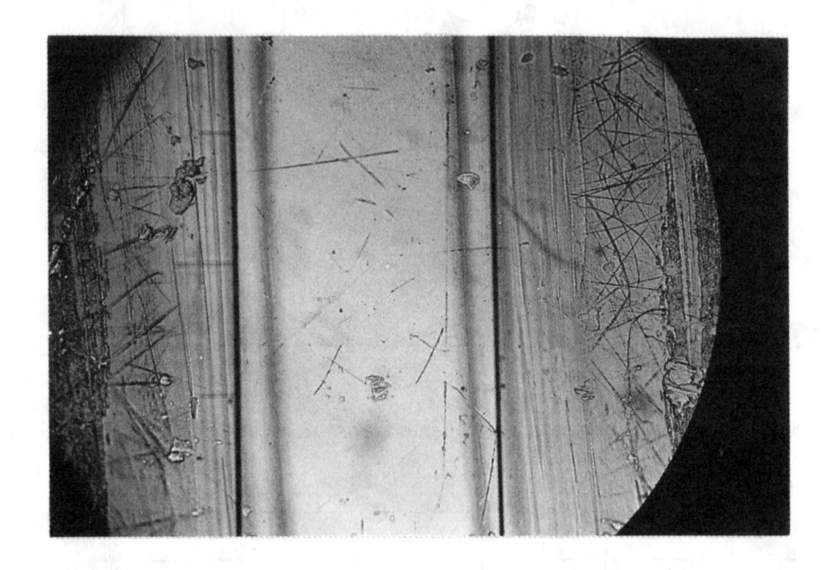

FIG. 14—*Micrograph of wear track on alumina coated CoCr ball*

References

[1] Schuller H.M., Marti R.K., "Ten-year socket wear in 66 hip arthroplasties - ceramic versus metal heads", *Acta Orthop Scand,* **61** (3): 240,1990

[2] Zichner L.P., Willert H.G., "Comparison of alumina - polyethylene and metal-polyethylene in clinical trials", *Clin Orthop,* 1992; **282**: 86-94

[3] Semlitsch, M. and Willert, H.B., "Clinical Wear Behavior of Ultra-High Molecular Weight Polyethylene Cups Paired with Metal and Ceramic Ball Heads in Comparison to Metal-on-Metal Pairings of Hip Joint Replacements," *Proc. Instn. Mech. Engrs./IMechE,* **211**, Part H (1997): 73-88.

[4] Oonishi, H., Igaki, H., and Takayama, Y. "Comparisons of Wear of UHMWPE Sliding Against Metal and Alumina in Total Hip Prosthesis", Bioceramics, 1(1989):272

[5] Semlitsch, M., Streicher, R.M., and Weber, H., *Orthopaede*, **18** (1989): 337-381

[6] Weber, B.G., "Total Hip Replacement: Rotating Versus Fixed and Metal Versus Ceramic Heads," *The Hip*, 1981: 264-275

[7] Bragdon, C.R., et al ., "Wear at the Ceramic on Polyethylene Articulation," *Trans. 21st Society for Biomaterials Meeting,* March 1995: 50.

[8] Livingston, B.J., Chmell, M.J., Reilly, D.T., Spector, M., and Poss, R., "The Wear Rate of Hylamer Cups is Higher Than Conventional PE and Differs with Heads from Different Manufacturers," *Trans. 43rd ORS*, February 1997: 141.

[9] Paschen U., "In-vivo-verschleib der gleitflachpaarung Al_2O_3 -keramic/polyethylen bei huftendoprosthesen", *Taf Der Mundlichen Parfung* 7: 1-15, 1986

[10] Selker J., Steinmann P.A., and Hintermann H.E., "The Scratch Test: Different Critical Load Determination Techniques", *Surface Coatings and Technology*, **36** (1988) 519-529

[11] Griffith M. et al., "Socket Wear in Charnley Low Friction Arthoplasty of the Hip", *Clin Orthop*, **137**, 37, (1978)

[12] McKellop H.A. and Clarke I.C., "Degradation and Wear of Ultra-High-Molecular-Weight Polyethylene", *Corrosion and Degradation of Implant Materials, 2nd Symp*, ASTM STP 859, A.C. Franker and C.D. Griffin Eds., ASTM, Philadelphia 1985 pp 351

[13] Dumbleton J.H., and Shen C., "The Wear Behavior of Ultra High Molecular Weight Polyethylene", *Wear,* **37**, 279 (1976)

[14] Bragdon C.R., et al, "The Importance of Multidirectional Motion for the Wear of Polyethylene in the Hip", *5th World Biomat. Cong.*, May 28, Toronto, Canada, I-582 (1996)

[15] Wang A., et al, "Wear Testing Based on Unidirectional Motion: Fact or Artefact?", *5th World Biomat. Cong.*, May 28 Toronto, Canada p I-583 (1996)

Alternative Polymeric Bearing Materials

Alain Meunier (1), Rémy Nizard (2), Pascal Bizot (2), Laurent Sedel (3)

Clinical results of alumina-on-alumina couple in total hip replacement.

REFERENCE: Meunier, A., Nizard, R., Bizot, P., and Sedel, L. "**Clinical Results of Alumina-on-Alumina Couple in Total Hip Replacement,**" *Alternative Bearing Surfaces in Total Joint Replacement, ASTM STP 1346*, J. J. Jacobs and T. L. Craig, Eds., American Society for Testing and Materials, 1998.

ABSTRACT :

Ceramic on ceramic bearings applications were developed, in Europe, 27 years ago. After the initial failures related to both manufacturing problems as well as the surgeons learning curve, these materials now appear to be very promising for total hip replacement surgery in young and active patients. Improvement of the material caracteristics has resulted in a higher toughness and reduced wear than that of the classical Metal on Ultra High Molecular Weight Polyethylene combination. Clinical results are now available from different centers, mainly situated in Germany, Austria, Italy, Spain, Finland and France. Although the initial total hip replacements sometimes gave socket loosening and some fracture, the clinical results are acceptable. Moreover the low rate of osteolysis observed may be a very promising long term advantage of this type of bearing surface.

KEYWORDS : surgery, total hip replacement, ceramics, clinical results, europe,

---

(1) PHD - Orthopaedic Research Lab.10, avenue de Verdun - 75010 - Paris- France
(2) MD - Orthopaedic Research Lab.10, avenue de Verdun - 75010 - Paris- France and Orthopaedic Department - Hopital Lariboisiere - 2 rue Ambroise Paré - 75010- Paris - France.
(3) Chairman- MD - Orthopaedic Research Lab.10, avenue de Verdun - 75010 - Paris- France and Orthopaedic Department - Hopital Lariboisiere - 2 rue Ambroise Paré - 75010- Paris - France.

Introduction

Osteolysis is now recognized as a major limiting factor for long term total hip implantation in young and active patients.
Many authors have stated that osteolysis is related to the generation of debris. The main source of debris is produced by the polyethylene rubbing against the metal. Increased wear due to the modularity of total hip replacements (THRs) may also be considered as a source of debris : morse taper corrosion related to fretting or polyethylene wear produced at the socket screw holes.
It is interesting to note that the original design and concept of J. Charnley are still in use and have been proved to give acceptable results for up to 20 years [1]. However, young, active, male, patients, for whom the results are significantly worse, are still a cause for concern.

History

In the early seventies, authors such as Ring and Boutin were looking for new bearing materials with a long life time. They selected the principle of two hard, frictional surfaces. It appeared that alumina ceramics could fulfill most of the requirements and could therefore be used as a bearing materials for total hip reconstruction. The first implantation was performed in 1970 by Pierre Boutin [2, 3, 4] following some biological studies in dogs. He implanted an alumina/alumina system which was cementless at the acetabular level and had a cemented stem. This material was manufactured by the Ceraver® company. He quickly changed to another socket design which could either be cemented or cementless (Table 1).

This system was considered as a potentially good one both by J. Charnley in his book on hip surgery and by Mac Kellop et al [5]. During this pioneering period, problems were related to the poor quality of the alumina. The risk of fracture and problems related to the fixation of the metallic stem and the alumina femoral head [6, 7].

The first generation of alumina had low mechanical properties, the head was glued or screwed on the stem and the socket was either cemented or cementless. In spite of many failures, this first experiment helped to develop a greater understanding of this new material and hence resulted in improved material characteristics and fixation devices. Also the histological sections obtained from samples retrieved from these first cases, demonstrated that alumina was highly biocompatible.

At this time, many other studies were being conducted around the world : Griss [8], Mittelmeier [9], Heimke [10, 11, 12] in Germany, Pizzoferato [13, 14] in Italy, Salzer [15] in Austria and Shikita [16] in Japan , who developed the concept of alumina/polyethylene bearings. The quality of the alumina employed in these THRs was variable. Many of the biological studies were conducted by Griss and Heimke [17, 8) who concluded the extreme tolerance of alumina both in bulk and particulate forms.

As socket loosening occurred repeatedly with the cemented, bulky acetabulum, different bone/alumina fixation systems have been evaluated since 1983 (Table 1). Our group experimented with a titanium alloy screw-in ring with an alumina liner Witvoet et al. [18], however in 1989, this trial was stopped due to excessive socket loosening related to the shape of the thread. Problems relating to the alumina liner were not experienced (fracture was not observed in more than 500 cases). For this reason, in 1989, we substituted a press fit titanium shell (with or without screws) with an alumina liner. Once again, in nearly 1000 implanted samples, alumina related problems were not encountered.

	year *Number*	**ceramic ball fixation**	**stem fixation**	**socket fixation**	**fractures (head and cup) %**
Boutin	1970	glued	cemented	cemented and cementless	unknown
Griss	1974	26/28 ceramic ball tapered	cementless	cementless	>10%
Sedel	1977-1983 *401*	32 ceramic ball tapered	cemented titanium alloy	cemented	1977-79: 4/401 (1%) 2 heads 2 cups
Sedel, Witvoet Acta Belg.	1983-1989 *560*	32 ceramic ball tapered	titanium alloy cemented	threaded titanium with alumina liner	no fracture
Salzer Symp. 96	1976-1979 *67*	32 ceramic ball tapered	cemented	cementless	9 /67: 13%
Mittlemeier Stuggart, 96	1974-1993 *6862*	Autophor tapered	cementless	cementless threaded	21/6862: 0,4%
Garcia Cimbrelo (J. Arthrop., 96)	Mittlemeier 1978-1984: *83*	Autophor tapered	cementless	threaded	3 cups :3,6%
Sedel and Witvoet Efort 97	1990-1995 *450*	tapered	cemented	cementless press-fit ti alloy shell alumina liner	no fracture

Table 1 : Published series of alumina/alumina couple (the number in italics refers to the number of cases)

Basics Properties of the Alumina Against Alumina Bearing System

Numerous research projects have been dedicated to the evaluation of alumina/alumina bearing systems. They have included mechanical simulator studies, implant retrieval analysis or tissues samples analyzed after revision surgery. Some of the data produced are summarized herein.

The Biological Characteristics

Alumina ceramics are highly oxidized. Their chemical inertness may explain the minimal reactions observed when the ceramic is in contact with living tissues or cells. A very high purity is important. If other phases, such as a glassy phase, are formed at the grain boundaries, alumina becomes susceptible to dissolution, even at body temperature. Various standards have been designed and published internationally (ISO 6474), and in the US (ASTM F-603), [20]. Biological performances of alumina ceramics in bulk and particulate forms were tested in vitro, in vivo and after human explantation [21]. Biological tolerance was tested in vitro on fibroblasts [10) lymphocytes or macrophages [22, 13] in muscle [22], in bone [17]. Carcinogenicity was tested in rats by Griss [17, 8]. One paper [23] described a clinical case of fibrosarcoma which developed ten months after the implantation of a ceramic against ceramic (Milttlemeier type) hip prosthesis. However, after examining this paper in greater detail, it appeared that the clinical case concerned a man operated on 12 years previously for a hip fracture using a cobalt chromium screw. Due to the long period of time necessary to develop a cancer induced by a material, it seems more likely that the cancer developed spontaneously or was caused by the screw. Griss [17, 8] experimented in a sheep, with a massive stem made of alumina ceramic. This presented very good bone/ceramic contact in the compressive zones whereas a considerable amount of fibrous tissue was detected at the interface under tension. Similar results were found in a retrieved post-mortem study performed by A.M. after 12 years of safe implantation [4].

Our team examined tissues retrieved from alumina/alumina THRs. In agreement with other studies, only a minute quantity of alumina particulate was found in the tissues. The biological reaction of the tissues in contact with the alumina particles was of a fibrocytic type, with neither macrophages nor giant cells. The majority of the alumina particles were situated outside the cells. Their mean size was 0.4 μm. In some samples, macrophagic reaction were observed. If these results are compared to other materials, there were statistically fewer macrophages than when evaluating tissues retrieved from a failed metal/polyethylene couple [26]. Quantification of PGE2 levels in these tissues revealed fewer inflammatory mediators than with the metal/polyethylene couple [24). In a recent study we also found that some of the ceramic particulates were not made of the alumina ceramic but were made of zirconia which was used as a radiological marker in the PMMA bone cement [25]. As some foreign body reactions were encountered in the tissues in contact with the zirconia particulates, it would be interesting to determine the role of the latter in the loosening of the alumina cemented component which was observed in our series.

The overall biological performances of alumina ceramics are so interesting that this material is often used as a negative control in material biocompatibility testing.

Mechanical Characteristics

Alumina ceramic is a stiff and brittle material. Alumina ceramic has an elastic modulus (380 GPa) when compared to that of cobalt chromium (220 Gpa), or to that of cortical bone (20 GPa) or to bone cement (2 GPa). Standard alumina ceramics require a bending strength of more than 400 MPa. Some of the better products exhibit a bending strength of 550 MPa.

Fracture toughness. The shock sensitivity of alumina ceramics is of concern. Many people believe that this brittle material will fracture under light impact loads. Alumina ceramics demonstrate a fracture toughness in the range of 5 MPa.$(m)^{1/2}$ which is lower than that of zirconia ceramics (9 MPa.$(m)^{1/2}$) [27, 29, 28].

Static and dynamic fatigue, aging. Ceramics undergo failure when tested under constant load or cyclic load. The size of the grains and their average distribution, as well as the presence of initial flaws in the material, are the critical factors governing the fatigue characteristics of alumina [28]. It is particularly important to minimize impurities such as SiO_2, Na_2O and CaO.

Many fatigue and aging tests have been conducted in aqueous environments [30]. For alumina ceramic either a small decrease or no decrease in fracture toughness were recorded even after very long periods.

In order to avoid excessive internal stresses the taper must be accurately machined. This accuracy must not only take into account the cone angle but also the cone circularity and linearity, as well as the surface roughness.

Head Fractures. Component fracture and especially head fracture, is one of the failure modes of alumina/alumina THAs. Fracture, because of its clinical consequences, is one of the major fears which limits the clinical application of this system. The frequency of fracture differs from one report to another, from 1/1200 up to 10/130 [32, 4, 33, 7, 19]. Alumina fracture is dependent on the quality of the alumina, the geometry of the taper junction and the applied load. Clinical cases of fracture were associated with (i) a small head diameter, [11] (ii) a poor quality of alumina with an especially large grain size of up to 40 μm, (iii) inborn stresses initiated during the material manufacturing process [7, 33], (iv) less than ideal fitting of the male and female taper and (v) short term subluxation and back to normal position [26].

Improved manufacturing processes, taper design and quality control have resulted in a considerable general decrease in the risk of fracture since the early 80s. Moreover, heads with a diameter of less than 28 mm are no longer employed in alumina/alumina prostheses. Due to these important improvements, it has become quite difficult to precisely assess the real current risk of fracture from historical records. According to Clarke and Willmann [19], given that the appropriate care is taken during surgery, the risk of fracture may be reduced to below 1 in 5000 cases.

From 1980 up until the present day, we have only documented two head fractures and no fractures of the socket component out of the 3000 alumina pieces which have been inserted, in our department, during this period.

Surface and wear performances. Alumina ceramics are extremely interesting materials with respect to wear resistance. This high resistance is related, in part, to the surface characteristics. With such a material, a very smooth surface (Ra = 0.02 μm) can be achieved, which is well below the best metallic surface finish obtainable.

Moreover, the wear properties of alumina are also related to its good wettability, which allows better in vivo lubrication. Due to the hardness of the material, cement or bone fragments caught between the ball and the socket do not present any risk of third body wear. This is not true for other bearing couples, including the metal on metal system.

Wear tests have been conducted using a large number of test configurations. The conventional wear tests included the pin on disc test or the disc on disc test, in either an oscillating or a reciprocating configuration. Hip simulator studies permitted more reliable tests to be conducted in conditions closer to the in vivo situation. These tests were dependent on the liquid used as a lubricant: demineralized water resulted in greater wear than bovine serum [34, 35].

The best results of the friction coefficient and wear were obtained with the alumina against alumina pairing. Boher (cited by Sedel [35]) published experimental work on clearance and the friction coefficient. It appeared that the best clearance obtainable with the alumina/alumina combination was between 10 and 50 μm. In France, this clearance was obtained by the Ceraver Osteal company using a special grinding process. The resulting ball and socket were sold as a non-interchangeable unit. Since 1993, manufacturing processes have permitted the use of independent components whilst retaining the appropriate clearance. Other companies sold have sold components which could be independently assembled since the early seventies.

Retrieval analysis of long term implanted material was conducted by J.M. Dorlot [36, 37] on 6 cemented implanted prostheses. He concluded that volumetric wear was very low in a normal configuration i.e. when the prosthesis did not tilt before retrieval. In this case, the estimated wear was 0,025 μm/year (about 4000 times less than that of the usual metal on polyethylene system). In two samples, after both loosening and tilting of the socket, gross wear (18 mm3 volumetric wear) was measured. Overall, the low wear in the standard position may explain the limited number of particles observed in the retrieved tissues obtained during the revision procedure and hence the minimal foreign body reaction.

Clinical Results of Alumina/Alumina THRs

Many papers have been published on the clinical results of alumina / alumina THRs

[40, 38, 41, 15, 42, 43], and our own team [33]. It appears that the results obtained in this study were comparable to other current materials. However when young and active patients were considered [44, 45], the results were favourable and compared well to similar series obtained with conventional couples. Moreover, in all the series available, osteolysis was not encountered.

In order to demonstrate the very long term results of the alumina/alumina couple, our longest term study is presented herein and considers a cemented alumina socket and a Ti6Al4V cemented stem.

Materials and Methods

The material examined includes the first 401 consecutive prosthesis implanted in primary cases between 1977 and 1982. There was not any patient selection at that time, all the patients had the same prosthesis implanted whatever their age, diagnosis or activity. Four hundred and one consecutive primary arthroplasties were performed in 351 patients in the orthopedic surgery department of the Lariboisière-Saint-Louis teaching hospital, in Paris (Table 2). Some patients had undergone conservative procedures including 6 femoral osteotomies, 3 shelf procedures, 3 femoral fractures, 1 shelf associated with a femoral osteotomy, and 1 Voss procedure. Three hips had a history of infection.

age	26 to 92	mean 66 ± 11.1
weight	39 to 123 kg.	mean 69 kg.
sex	221 females	180 males
primary arthritis	231	57.6%
inflammatory diseases (RA and AS)	56	13.9%
CDH or subluxation	46	11.4%
AVN	38	9.5%
miscellaneous	30	7.6%
past history	none : 382	conserv.surgery : 16 previous infection : 3

Table 2 : Characteristics of the patients

The prosthesis. The prosthesis was manufactured by Ceraver Osteal* (Roissy, France). The stem was made of annealed titanium alloy (Ti6Al4V) which was anodized to produce a 5000 A thick layer of titanium oxide. It was a collared and cemented stem. Twelve different sizes were available to allow optimal filling and fitting of the medullary canal.

The head and the socket were made of pure, medical grade, dense alumina. To obtain a low clearance between the components and hence a large contact area, the head and socket were paired and were available as a unit. The 32 mm head was inserted on a Morse taper. The cemented acetabular component was hemispherical with 1mm grooves on the outer surface.

Surgical Technique. The operation was performed under general anesthesia. Both the approach and the cementing technique are summarized in Table 3.

approach	**transtroch.:129**	**posterior : 270**	**Hardinge : 2**
technique for cementing the stem	**finger packing : 305**	**low-viscosity, seringe and Pe plug : 96**	

Table 3 : Surgical technique

We were concerned by the quality of the position of the components. The socket had to be placed at a 45° inclination angle and 25° anteversion. The cementing technique was not the same in every case. In some cases a small socket was inserted in a large amount of cement. Sometimes the socket was press fitted resulting in a thin cement mantle. It is difficult in a retrospective study to assess which technique was employed in each case and therefore we will not make further reference to it. The results were considered with respect to the socket size used. In the femur, we tried to obtain good collar-calcar contact in order to improve proximal stress transfer and rotational stability. The largest stem was always chosen in order to obtain bone contact. No long term consequence were observed when bone contact was not achieved or when a proximal crack was noticed.

A conventional **rehabilitation program** was used initially, however several years after surgery, the patients were asked to perform any activity, including strenuous exercises and sports, as we assumed that this would not impair the results.

Evaluation

Clinical pre and post operative assessment of the results was performed using the Postel Merle D'aubigné grading system.

A radiological evaluation was completed by an independent observer ie someone other than the operating surgeon. All the measurements were scaled, when necessary, to the known diameter of the prosthetic head in order to compensate for the enlargement of the radiographs. **For the stem**, the parameters evaluated were : the stem angle, filling of the canal, radiolucent lines according to Gruen et al, collar/calcar contact, subsidence, osteolysis, calcar resorption, and cement mantle fracture. The most recent follow-up radiograph was then classified according to Harris as either possible, probable, or definite loosening and then according to Gruen et al. if loosening had occurred. **For the socket**, any radiolucent line were recorded according to Charnley and De Lee on AP and Profile view. The socket angle was measured between the equatorial and the horizontal lines of the prosthesis. Protrusio and vertical migration were also recorded.

The data was stored and analyzed on a personal computer using statistical software. The relationship between the categorical data was assessed with the $\chi 2$ test and the continuous data was evaluated using the t-test. The Kaplan-Meier method was used to evaluate the survivorship function and comparisons of survivorship functions were carried out using the Log-rank test. A probability level of $p<0.05$ was chosen to indicate a significant difference.

Results

Complications. Post-operative complications occurred in 51 patients, 5 of which were fatal : one being a large myocardial infarction and 4 fatal pulmonary embolisms. Twenty-four deep vein thromboses occurred, and were associated with symptomatic or asymptomatic pulmonary embolism in 16 patients. Three patients developed an early infection and hence underwent revision. Dislocation of the prosthesis occurred in 13 of the hips, and a component exchange was required for one of them. The others were treated with closed reduction and immobilization. A common peroneal nerve palsy occurred in 6 hips, 4 of which completely recovered and the other two partially recuperated. This complication rate corresponds to the state of the art during the early eighties.

Follow-up (Table 4). Eighty-five patients died (21.2%), 80 before the ten-year end point and 5 afterwards. During the observation period, 60 revisions were performed, and they are presented separately. One hundred and twenty-nine hips were lost to follow-up after an average period of 4.3 ± 3.2 years. These patients were significantly older (69.6 years versus 65.1 years, p=0.0002).

One hundred and fifty six femoral components had a minimum follow-up of 10 years, these included 127 hips which had not been revised and 29 hips which underwent an acetabular revision without the removal of the femoral component ; the mean follow-up period of these hips was 12.2 ± 1.8 years.

Deceased	**85 (80 before 10 years)**
Revised	**60**
Lost before 10 years	**129 (average follow-up : 4.3±3.2 years)**
Followed for more than 10 years	**156**
Phone	**10**
Clinically evaluated	**146**
Radiographic evaluation	**126**

Table 4: Follow-up

Results at the latest follow-up evaluation

Clinical Results. We tried to contact all the living patients. Most of them were reviewed in the institution although 10 patients refused to participate and therefore an adequate clinical evaluation of these cases was impossible. 146 hips were clinically evaluated 10 years or more after the index arthroplasty, the hip score improved from a pre-operative mean of 10.3 (range, 0-14 points) to a last follow-up post-operative mean of 17 (range, 9-18 points). Initially, 93.6% of these hips were graded as poor and 6.4% as fair. At the latest follow-up 56.1% were classed as excellent, 23.3% as very good, 12.3% as good, 2.1% as fair and 6.2% as poor (9 hips). All but one of the poor results were associated with cup loosening, the exception was associated with femoral loosening. Improvement of the hip score was statistically significant ($p<0.0001$).

Radiographic Results (Fig. 1 and 2). Measurements were made on the latest radiograph available and were compared to the immediate post operative X-ray. When necessary all the intermediate radiographs were also examined in order to determine, as precisely as possible, the moment when the implant underwent a change.

One hundred and twenty-six femoral stems were radiographically examined 10 years or more after the index operation. For 30 hips radiographs were not avalaible, as these patients either only responded to a questionnaire, or refused to undergo an x-ray.

Using the radiographic criteria described by Harris et al. 4 of the femoral components were definitely loose, with migration, none were probably loose with a complete radiolucent line, either at the bone-cement interface or at the cement-stem interface, and 4 were possibly loose, with evidence of a radiolucent line that occupied over 50% but less that 100% of either the bone-cement interface or the cement-stem interface. Two of the four definitely loose stems were symptomatic of a Postel Merle D'Aubigné score of 12 and 15.

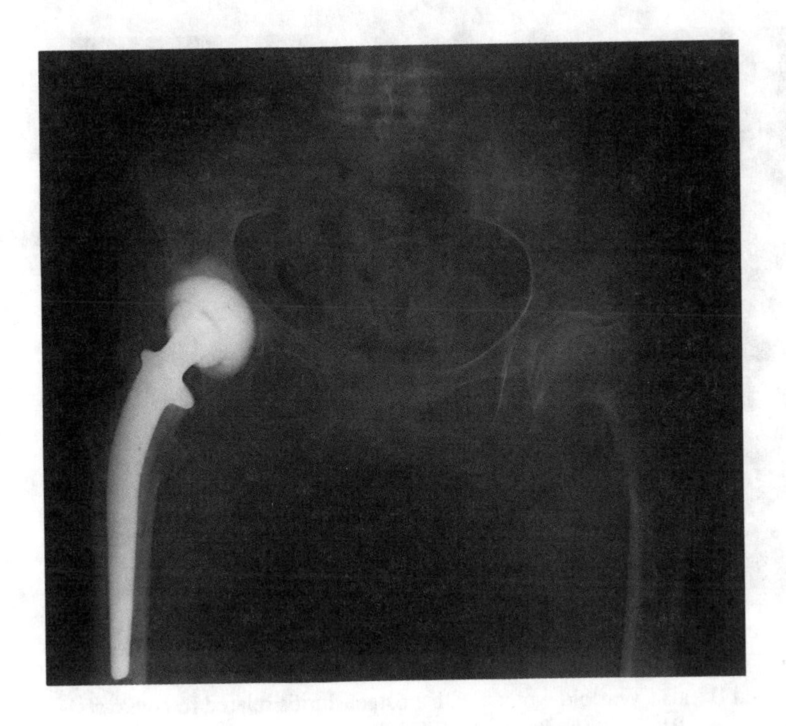

[1] Aspect after 18 years in a 27 year old woman presenting a severe avascular necrosis of the right femoral head. This was a revision from a cup arthroplasty. The clinical result is excellent despite the slight pain in the left hip that had not been operated on.

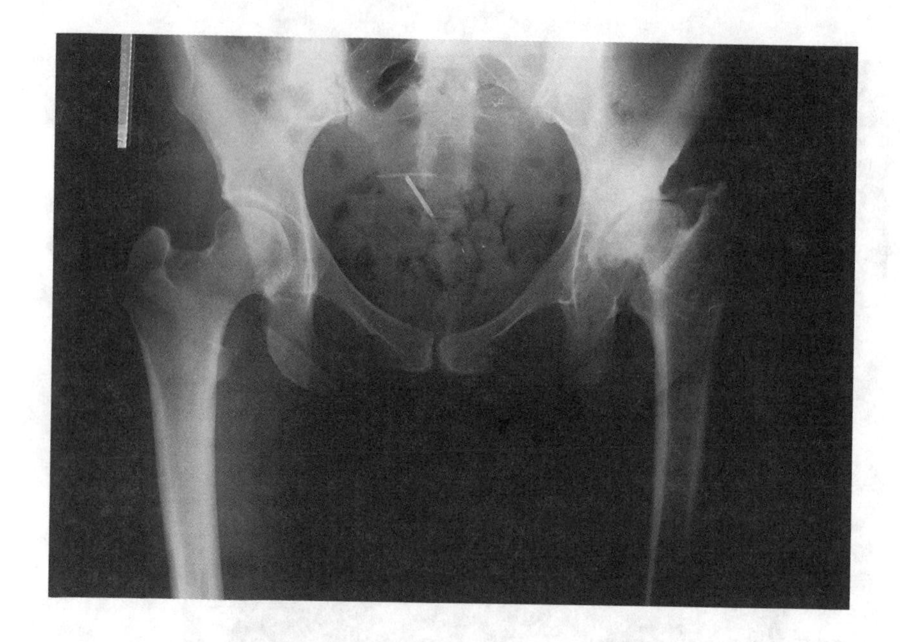

[2] A and B : a 31 year old woman with a osteoarthritis related to congenital coxa vara. Radiograph after 8 years. She has no pain, full range of motion and had a pregnancy 3 years ago without any problem.

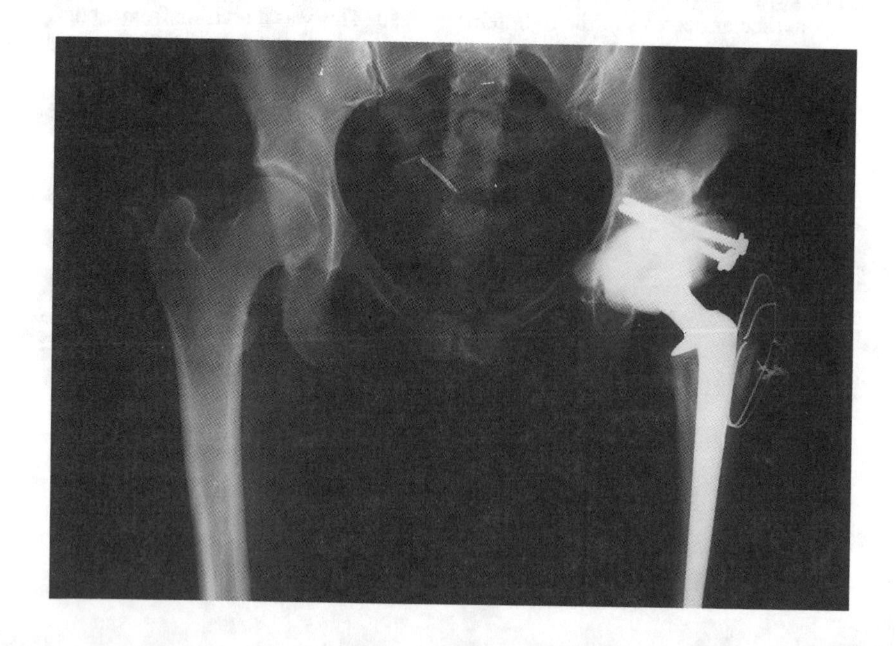

Significant calcar resorption was seen in 21 patients (5-20 mm), it exceeded 10 mm in 4 of the hips.

Endosteal erosion was seen in 4 hips, in 3 cases it was limited to one or two zones, and in the last case it was extensively observed in seven zones. This case had socket loosening and refused to be revised for 12 years. At revision there was massive metallic wear resulting from the tilted alumina socket rubbing on the titanium stem. There was also massive wear of the alumina head. This was considered to result from friction between the ceramic head and the socket rim, after the latter tilted.

Six of the sockets were considered as impending failures as either tilting of the socket or protrusion were observed.

Heterotopic Ossifications. The incidence of heterotopic ossification according to Brooker, at the latest follow-up available was : none in 69.5%, grade 1 in 18.2%, grade 2 in 4.4%, grade 3 in 6.6%, and grade 4 in 1.3%.

Revisions. Among the sixty revisions, one was performed outside of our institution and was considered as a « worst case » i.e. a bipolar aseptic loosening with the removal of both the femoral and acetabular components. Amongst the other 59 revisions (Table 5), 1 was carried out for recurrent dislocation, 1 for femoral shaft fracture below the tip of the stem, 4 for septic loosening, 4 for alumina fractures (2 cups and 2 heads) and 49 for aseptic loosening. Forty-three of the 49 aseptic loosenings were isolated acetabular loosenings, 5 were bipolar loosenings and 1 was an isolated femoral loosening. As it can be observed in Table 5, socket loosening represents the majority of the reasons for revision . Sometimes loosening occurred suddenly due to acute tilting of the socket. Sometimes the loosening occured progressively. Initially a radiolucent line was noticeable not only at the bone/cement interface but also at the cement/prosthesis interface, especially at the lower aspect (Charnley zone 3). When pain or acute tilting occurred revision was advised.

Acetabular loosening occurred after an average of 7.1 years (range 0.7 to 15.4 years), bipolar loosening after an average of 10.4 years, and the femoral loosening after 1.5 years.

Only 6 stems were removed for stem loosening and in 2 of these cases loosening was related to an inadequate initial technique and in one case it was due to a foreign body reaction. The latter was resulted from long term socket loosening with an associated massive generation of debris which was created by the contact between the ceramic and the titanium.

Revision procedures were adapted with respect to the origin of the loosening. As shown in table 5, most of the acetabular loosening had a cup revision leaving the femoral component unchanged. In a case of isolated acetabular loosening, when the femoral component was changed, this procedure was due to either a difficult exposure necessitating removal of the femoral component, to an involuntary stem extraction when trying to remove the head from the Morse taper, to deterioration of the cone during ball withdrawal or because the revision was carried out outside our institution. Twenty-four femoral components were extracted : 1 for femoral shaft fracture, 1 for recurrent dislocation, 1 for isolated femoral loosening, 4 for bipolar septic loosening, 9 for isolated acetabular component loosening, 3 for alumina fractures, and 5 for aseptic bipolar loosening.

Interestingly, the majority of these revisions were considered as a relatively simple procedure because the bone stock was retained. There was no osteolysis except in one case which has already been described. Socket reconstruction was simple.

	number	**socket and stem exchange**	**socket exchange**	**stem exchange**	**Girldstone**
infection	**4**	**2**	**-**	**-**	**2**
socket loosening	**43**	**9**	**34**	**-**	**-**
stem loosening	**1**	**-**	**-**	**1**	**-**
bipolar L.	**5**	**5**	**-**	**-**	**-**
Recurrent dislocat.	**1**	**1**	**-**	**-**	**-**
Alumina fracture	**4**	**3**	**1**	**-**	**-**
femoral fracture	**1**	**-**	**-**	**1**	**-**

Table 5 : Reasons for revision and for the procedures performed at revision

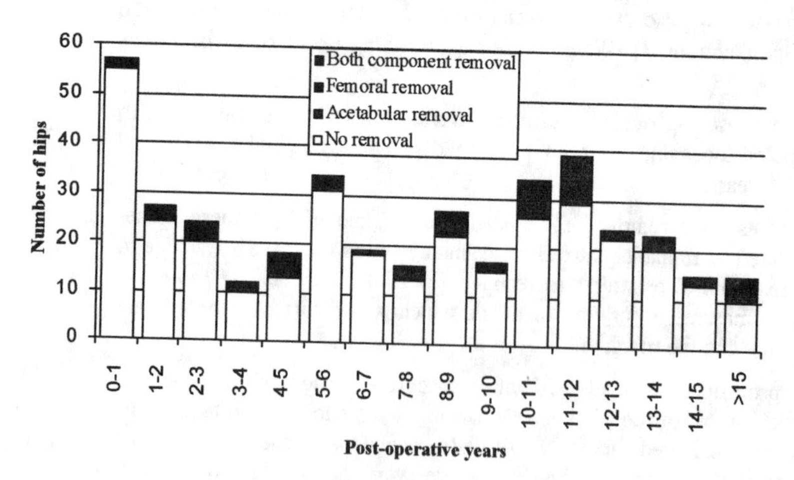

Figure 3 : Period and type of revision performed

Survival Analysis. The results were evaluated using the actuarial method. The definition for failure was the removal of the components for whatever reason. These could be infection, recurrent dislocation, or the aseptic loosening of the socket, the stem or both components. We also examined revision for aseptic loosening. In the results section it has already been noted that the main reason for revision was socket loosening.

If we consider failure as **implant removal whatever the reason** the survivorship analysis depicted 70 % (± 4.3) survivors at 14 years. The results for patients below and above 60 years old are as follows: 66.8 % (±7.3) compared to 73.2 % (± 4.3) respectively. This is not statistically significant. If we compare survivorship for patients younger than 50 years old (35 patients) and older (364) then these percentages are 86.2 ± 7.6 % and 66.9 % (± 5.1) respectively. the difference is now statistically significant.

If we now consider failure as the removal of an implant for **aseptic loosening** we can see that there are still no differences between the patients of over and under 60 years of age. For the patients under 50 years of age there is 100% survival. We had already observed these very surprising results in a younger age group [45].

When failure was defined as **removal of the femoral component,** regardless of the cause of removal, the survival of the femoral component was 92.9% ±3.2 at the ten-year review and 85.4% ± 9.2 at the fifteen-year review. When failure was defined by the removal of the femoral component for **isolated femoral loosening or bipolar loosening**, the survival of the femoral component was 98.1% ± 2 at the ten-year review and 97.4 ± 2.4 at the fifteen-year review. When failure was defined as definite or probable radiological loosening or the removal of the femoral component for aseptic loosening, the survival analysis depicted a 98.1 ± 2% rate at ten years and a 86.8 ± 8.6% at fifteen years.

Neither demographic (age, gender, weight) nor technical parameters (component position, filling of the medullary canal, cementing technique) were found to be predictive of the survival of the femoral component.

Discussion

In order to address the **failures** related to the alumina fractures, which were encountered 4 times in the first 401 cases, and are now observed in less than 1/3000 cases, we have to compare these figures to the failure rate of other components.

In a recent publication, D. Deck et al. [46] quantified the prosthetic component failures in a five year period for the entire membership of the American Association of Hip and Knee Surgeons (Table 6).

metal backed socket : complete polyethylene failure	**172/60115**	**0.29%**
all polyethylene failure	**77/3219**	**2.4%**
modular acetabular dissociation	**87/60115**	**0.15%**
metal stemmed fracture	**172/64483**	**0.27%**
dissociation of a modular head	**15/66888**	**0.03%**
fracture of ceramic head	**11/5023**	**0.22%**

Table 6 : Number and percent of material failures of different components

According to this recent work, ceramic fracture, although possible, is less frequent than stem fracture or polyethylene rupture. We must also emphasize that 3 of the 11 fractures observed were with the same product at the same institution.

The reasons for revision in our institution are now considered. The most common reason for revision was acetabular aseptic loosening of the first generation implant.

Revision was more frequent for the older patients because in the patient aged 50 or less the revision rate was quite acceptable. Osteolysis was only encountered in one case in which it could be related the generation of metallic debris.

We improved the socket fixation using either the direct interference fit of a plain alumina socket, since 1983 (Fig. 4), or a metal-backed alumina liner, since 1990. These materials are still under trial but revision rate at 5 years is very low.
It appears that an alumina/alumina sliding system, if well produced and controlled, has attained a good level of security. The fracture risk is below 1/3000, and material-related osteolysis has been advoided in every series employing this material. Therefore revision almost immitates a primary procedure. For all of these reasons we consider that this material is particularly appropriate for young, active people, even when performing strenuous activities including sports

References

[1] Schulte, K.R., Callaghan, J.J., Kelley, S.S., Hill, C., Johnston, R.C., 1993, « **The Outcome of Charnley Total Hip Arthroplasty with Cement After a Minimum Twenty Year Follow-Up** », *Journal of Bone and Joint Surgery,* Vol. 75 A, pp.961-975.

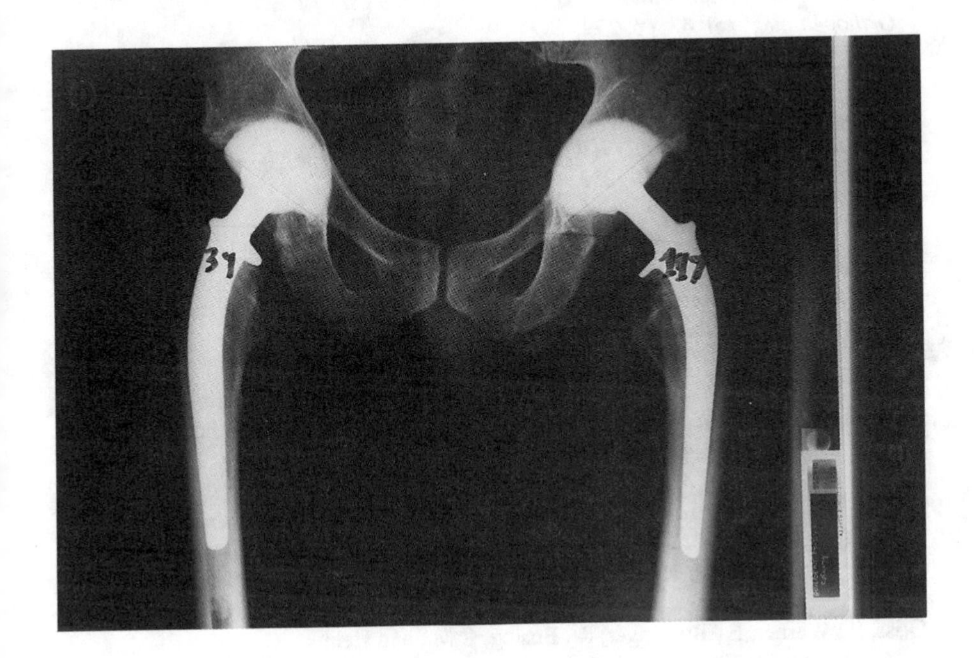

[3] A 47 year old man with a bilateral avascular necrosis operated on 3 and 11 years ago with a cemented femoral stem and a cementless plain bulky ceramic acetabulum. Excellent results were obtained on both sides.

[2] Boutin, P., 1972, « **Arthroplastie Totale de Hanche par Prothèse en Alumine Frittée** », *Revue de Chirurgie Orthopédique,* Vol.58, pp.229-246.

[3] Boutin, P., Blanquaert, D., 1981, « **Le Frottement Al/Al en Chirurgie de la Hanche : 1205 Arthroplasties Totales** », *Revue de Chirurgie Orthopédique,* Vol. 67, pp. 279- 287.

[4] Boutin, P., Christel, P., Dorlot, J.M., Meunier, A., de Roquancourt, A., Blanquaert, D., and al, 1988, « **The Use of Dense Alumina-Alumina Ceramic Combination in THR** », *Journal of Biomaterial Materials Research,* V. 22, pp. 1203-1232.

[5] McKellop, H., Clarke, I., Markolf, K., and Amstutz, H., 1981, « **Friction and Wear. Properties of Polymer, Metal and Ceramic Prosthetic Joint Materials Evaluated on a Multichannel Screening Device** », *Journal of Biomedical Materials Research,* Vol.15, pp. 619-653.

[6] Walter, A. and Plitz, W., « **Wear Characteristics of Ceramic-to-Ceramic Hip. Joint Endoprostheses** », 11th Annual Meeting of the Society For Biomaterials, 1985, pp.178.

[7] Walter, A., 1992, « **On the Material and the Tribology of Al/Al Coupling for Hip Joint Prostheses** », *Clinical Orthopaedic and Related Research,* Vol. 282, pp.31-46.

[8] Griss, P., Werner, E., Buchinger, R., Busing, C.M., and Heimke, G., 1977, « **Zur Frage der Unspezifischen Sarkomenststehung um Al2O3-Keramischee Implantate** », *Archiv fur Orthopädische und Unfall-Chirurgie,* Vol. 90, pp. 29-40.

[9] Mittelmeier, Th., and Walter, A., 1987, « **The Influence of Prosthesis Design on Wear and Loosening Phenomena** », *CRC Critical Reviews in Biocompatibility,* Vol. 3, pp. 319.

[10] Heimke, G. and Griss, P., 1981, « **Five Years Experience with Ceramic-Metal-Composite Hip Endoprostheses II. Mechanical Evaluations and Improvements** » *Archives of Orthopaedic and Traumasurgery,* Vol. 98, pp. 165-171.

[11] Heimke, G, « **Bioinert Ceramics** », P. Vincenzini, Ed., *Ceramics in Surgery,* Elsevier Science, Amsterdam, 1983, pp. 33-47.

[12] Heimke, G., « **Biomechanically Controlled Tissue Reactions** », H. Oonishi, H. Aoki, Sawai, Ed., *Bioceramics 1,* Proceedings of the 1st International Symposium on Ceramics in Medicine, Kyoto, Japan, 1989, pp. 213-218.

[13] Pizzoferrato, A., Vespucci, A., Ciapetti, G., and al, 1987, « **The Effect of Injection of Powdered Biomaterials on Mouse Peritoneal Cell Populations** », *Journal of Biomedical Materials Research.*, Vol. 21, No. 4, pp. 419-428.

[14] Pizzoferrato, A., Cenni, E., Ciapetti, G., Savarino, L. and Stea, S., « **In Vitro Cytocompatibility and Tissue Reaction to Ceramics** », A. Ravigliolі, A. Krajewski, Ed., *Bioceramics and the human body*, Elsevier, The Netherlands, 1992, pp. 288-291.

[15] Böhler, M., Mayr, G., Goria, O., Frzank, E., Mühlbauer, M., Salzer, M. « **Ergenisse mit der Keramik-Kezramik Gleitpaarung in der Hüftendoprothetik** », *Proceedings CERASIV Symposium,* Stuttgart, March 1996, pp.33-38.

[16] Shikita, K., Oonishi, H., 1983, « **Alumina Ceramics Artificial Hip Joint Orthopaedic Surgery** », *Orthopaedic Surgery*, Vol. 3, pp. 263-279.

[17] Griss, P., Von Andrian-Werburg, H., Krempien, B., and Heimke, G, 1973, « **Biological Activity and Histocompatibility of Dense Al2O/MgO Ceramic Implants in Rats** », *Journal of Biomedical Materials Research Symposium.*, Vol. 4, pp. 453-462.

[18] Witvoet, J., Darman, Z., Christel, P., Fumery, P., 1993, « **Arthroplastie Totale de la Hanche avec Anneau Cotyloïdien en Titane Vissé** », *Revue de Chirurgie Orthopdique.*, Vol. 79, pp.484-489.

[19] Clarke, I.C., and Willmann, G., 1994, « **Structural Ceramics in Orthopedics** », Cameron, Ed., *Bone Implant Interface*, Mosby, 1994, pp. 203-252.

[20] Christel, P., Dorlot, J.M., and Meunier, A., 1989, « **On the Specifications for the Use of Bioinert Ceramics in THR** », *Bioceramics*, Vol.1, pp. 266-271.

[21] Christel, P., 1992, « **Biocompatibility of Surgical-Grade Sense Polycrystalline Alumina** », *Clinical Orthopaedic and Related Research*, Vol. 282, pp.10-18.

[22] Harms, J., and Mäusle, E., 1979, « **Tissue Reaction to Ceramic Implant Material** », *Journal of BiomedicalMaterials Research,* Vol. 13, pp.67-87.

[23] Ryu, R.K., Edwin,,E.G., Skinner, H.B., and Murray, W.R., 216, « **Soft Tissue Sarcoma Associated with Aluminium Oxide Ceramic Total Hip Arthroplasty. A Case Report** », *Clinical Orthopaedic and Related Research,* Vol. 216, pp.207-212.

[24] Sedel, L., Simeon, J., Meunier, A., Villette, J.M., and Launey, S.M., 1992, « **Prostaglandin E2 Level in Tissue Surrounding Aseptic Failed Total Hips : Effects of Materials** », *Archives of Orthopaedic and Traumasurgery,* Vol. 111, pp. 255-258.

[25] Lerouge, S., Huk, O., Yahia, L'h., Witvoet, J., Sedel, L., 1997, « **Ceramic-Ceramic vs Metal-Polyethylene : a Comparison of Periprosthetic Tissus from Loosened Total Hip Arthroplasties** », *Journal of Bone and Joint Surgery,* Vol. 79 B,. No 1, pp. 135-139.

[26] Lerouge, S., Huk, O., Yahia, L'h., Sedel, L., 1996, « **Characterization of in Vivo Wear Debris From Ceramic-Ceramic Total Hip Arthroplasties** ». *Journal of Biomedical and Materials Research,* Vol.32, pp. 627-633.

[27] Osterholm, H.H., and Day, D.E., 1981, « **Dense Alumina Aged in Vivo** », *Journal of Biomedical Materials Research,* Vol. 15, pp. 279-288.

[28] Wu, C., Rice, R.W., Johnson, D., and Platt, B.A., 1985, « **Grain Size Dependence of Wear in Ceramics** », *Ceramic Engineering and Science Proceedings,* Vol. 6, pp. 995-1011.

[29] Zeibig, A., and Luber, H., « **Bioceramic Hip Joint Components-Industrial Production and Testing Procedures to Ensure High Functional Reliability** », P. Vincenzini Ed., *Ceramics in Surgery,* Elsevier, Amsterdam, 1983, pp. 267-275.

[30] Sinharoy, S., Levenson, I., and Day, D., 1979, « **Influence of Calcium Migration on the Strength Reduction of Dense Alumina Exposed to Steam** », *Ceramic Bulletin,* Vol. 58, No. 4, pp. 231-233.

[31] Sudanese, A., Toni, A., Catteno, G.L., Ciaroni, D., Greggi, T., Dallari, D., and al, « **Alumina vs Zirconium Oxide: a Comparative Wear Test** », H. Oonishi, H. Aoki, Sawai, Ed., *Bioceramics 1,* Proceedings of the 1st International Symposium on Ceramics in Medicine, Kyoto, Japan, 1989, pp. 237-240.

[32] Plitz, W., and Griss, P., « **Clinical, Histomorphological and Material Related Observations on Removed Alumina-Alumina Hip Joint Components »,** pp. Weinstein, Gibbons, Brown and Ruff, Ed., *Implant Retrieval: material and biological analysis,* NBS Special Publication 601, US Dept of Commerce, New York, 1981, pp. 131-156.

[33] Nizard, R., Sedel, L., Christel, P., and al, 1992, « **Ten-Year Survivorship of Cemented Ceramic-Ceramic Total Hip Prosthesis »,** *Clinical Orthopaedics and Related Research,* Vol. 282, pp. 53-63.

[34] Sedel, L., 1992, « **Ceramic Hips »,** *Editorial Journal of Bone and Joint Surgery,* Vol. 74B, pp. 331-332.

[35] Sedel, L. « **The Tribology of Hip Replacement »,** *European Instructional Course Lectures,* J. Kenwright, J. Duparc, P. Fulford Ed.,Vol. 3, 1997, pp. 25-33.

[36] Dorlot, J.M., Christel, P., and Meunier, A., 1989, « **Wear Analysis of Retrieved Alumina Heads and Sockets of Hip Prostheses »,** *Journal of Biomedical and Materials Research : Applied Biomaterials,* Vol. 23, No. A3, pp.299-310.

[37] Dorlot, J.M., 1992, « **Long-Term Effects of Alumina Components in Total Hip Prostheses »,** *Clinical Orthopaedic and Related Reseach,* Vol. 282, pp. 47-52.

[38] Mahoney, O.M., and Dimon, J.H., 1990, « **Unsatisfactory Results with a Ceramic Total Hip Prosthesis »,** *Journal of Bone and Joint Surgery,* Vol. 72A, pp. 663-671.

[39] Toni, A., Terzi, S., Sudanese, A., Tabarroni, M., Zappoli, F.A., Stea, S. Giunti, A., 1995, « **The Use of Ceramic in Prosthetic Hip Surgery. The State of the Art »,** *Chirurgia Degli Organi di Movimento,* No. LXXX, pp. 125-137.

[40] Riska, E.B., 1993, «**Ceramic Endoprosthesis in Total Hip Arthroplasty »** *Clinical Orthopaedics,* 297, pp.87-94

[41] Ivory, J.P., Kershaw, C.J., Choudry, R., Parmar, H., Stoyle, T.F., 1994, « **Autophor, Cementless Total Hip Arthroplasty for Osteoarthrosis Secondary to congenital hip dysplasia »,** *The Journal of Arthroplasty,* Vol 9, No. 4, pp. 427-433.

[42] Garcia-Cimbrelo, E., Sayanes, J.M., Minuesa, A., Munuera, L., Mittlemeier, Th., 1996, « **Ceramic-Ceramic Prosthesis after 10 Years** », *The Journal of Arthroplasty* Vol 11, No. 7, 773-781.

[43] Huo, M.H., Martin, R.P., Zatorski, L.E., Keggi, K.J., 1996, « **Total Hip Replacements Using the Ceramic Mittlemeier Prosthesis** », *Clinical Orthopaedic and Related Research*, Vol.332, pp. 143-150.

[44] Sedel, L., Kerboull, L., Christel, P., Meunier, A., Witvoet, J. 1990, « **Alumina-on-Alumina Hip Replacement : Results and Survivorship in Young Patients** », *Journal of Bone and Joint Surgery,* Vol.72-B, n° 4, pp. 658-663.

[45] Sedel, L., Nizard, R., Kerboull, L., and Witwoet, J., 1994, « **Alumina-Alumina Hip Replacement in Patients Younger Than 50 Years Old** », *Clinical Orthopaedics and Related Research,* Vol. 298, pp. 175-183.

[46] Heck, D.A., Partridge, C.M., Reuben, J.D., Lanzer, W.L., Lewis, C.G., Keating, E.M., 1995, « **Prosthetic Component Failures in Hip Arthroplasty Surgery** », *The Journal of Arthroplasty*, Vol.10, No. 5, pp. 575-580.

Spiro J. Megremis[1], Steven Duray[2], and Jeremy L. Gilbert[1]

SELF-REINFORCED COMPOSITE POLYETHYLENE (SRC-PE): A NOVEL MATERIAL FOR ORTHOPEDIC APPLICATIONS

REFERENCE: Megremis, S. J., Duray, S., and Gilbert, J. L., **"Self-Reinforced Composite Polyethylene (SRC-PE): A Novel Material for Orthopedic Applications,"** *Alternative Bearing Surfaces in Total Joint Replacement, ASTM STP 1346,* J. J. Jacobs and T. L. Craig, Eds., American Society for Testing and Materials, 1998.

ABSTRACT: An approach to fabricating high fiber volume fraction UHMWPE composites where the reinforcing phase and the matrix phase are of identical composition, and the matrix derives directly from the fiber is characterized. The processing method utilizes a hot compaction technique. During hot compaction, UHMWPE fibers are heated in a constrained mold under pressure to allow diffusion bonding of adjacent fibers. Thus, a composite results where the matrix comes from the fibers; however, the fibers themselves retain much of their original mechanical properties. This material is referred to as self-reinforced composite polyethylene (SCR-PE). Preliminary processing methods are described, and the morphology of the unidirectional SRC-PE composites are examined along with their thermal and mechanical properties. SEM micrographs of etched cross-sections of the composites exhibit fully consolidated specimens in which the fibers are still easily distinguishable and areas of fiber-fiber bonding are revealed. DSC plots show that the composites have very similar thermal properties to the original fibers. The composites also exhibit substantial unidirectional strength in the fiber direction with an approximately ten fold increase in modulus (9.99 ± 1.06 GPa) and strength (506 ± 139 MPa) in tension as compared to reference UHMWPE. However, wide variations in mechanical properties with the type of loading (tension, compression, or bending) were observed. For instance, when compression tests were performed in the fiber direction, the unidirectional specimens exhibited low modulus (1.74 ± 0.46 GPa) and strength (33.8 ± 4.8 MPa), relative to tension and bending, which may be beneficial in orthopedic load bearing applications by allowing for more

---

[1]Research Fellow and Associate Professor, respectively, Division of Biological Materials, Northwestern University, Chicago, IL 60611.

[2]Research Scientist, Bisco Inc., Schaumburg, IL 60193.

deformation during contact resulting in a lowering of contact stresses. However, the high tensile and bending strengths in the fiber direction can be advantageous in providing resistance to microfracture events associated with debris generation.

KEYWORDS: self-reinforced composite, UHMWPE, UHMWPE fibers, reference UHMWPE, hot compaction, DSC, mechanical properties

---

Introduction

Ultra-high-molecular-weight polyethylene (UHMWPE) has been used as a bearing material in total joint arthroplasty for almost forty years. Its superior frictional properties and excellent wear properties have made it the most acceptable polymer for orthopedic wear applications to date. However, even with the recognized success rate of this material, wear of UHMWPE, particularly the generated submicron wear debris, has been identified as a primary materials based complication of total joint prostheses [*1-6*].

In recent years there have been many studies investigating the deleterious effects of UHMWPE debris, such as its association with particulate-based osteolysis [*7-15*]. Therefore, even though UHMWPE is an excellent wear material, the byproducts of the inevitable wear process have been a cause for concern. This has prompted a search for alternative bearing surfaces that reduce the overall burden of particulate debris present in local tissues.

One approach which has received some attention is composites made with UHMWPE as the matrix. For instance, carbon fiber reinforced UHMWPE was introduced into the orthopedic market in an attempt to reduce creep and increase the strength of UHMWPE used in load bearing applications. However, it was soon discovered that the composite had poor wear characteristics [*16*]. Furthermore, it was also observed that the fatigue crack propagation resistance of the composite was significantly worse than that of bulk UHMWPE. This was attributed in part to inferior adhesion between the UHMWPE matrix and the carbon fibers [*17*].

More recently, composites which were not developed with medical devices in mind have been fabricated in which both the matrix and the reinforcing fibers are made of polyethylene. Generally, the principle behind the formation of these composites is that the polyethylene matrix is able to be recrystallized from the melt state onto the reinforcing fibers. This requires that the melting points of the matrix and the reinforcing fibers be different. This can be achieved by using polyethylenes of different types: low density, high density, and UHMWPE. For example, a polyethylene composite composed of high density polyethylene, with a melting point that ranges from about 130 to 137°C, and UHMWPE fiber, with a melting point of approximately 147°C, can be melt processed without any melting of the UHMWPE fibers [*18*]. Composites such as these have been fabricated by Teishev et al. and Ajji et al. [*19,20*].

It has also been shown that composites can be fabricated in which both the fibers and matrix consist of UHMWPE. For example, in 1992, Zachariades patented a method of producing a composite structure of UHMWPE in which a UHMWPE "pseudo-gel"matrix is applied onto UHMWPE fibers [*18*]. Furthermore, Shalaby and Deng have published work on a composite (developed for medical use) comprised of a low volume fraction of UHMWPE reinforcing fibers in a matrix of bulk UHMWPE. This is accomplished by first melting virgin UHMWPE powder and then pressing it into films. When the film is reheated, its melting temperature is about 10°C less than the virgin powder and, consequently, the fibers. Therefore, the film can be heated to its melting point and made to flow around the fibers without melting the fibers themselves [*16,21*].

The current paper presents an approach to fabricating high fiber volume fraction UHMWPE composites where the reinforcing phase and the matrix phase are of identical composition, and the matrix derives directly from the fibers. The processing method utilizes a hot compaction technique. During hot compaction, UHMWPE fibers are heated in a constrained mold under pressure to allow diffusion bonding of adjacent fibers. Thus, a composite results where the matrix comes from the fibers; however, the fibers themselves retain much of their original mechanical properties. This material is referred to as self-reinforced composite polyethylene (SRC-PE). Researchers at the University of Leeds have also been working on the hot compaction of high-modulus melt-spun polyethylene fibers [*22-26*]. And Harpell et al. have patented a processing method that entails consolidating UHMWPE fibers into a film [*27*].

This paper presents the initial results from an effort to produce high fiber volume fraction SRC-PE materials, where the matrix is derived directly from the UHMWPE fibers themselves. Preliminary processing methods, material structure, thermal properties, and mechanical properties are presented.

Experimental Procedure

UHMWPE fibers (Spectra 900, Allied Signal Inc., Petersburg, VA) were used in this study and were made using a gel-spinning technique. These fibers have a nominal weight average molecular weight of 1 to 5 million g/mole and a specific gravity of 0.97 [*28*].

Typically, the manufacturing process of the SRC-PE composites is comprised of the following steps. The UHMWPE fibers are wrapped around a "C" shaped frame. Anywhere from 100 to 200 wraps are made around the frame, resulting in 200 to 400 unidirectionally aligned strands of fibers (there are 118 filaments in a strand). The fibers are then placed in an aluminum channel mold with three sides fixed to constrain the fibers from deforming macroscopically in those directions. An aluminum bar is then applied so that only the fiber ends are unconstrained. The mold is then placed in a spring loaded press, and the desired pressure is applied (see Fig. 1). The entire press with the mold is then inserted into a furnace, set at the required temperature (ranging between 145°C and 155°C, see Table 1), and heated for an appropriate amount of time. At the end of this

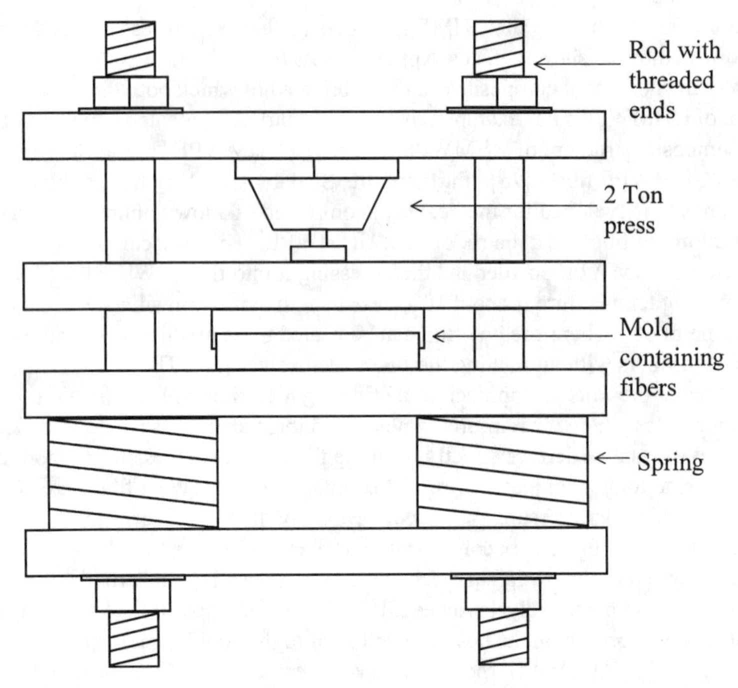

FIG. 1--*UHMWPE fiber mold and spring loaded press assembly.*

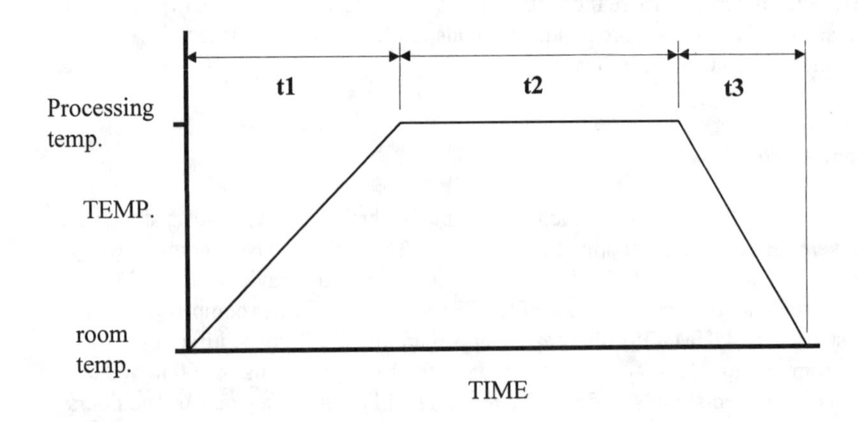

FIG. 2--*Temperature versus time curve (pressure is constant) representing the heating process for the UHMWPE fibers.*

time, the press assembly is removed from the furnace and allowed to air cool to around room temperature. The mold is then removed from the press, and the composite withdrawn from the mold. During this process, the temperature of the fibers is monitored directly using a thermocouple placed into the unconstrained end of the fibers. Therefore, the actual fiber temperature can be well controlled and monitored. The dimensions of the resulting composites are approximately 1.6 x 4.4 x 0.25 cm.

When the mold assembly is placed in the oven, it and the oven are approximately at room temperature. The assembly is then slowly heated to the desired processing temperature so that the temperatures of the press, mold, and fibers have time to equilibrate. Therefore, the temperature versus time curve of the heating process resembles Fig. 2. In this figure, **t1** is the time required to reach the desired processing temperature (note that much of this time can be attributed to heating the spring loaded press of Fig. 1 from room temperature to processing temperature); **t2** is the amount of time that the sample remains at the desired processing temperature; and **t3** is the time needed to air cool to approximately room temperature. Table 1 lists the processing variables for some of the composites used to assess structural and thermal properties. Note that sample 5 was processed such that discrete recrystallization fronts developed from the unconstrained ends of the mold toward the middle. The recrystallization fronts proceeded about one third of the way into the constrained area of the mold from each end; therefore, the final sample consisted of about two thirds recrystallized material and one third fiber/matrix composite. It is not entirely clear while sample 5 exhibited a recrystallization front. However, possible reasons for this phenomenon include the existence of pressure and temperature gradients along the length of the sample (see Discussion section). It is interesting to note that even though the results of sample 5 were not the desired ones, a composite that is comprised of regions possessing different material properties could have some interesting applications.

TABLE 1--*Processing parameters for SRC-PE composites.*

Sample #	Pressure (MPa)	**t1**	**t2**	Temp. range at T2 (°C)	Max. Temp. (°C)
1	21.8	6 hrs	17 hrs 7 min	145 -148	148.4
2	21.8	3 hrs 24 min	2 hrs	149 -150	150.2
3	21.8	4 hrs 6 min	1 hr 1min	150 - 154.9	154.9
4	21.8	6 hrs 16 min	1 hr 22 min	148 - 149	149.2
5	21.8	2 hrs 45 min	1 hr 10 min	153 - 154	154.2

In order to evaluate the microstructure of the SRC-PE composites in Table 1, an etching technique similar to that used by Olley et al. [*24*] was used on samples sectioned using an Isomet low speed saw (Buehler Inc.) with a diamond blade. The etchant consisted of the following ingredients: 1% wt/vol potassium permanganate, 10 volumes sulfuric acid (Analar grade-minimum 98%), 4 volumes phosphoric acid (approximately

92%), and 1 volume water. The potassium permanganate was added to the sulfuric acid mixture while rapidly mixing the solution using a magnetic stirrer. The samples were left in the mixture for approximately four hours while being continuously stirred. The samples were then rinsed in successive washes of chilled sulfuric acid, hydrogen peroxide, distilled water, and acetone as described by Olley and Bassett [*29*]. After etching, the samples were sputter coated with gold for examination in a scanning electron microscope (SEM). Samples that were sectioned both transverse and longitudinal to the fiber direction were evaluated.

The melting behavior of the SRC-PE composites in Table 1 was evaluated using differential scanning calorimetry (Perkin Elmer DSC-2 differential scanning calorimeter, Norwalk, Conn.), DSC, in accordance with ASTM Test Method for Transition Temperatures of Polymers by Thermal Analysis (D-3418) guidelines. The DSC was calibrated using indium and lead samples. All DSC scans were performed in argon at atmospheric pressure. Samples weighing 5 to 10 mg (except when noted otherwise) were heated at a rate of 10°C/min over a temperature range of 50 to 200°C for all tests. A cooling rate of 80°C/min was used for specimens that were scanned more than once. The melt transition temperatures as well as the peak melting temperatures were determined from all DSC scans. Furthermore, for comparison with the SRC-PE composites, DSC scans of both constrained and unconstrained UHMWPE fibers were performed. Fibers were constrained by either tying them in knots or laying them over the sides of the aluminum pans and then crimping them, with the excess fibers extending out of the crimped pans being trimmed. Unconstrained fibers were fibers that were rolled into balls and then placed in the middle of the aluminum pans.

Early processing of the SRC-PE composites was not as well controlled in pressure or temperature as those in Table 1. Initially, a minimal amount of pressure was applied to the fibers, just enough to prevent them from shrinking. The pressure was applied using "C" clamps instead of the spring loaded press of Fig. 1. Furthermore, temperatures were monitored by a thermometer at the front of the oven instead of a thermocouple placed directly in the fibers. Therefore, the recorded processing temperatures, which ranged from approximately 166 to 172°C, are not indicative of the processing temperatures of Table 1. The processing times, which ranged from approximately 39 to 45 minutes, are also not characteristic of those listed in Table 1. This is because the fiber-filled mold and "C" clamps were placed in the oven with the oven already at the desired processing temperature. Furthermore, the "C" clamps were not nearly as massive as the spring loaded press and, therefore, did not require the same amount of time to heat up. Nevertheless, some of these composites were well consolidated and were used for preliminary mechanical property assessment. Mechanical properties were measured using three point bending, compression, and tension testing.

Three-point flexural tests were performed on an electrohydraulic mechanical test system (Instron, Model 1350, Canton, MA). Samples with nominal dimensions of 4 x 1.275 x 0.23 cm were loaded at a nominal cross-head speed of 0.94 mm/min in air at room temperature. The unidirectional test specimens were tested such that stresses were developed in the fiber direction. The maximum outer fiber stress and the flexural modulus were determined according to the following equations:

$$\sigma = \frac{3Pl}{2bh^2} \qquad (1)$$

$$E = \frac{\sigma}{\varepsilon} = \frac{Pl^3}{4bh^3\delta} \qquad (2)$$

where P = load, l = span length between the lower supports, b = sample width, h = sample thickness, ε = the outer fiber strain, and δ= the mid-span deflection.

The compressive and tensile tests were performed on a screw-driven mechanical test system (Instron, Model 1114). A cross-head speed of 0.508 mm/min was used for both the compression and tension tests. The unidirectional SRC-PE specimens were stressed in the fiber direction for both sets of tests, and the stress at failure and modulus of elasticity were calculated for all of the specimens tested. The nominal dimensions of the compression samples were 2 x 2 x 5 mm; and the nominal dimensions of the gage section of the tensile specimens were 3.3 x 2.2 x 30 mm. Note that the tensile specimens were difficult to grip and tended to fracture (split longitudinally) in the grip section.

For comparison purposes, this paper includes data from the Hospital for Special Surgery, Poly Hi Solidur, Hoechst Celanese reference UHMWPE material (reference # MB948-1459) [*30*]. The resin used in this material is 4150 UHMWPE powder (lot 8544858) that was then ram extruded. The material was used to perform DSC tests for comparison with the SRC-PE composites. Also, the material properties provided by the Hospital for Special Surgery were used for mechanical property comparisons [*30*].

Results

Morphology

Figures 3a and 3b show SEM micrographs at two different magnifications of a segment of sample 1 that was sectioned transverse to the fiber direction and etched. It can be seen from these figures that substantial deformation of the fibers has taken place. The fibers are polygonal in shape instead of their original circular form. For the most part, distinct boundaries are visible between the misshapen fibers, suggesting that substantial melting of the surface of the fibers has not occurred.

Figures 4a-c show a series of SEM micrographs at progressively higher magnifications of a segment of sample 2 that was again sectioned transverse to the fiber direction. It can also be seen in these figures that the fibers are polygonal in shape. Figure 4c details the boundaries between some adjacent fibers. It can be seen that the boundaries between the fibers are not as distinct as those from sample 1. It can also be observed that in certain areas the boundary between the fibers seems to have disappeared. In these areas it appears that the fibers have been diffusion bonded together.

Figure 5a shows a cross-section of sample 3 parallel to the fiber direction. Notice that there is not a continuous bead of melt between fibers. Instead, the surfaces of adjacent fibers seem to preferentially melt together at certain locations, appearing similar to spot welds. Figure 5b, a higher magnification of Figure 5a, shows the bonding which takes place at these fiber-fiber junctions in greater detail. Interdiffusion and entanglement of adjacent polymer is taking place across fiber boundaries.

Figure 6 is a cross-section of the recrystallized area of sample 5. It was sectioned perpendicular to the axes of the original fibers. The original structure of the fibers is no longer present. However, recrystallized lamella are clearly visible. Even though the lamellar regions are not of the same dimensions as the original fibers, it can be seen that recrystallization occurs such that structure from the prior fiber boundaries is still present.

DSC Results

In this paper, the transition temperature (or melting onset temperature) is defined as the intersection of the extrapolated lines of both the DSC baseline and the leading edge of the DSC endotherm. Furthermore, all temperatures that are presented in this paper are the average of three or more DSC runs.

Figure 7 shows typical DSC melting endotherms for UHMWPE fiber. It can be seen from this figure that the fiber produces three different DSC curves. Table 2 summarizes the peak and onset melting temperatures of these three curves and the conditions under which they were obtained. As stated in the procedure section, the fibers were tested either in a constrained or unconstrained state. It was discovered that whether or not the fibers were constrained did indeed influence the resulting DSC curves. As shown in Fig. 7, the plot of the constrained fibers exhibits three distinct melting peaks, whereas the plot of the unconstrained fibers exhibits four discrete melting peaks. It was also discovered during testing that the mass of the sample tested, likewise, had an effect on the resulting DSC plot. For samples with masses ranging from 4.8 to 6.1 mg, the DSC plots exhibited only two distinct melting peaks regardless of whether the fibers were constrained or unconstrained, as exemplified in Fig. 7. Note that the method of constraint did not appear to influence the results.

TABLE 2: *Peak and onset melting temperatures for curves of Fig. 7 and the conditions under which they were obtained. The temperatures quoted are avg. ± standard deviation.*

DSC Curve	Type of fiber sample	Sample Mass (mg)	Transition Temp. (°C)	Peak 1 (°C)	Peak 2 (°C)	Peak 3 (°C)	Peak 4 (°C)
A	constrained	0.7 - 1.9	142.3 ± 0.4	144.6 ± 0.5	NA	153.8 ± 0.2	156.7 ± 0.2
B	unconstr.	1.1 - 2.2	142.7 ± 0.4	144.5 ± 0.5	147.3 ± 0.6	153.8 ± 0.3	156.8 ± 0.2
C	both	4.8 - 6.1	142.7 ± 0.3	NA	147.7 ± 0.7	NA	156.8 ± 1.2

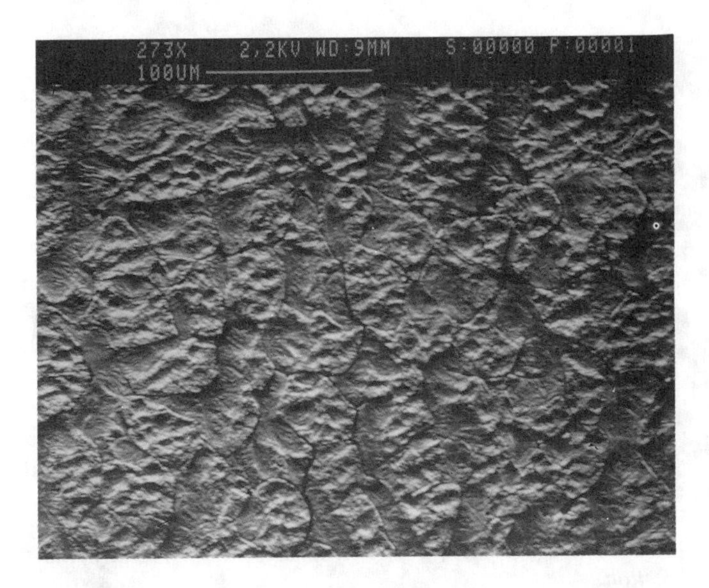

FIG. 3a--*SEM micrograph of a segment of sample 1 that was sectioned transverse to the fiber direction and etched showing the polygonal shape of the fibers.*

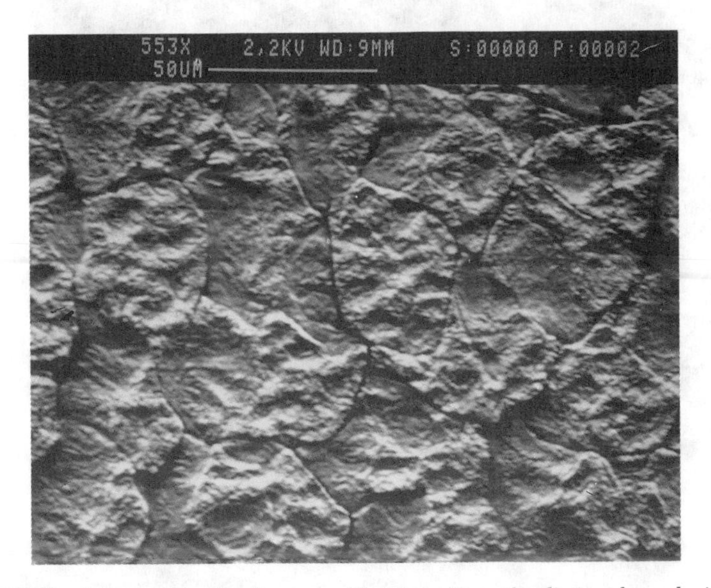

FIG. 3b--*Sample 1 at a higher magnification. Note the distinct boundaries between the misshapen fibers.*

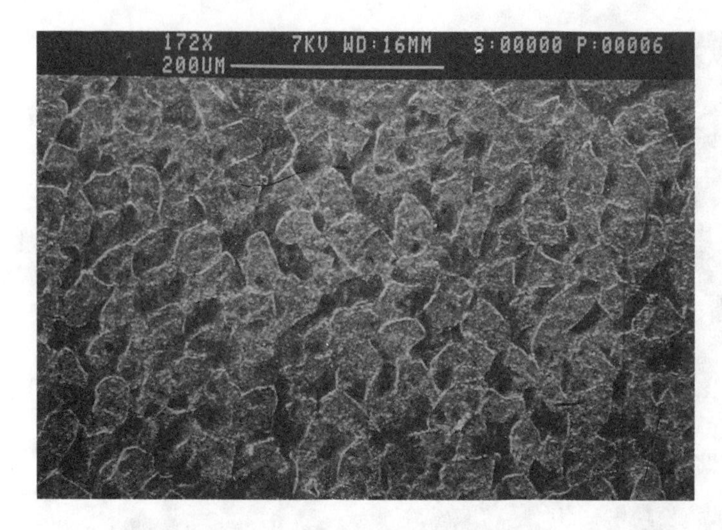

FIG. 4a-- *SEM micrograph of a section of sample 2 transverse to the fiber direction.*

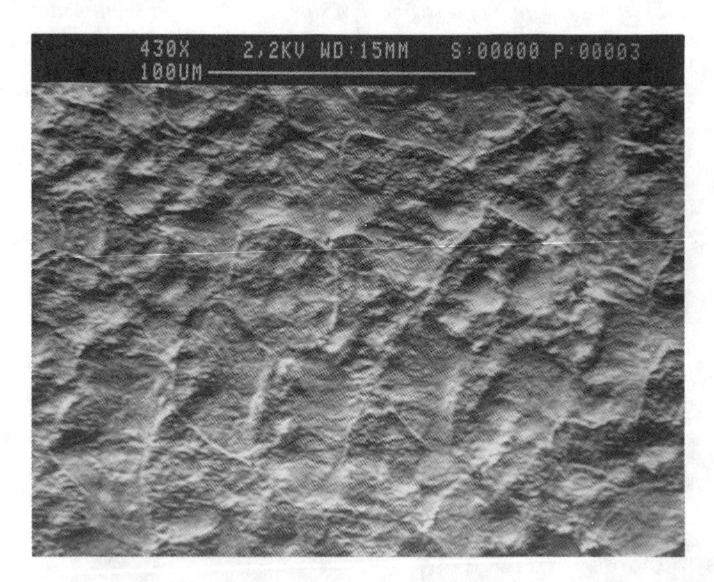

FIG. 4b--*SEM micrograph of sample 2 at higher magnification. Note the tight junctions between fibers.*

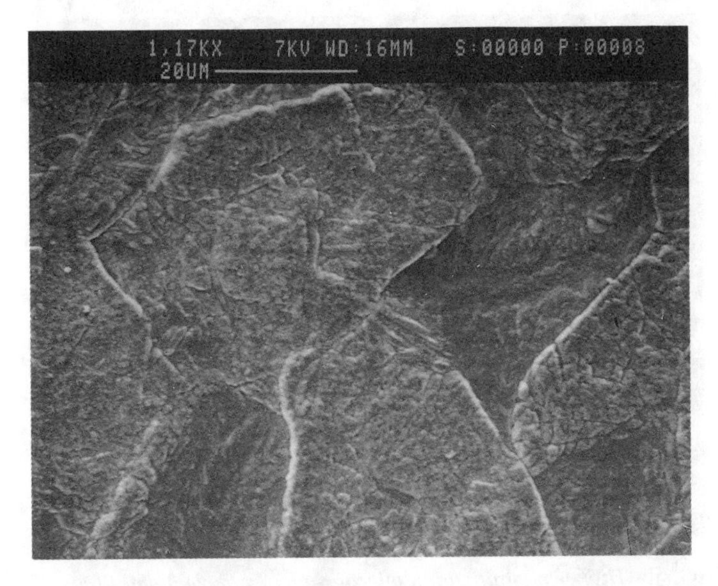

FIG. 4c--*Detail of the boundaries between adjacent fibers of sample 2. There is a lack of substantial amounts of melt between fibers and in certain areas the boundary between the fibers seems to have disappeared.*

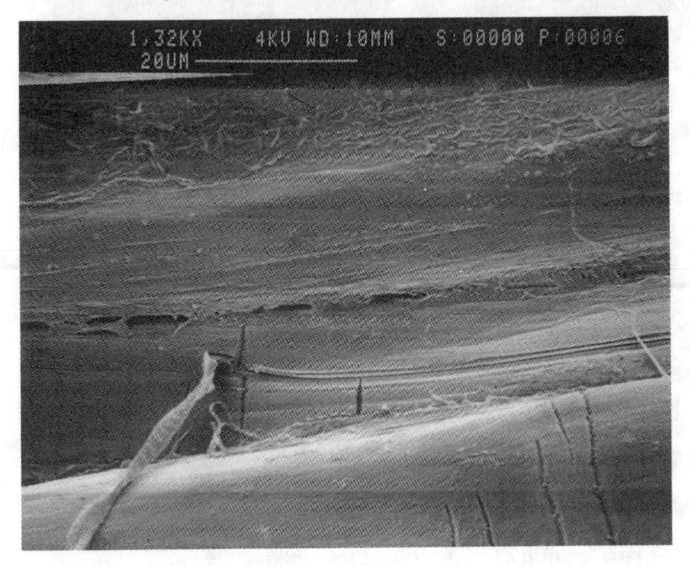

FIG. 5a--*Cross-section of sample 3 parallel to the fiber direction.*

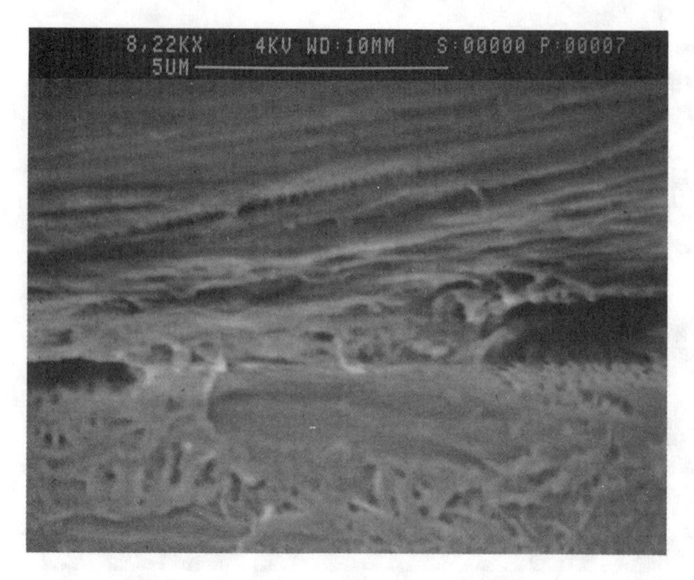

FIG. 5b--*Higher magnification micrograph of sample 3 detailing a fiber-fiber junction.*

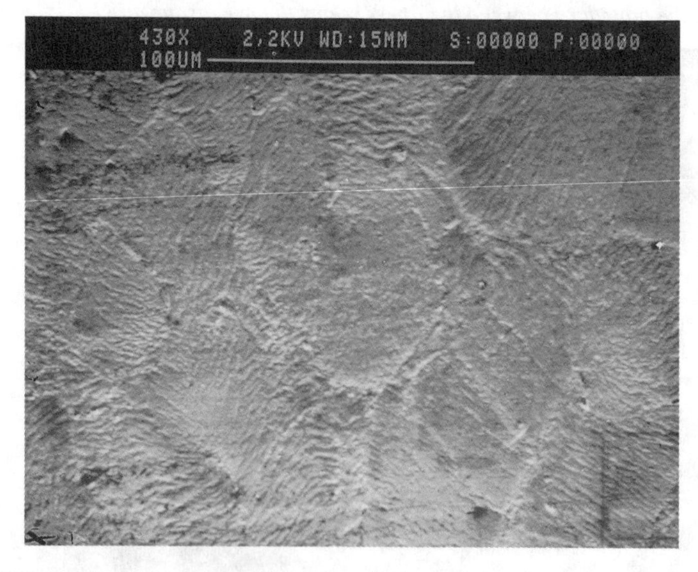

FIG. 6--*Cross-section of the recrystallized area of sample 5. Note the the clearly visible lamellar regions.*

Figure 7 also shows a typical DSC melting endotherm for the second scans, or remelts, of the UHMWPE fiber. The one remelt curve is typical of the remelt curves of all three of the different DSC curves for the fiber. It can be seen that the remelt curve contains only a single melting endotherm at a much lower temperature (ca. 133°C) than any of the melting endotherms from the original scans.

Figure 8 contains a DSC plot of an SRC-PE composite along with DSC plots of the UHMWPE fiber and the UHMWPE reference material. Note that the DSC plots of samples 1 through 4 all had similar melt characteristics; therefore, the DSC run illustrated in Fig. 8 is typical of all of the SRC-PE composites, except for sample 5. Because sample 5 was multiphased, the melt characteristics of the sample were dependent on where on the sample the DSC specimens were retrieved. Further note that the DSC plot of the fiber in Fig. 8 is typical of curve B of Fig. 7. This curve was chosen for comparison because it contains all four of the melting peaks of Table 2.

It can be seen that both the transition temperature and the peak melting temperature of the reference material are much lower than those for the SRC-PE composite and the UHMWPE fiber. However, the melting peak of the SRC-PE composite (ca. 148°C) corresponds well with peak 2 of Table 2. Furthermore, the transition temperature (ca. 143 - 144°C) of the SRC-PE composite compares well with the transition temperatures listed in Table 2.

Figure 9 contains a DSC plot of the UHMWPE reference material along with the DSC plot of the recrystallized region of sample 5. It can be seen from the figure that both the transition temperatures (ca. 128°C) and peak melting temperatures (ca. 138°C) coincide. This indicates that a phase transition has taken place within the UHMWPE fibers that is more representative of bulk UHMWPE.

Figure 10 shows typical DSC runs of the second scans of the SRC-PE composites, the UHMWPE fibers, and the reference material. It can be seen that the DSC plots of all three materials are very similar. Furthermore, the peak melting temperature for all three materials is approximately 133-134°C.

Mechanical Property Results

The results of the mechanical tests are shown in Table 3. As stated previously, the SRC-PE composites on which the mechanical tests were performed were some of the first composites produced and, therefore, not the most optimal. However, in tensile properties alone, it can be observed from Table 3 that the SRC-PE composites exhibit greatly enhanced strength over the reference UHMWPE.

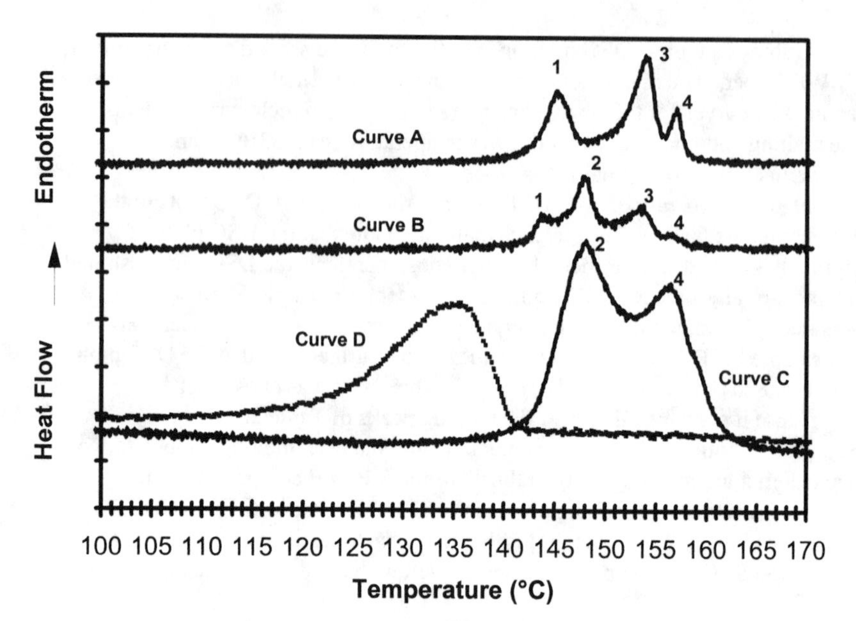

FIG. 7--DSC melting endotherms of unconstrained UHMWPE fiber (curve A), constrained UHMWPE fiber (curve B), large mass samples of constrained and unconstrained UHMWPE fiber (curve C), and rescanned UHMWPE fiber of curve C (curve D). See Table 2 for further explanation of curves A-D.

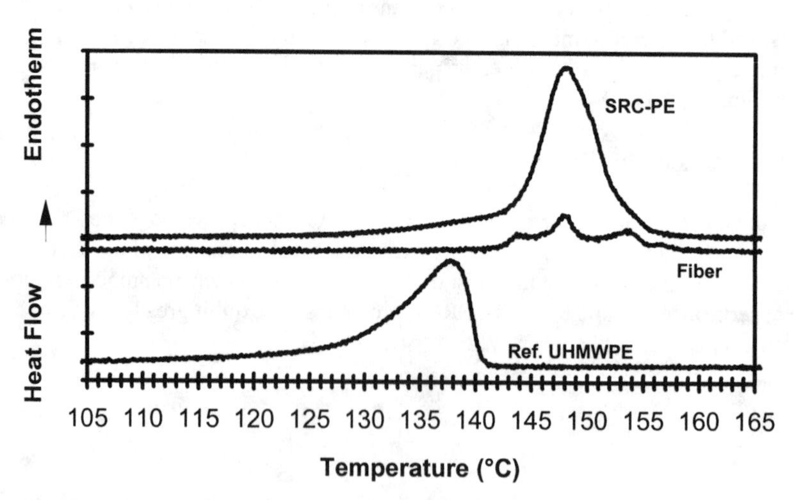

FIG. 8--DSC melting endotherms of an SRC-PE composite, UHMWPE fiber, and UHMWPE reference material.

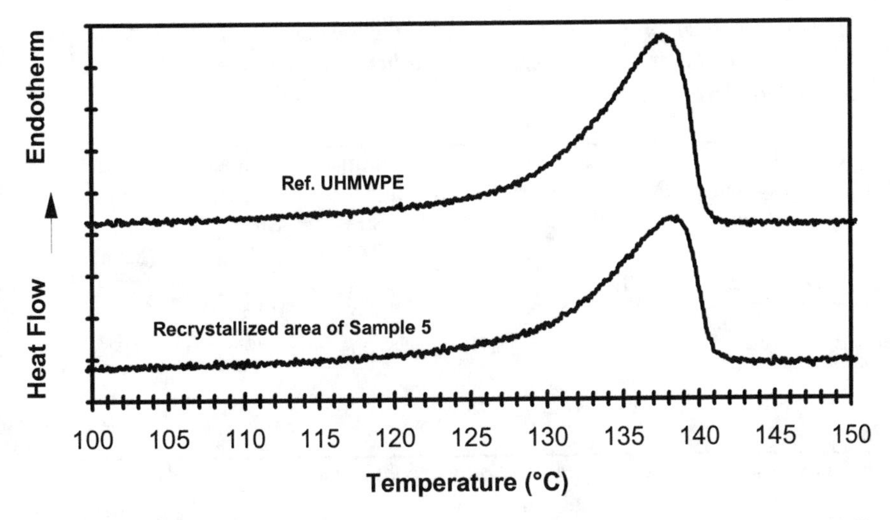

FIG. 9--DSC melting endotherms of UHMWPE reference material and recrystallized area of sample 5.

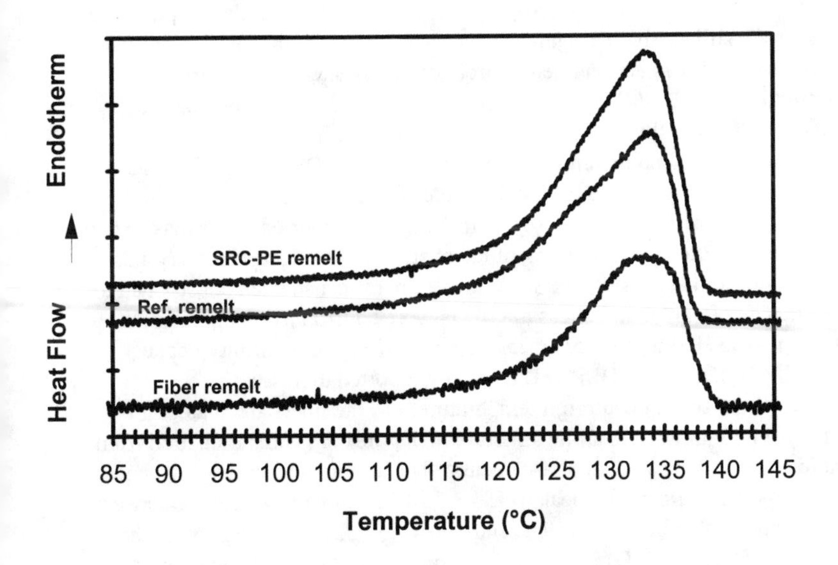

FIG. 10--DSC melting endotherms of the second scans of an SRC-PE composite, UHMWPE fiber, and reference UHMWPE.

TABLE 3--*Mechanical properties for SRC-PE, the reference UHMWPE, and the UHMWPE fiber. NR stands for not reported in the literature, and the numbers quoted are avg. ± standard deviation.*

Sample Type	Flexural Modulus (GPa)	Tensile Modulus (GPa)	Compress. Modulus (GPa)	Ultimate Flexural Stress (MPa)	Ultimate Tensile Stress* (MPa)	Ultimate Compress. Stress (MPa)
SRC-PE	10.5 ± 3.4	9.99 ± 1.06	1.74 ± 0.46	105 ± 9	506 ± 139	33.8 ± 4.8
Ref. PE [*30*]	NR	0.916 ± 0.076	NR	NR	49 ± 1.7	NR
Fiber [*28*]	NR	NR	NR	NR	2586	NR

**Ultimate tensile stress is stress in gage section when failure in grip occurred*

Discussion

The fabrication of self-reinforced composites of UHMWPE has been successfully accomplished in this study. The SEM micrographs exhibit fully consolidated specimens in which the fibers are still easily distinguishable. Also, enough of the mechanical properties of the original fibers are retained to produce composites with superior mechanical strength to bulk UHMWPE. Furthermore, the DSC plots show that the composites have very similar thermal properties to the original fibers.

Many other interesting phenomenon were observed from the DSC plots. The multiple endothermic peaks of the DSC curves of Fig. 7 are consistent with literature [*20,21,31,32*]. Peak 1 corresponds to the 145°C melting peak reported by Tsubakihara et al. [*31*], which they attributed to the melting of unconstrained extended-chain crystals. The researchers achieved these results on Spectra 900 fiber that had been constrained to varying amounts. They found that the less the fibers were constrained the greater the latent heat of the peak [*31*]. Furthermore, peaks 3 and 4 of Fig. 7 are also typical of published research [*31,32*]. The UHMWPE fibers are reported to possess an orthorhombic crystalline structure at room temperature. As the fibers are heated, it is believed that the orthorhombic crystalline structure melts (peak 3) and a transition from an orthorhombic phase to a hexagonal phase occurs. Then, upon further heating, the hexagonal crystalline structure melts (peak 4) [*31,32*]. Literature places peak 3 between 150°C and 155°C and peak 4 between 159°C and 160°C [*31,32*]. The single endothermic peak of the remelted fiber (curve D) is also well documented [*23,31,32*] and coincides well with the reported melting peak (ca. 131°C) for folded-chain crystals [*31*].

The difference between curves A and B and curve C may be due to the fact that DSC curves are the summation of all thermal events at each given time (temperature). Therefore, if two different thermal events are occurring simultaneously, one event may mask the other. The amount of heat generated (size of the endotherm) by a sample is dependent on its mass. Thus, the larger the endotherm the less the overall peak may be affected by individual thermal events. Performing the DSC runs for the larger mass samples at lower scan rates may resolve the larger peaks more effectively.

Research by Hsieh and Ju [*32*] reinforces the notion that the mass of the fibers may affect the resulting DSC curve. The researchers observed only two peaks, one at 150°C and another at 160°C, on their DSC curves when using 3.5 to 4 mg of Spectra 1000 fibers wound into small loops and placed at the bottom of aluminum sample pans. Note that the authors used a slower heating rate of 5°C/min and still only observed two peaks. Furthermore, Deng and Shalaby observed two peaks (about 146 and 153°C) when scanning 4 mg samples of Spectra 1000 fiber at 10°C/min [*21*]. Likewise, Ajji et al. reported two peaks when scanning Spectra 1000 fiber at 10°C/min [*20*]. Since the above mentioned studies all used Spectra 1000 fibers and Tsubakihara et al. [*31*] and the current study used Spectra 900 fibers, it is possible that a difference exists between the thermal properties of Spectra 900 and Spectra 1000 fibers.

The fact that peak 2 of curve B of Fig. 7 does not appear in curve A implies that constraining the fibers does affect their melting behavior. Furthermore, it does not seem that the mass of the samples is a factor in the difference between these two curves, since the masses used to generate each of the curves are similar in range (see Table 2).

As shown in Fig. 8, the single peak of the SRC-PE composites compares with peak 2 of Fig. 7. It is possible that peak 2 may be the melting point of the orthorhombic crystalline structure and not peak 3. The existence of the single endothermic peak of the SRC-PE composites is consistent with literature indicating the crystal transformation from an orthorhombic phase to a hexagonal phase is suppressed or eliminated by stress applied perpendicular to the fiber axis, as is the case in the preparation of the SRC-PE composites [*32*]. The origin of this peak needs to be further investigated.

In comparing the hot compacted, polyethylene fiber composites produced at the University of Leeds, the SRC-PE composites exhibit different thermal properties. The Leeds composites displayed two distinct endothermic peaks during melting [*23*]. The lower melting peak was attributed to the melting of small amounts of the original fiber during processing of the composites which upon cooling changed form into a material with a lower melting point [*23*]. The SRC-PE composite in Fig. 8 shows the semblance of a lower melting peak; however, it is minimal and not nearly as distinctive as the peaks shown in the Leeds composites. This fact coincides with the small amounts of melt surrounding the deformed fibers shown in Figs. 3 and 4 and the noncontinuous bead of melt between fibers in Fig. 5. This is in contrast to the Leeds composites which exhibit transverse sections of circular fibers surrounded by recrystallized material and longitudinal sections with continuous junctions of recrystallized material between adjacent fibers [*23-26*].

The Leeds researchers further observed fluctuations in the size of the lower melting peak with processing temperature [*23*]. This was not the case with the SRC-PE composites. As stated previously, samples 1 through 4 all exhibited similar DSC curves. Nonetheless, many of the differences in thermal properties between the Leeds composites and the SRC-PE composites can be attributed to the fact that the Leeds composites are comprised of melt-spun polyethylene fibers with a weight-average molecular weight of

150000 g/mole [*23*]; however, the SRC-PE composites are comprised of gel-spun fibers with a nominal weight-average molecular weight of 1 to 5 million g/mole.

When fabricating SRC-PE, three parameters are essential to the characteristics of the composite: time, temperature, and pressure. The optimization of these parameters is dependent on the application of the final product, which in this instance is as an orthopedic bearing surface, and is still being investigated. However, it is believed that the processing pressure of 21.8 Mpa is too high for proper consolidation of the composite. There are several observations that support this assertion.

For instance, the unconstrained fiber ends that protrude from the mold have been observed to melt into a translucent, gelatinous mass; however, when some specimens were removed from the mold, the fibers that were under pressure remained relatively distinct and not optimally consolidated. This is most likely due to the high level of constraint imposed by the pressure which inhibits polymer relaxation and motion from taking place in the interior fibers, not the fiber ends. That is, a pressure gradient exists in these samples. Note that the researchers at the University of Leeds found that too high a pressure also resulted in poor consolidation of their hot compacted, polyethylene fiber composites [*23*].

Also, with the high pressures being applied before heat, it is evident that heat transfer between the fibers is conductive in nature with no convective component. Therefore, the fibers are being heated from the transfer of heat from the metal mold to the fibers, except for the case of the unconstrained ends of the fibers, which are being heated by the ambient air in the oven. Therefore, temperature gradients may result in uneven heating of the fibers. These temperature and pressure gradients may be the source of the recrystallization front in sample 5.

Finally, samples made for mechanical testing had much lower pressures applied to them; however, these samples appeared (qualitatively) to have better fiber-fiber bonding taking place. Currently, specimens are being fabricated at different pressures and evaluated. Furthermore, there are plans of trying different methods of applying pressure, such as allowing the fibers to attain the desired processing temperature and then applying pressure.

The mechanical tests performed on preliminary SRC-PE composites revealed an approximately 10 fold increase in modulus and strength in tension (see Table 3). However, it is important to note that these SRC-PE composites were unidirectional and tested in the fiber direction. The mechanical properties of a unidirectional form of the SRC-PE composite are very dependent on the orientation of the fibers to the principal stress direction. Tests were not performed to quantitatively evaluate the mechanical properties of the composites transverse to the fiber direction, although it was apparent from qualitative tests that the transverse strength of the composites was not as good as the longitudinal strength. However, as the optimization process of the composites progresses and fiber bonding increases, the transverse strength of the composites should increase.

It is also important to note the wide variations in mechanical properties with the type of loading: tension, compression, or bending. The low modulus and strength in compression (relative to tension and bending) may be advantageous for orthopedic load bearing applications allowing for more deformation during contact and a lowering of contact stresses. However, the high tensile and bending strengths can be beneficial in providing resistance to microfracture events associated with debris generation.

The fact that a UHMWPE composite where the matrix comes from the fibers has been successfully fabricated with excellent mechanical properties is significant. However, ultimately, it is the SRC-PE composite's ability to resist wear processes that will dictate its success as an orthopedic bearing material. These tests are currently being performed.

Acknowledgments

The authors would like to thank Allied Signal Inc. for providing the UHMWPE fibers, Stephen Li for providing the Hospital for Special Surgery, Poly Hi Soldur, Hoechst Celanese Reference UHMWPE Material, and NIDR (T32 DEB7042) for their financial support of this work.

References

[*1*] McKellop, H., Campbell, P., Park, S-H., and Grigoris, P., "Morphology of UHMW Polyethylene Wear Surfaces and Debris," 198. Report presented at the 20th Annual Meeting of the Society for Biomaterials, Boston, Massachusetts, April 1994.

[*2*] McKellop, H. A., Schmalzried, T., Park, S-H., and Campbell, P., "Evidence for the Generation of Sub-Micron Polyethylene Wear Particles by Micro-Adhesive Wear in Acetabular Cups," Report presented at the 19th Annual Meeting of the Society for Biomaterials, Birmingham, Alabama, April 1993.

[*3*] Schmalzried, T. P., Jasty, M., Rosenberg, A., and Harris, W. H., "Histologic Identification of Polyethylene Wear Debris Using Oil Red O Stain," *Journal of Applied Biomaterials,* Vol. 4, 1993, pp. 119-125.

[*4*] Kobayashi, A., Bonfield, W., Kadoya, Y., Al-Saffar, N., Scott, G., Freeman, M. A. R., and Revell P. A., "Size and Shape of Particulate Polyethylene Wear Debris in Conforming Tribiofemoral Prostheses," 316. Report presented at the 21st Annual Meeting of the Society for Biomaterials, San Francisco, California, March 1995.

[*5*] Shanbhag, A. S., Rubash., H. E., Bailey, H. O., Crossett, L. C., and Herndon, J. H., "Characterization of Polyethylene Wear Debris Associated with Failed Total Knee Replacements," 328. Report presented at the 21st Annual Meeting of the Society for Biomaterials, San Francisco, California, March 1995.

[*6*] Morrey, B. F., Ed. *Biological, Material, and Mechanical Considerations of Joint Replacement*, New York: Raven Press, 1993.

[*7*] Willert, H. G. and Semlitsch, M., "Reactions of the Articular Capsule to Wear Products of Artificial Joint Prostheses," *Journal of Biomedical Materials Research,* Vol. 11, 1977, pp. 157-164.

[*8*] Bragdon, C. R., Fahmy, J. N., Jasty, M., Lowenstein, J. D., and Harris, W. H., "Role of Polyethylene Debris Migration on Osteolysis with Cementless THA," 185. Report presented at the 19th Annual Meeting of the Society for Biomaterials, Birmingham, Alabama, April 1993.

[*9*] Shanbhag, A. S., Black, J., Jacobs, J. J., Galante, J. O., and Glant, T. T., "Human Monocyte Responses to Sub-micron Titanium -6% Aluminum -4% Vanadium, Titanium and Polyethylene Particles," 79. Report presented at the 20th Annual Meeting of the Society for Biomaterials, Boston, Massachusetts, April 1994.

[*10*] Shanbhag, A. S., Jacobs, J. J., Glant, T. T., Talbert, L. F., Leigh, H. D., and Black, J., "Submicron Particulate Polyethylene and Titanium-Alloy Simulated Bone Resorptive and Fibroblast Stimulatory Activity," 242. Report presented at the 19th Annual Meeting of the Society for Biomaterials, Birmingham, Alabama, April 1993.

[*11*] Goodman, S. B., Aspenberg, P., Song, Y., Doshi, A., Regula, D., and Lidgren, L., "The Effects of Particulate Cobalt Chrome Alloy and High Density Polyethylene on Tissue Ingrowth into the Bone Harvest Chamber in Rabbits," 78. Report presented at the19th Annual Meeting of the Society for Biomaterials, Birmingham, Alabama, April 1993.

[*12*] Goodman, S. B., Knoblich, G., Song, Y., Hule, P., Regula, D., Aspenberg, P., and Lidgren, L., "Tissue Ingrowth and Differentiation in the Bone Harvest Chamber in the Presence of Polyethylene Particles," 171. Report presented at the 21st Annual Meeting of the Society for Biomaterials, San Francisco, California, March 1995.

[*13*] Goodman, S. B., Aspenberg, P., Song, Y., Doshi, A., Regula, D., and Lidgren, L., "Tissue Differentiation in the Presence of Different Concentrations of Phagocytosable Polyethylene and Titanium Alloy Particles," 169. Report presented at the 21st Annual Meeting of the Society for Biomaterials, San Francisco, California, March 1995.

[*14*] Benz, E., Sherburne, B., Hayek, J., Falchuk, K., Godleski, J. J., Sledge, C. B., and Spector, M., "Migration of Polyethylene Wear Debris to Lymph Nodes and Other Organs in Total Joint Replacement Patients," 83. Report presented at the 20th Annual Meeting of the Society for Biomaterials, Boston, Massachusetts, April 1994.

[*15*] Schmalzried, T. P., Jasty, M., Rosenberg, A., and Harris, W. H., "Polyethylene Wear Debris and Tissue Reactions in Knee as Compared to Hip Replacement Prostheses," *Journal of Applied Biomaterials,* Vol. 5, 1994, pp. 185-190.

[*16*] Shalaby, W. S. and Deng, M., World International Property Organization, International Patent WO 95/06148; Application PCT/US94/09381; International Publication Date: 2 March 1995.

[*17*] Connelly, G. M., Rimnac, C. M., Wright, T. M., Hertzberg, R. W., and Manson, J. A., "Fatigue Crack Propagation Behavior of Ultrahigh Molecular Weight Polyethylene," *Journal of Orthopaedic Research,* Vol. 2, 1984, pp. 119-125.

[*18*] Zachariades, E. A., US Patent US005160472A (1992); Application No.: 447,628; Patent Number: 5,160,472; Date of Patent: 3 November 1992.

[*19*] Teishev, A., Incardona, S., Migliaresi, C., and Marom, G., "Polyethylene Fibers-Polyethylene Matrix Composites: Preparation and Physical Properties," *Journal of Applied Polymer Science,* Vol. 50, 1993, pp. 503-512.

[*20*] Ajji, A., Ait-Kadi, A., and Rochette, A., "Polyethylene-Ultra High Modulus Polyethylene Short Fibers Composites," *Journal of Composite Materials,* Vol. 26, No. 1, 1992, pp. 121-131.

[*21*] Deng, M. and Shalaby, W. S., "Properties of Self-Reinforced Ultra-High-Molecular Weight Polyethylene Composites," *Biomaterials,* Vol. 18, No. 9, 1997, pp. 645-655.

[22] Tissington, B., Pollard, G., and Ward, I. M., "A Study of the Influence of Fibre/Resin Adhesion on the Mechanical Behavior of Ultra-High-Modulus Polyethylene Fibre Composites," *Journal of Materials Science,* Vol. 26, 1991, pp. 82-92.

[23] Hine, P. J., Ward, I. M., Olley, R. H., and Bassett, D. C., "The Hot Compaction of High Modulus Melt-Spun Polyethylene Fibres," *Journal of Materials Science*, Vol. 28, 1993, pp. 316-324.

[24] Olley, R. H., Bassett, D. C., Hine, P. J., and Ward, I. M., "Morphology of Compacted Polyethylene Fibres," *Journal of Materials Science,* Vol. 28, 1993, pp. 1107-1112.

[25] Kabeel, M. A., Bassett, D. C., Olley, R. H., Hine, P. J., and Ward, I. M., "Compaction of High-Modulus Melt-Spun Polyethylene Fibres at Temperatures Above and Below the Optimum," *Journal of Materials Science*, Vol. 29, 1994, pp. 4694-4699.

[26] Kabeel, M. A., Bassett, D. C., Olley, R. H., Hine, P. J., and Ward, I. M., "Differential Melting in Compacted High-Modulus Melt-Spun Polyethylene Fibres," *Journal of Materials Science,* Vol. 30, 1995, pp. 601-606.

[27] Harpell, A. G., Kavesh, S., Palley, I., and Prevorsek, D. C., US Patent US005135804A (1992); Application No.: 529,673; Patent Number: 5,135,804; Date of Patent: 4 August 1992.

[28] Allied Signal, Inc., *Spectra Fibers*, Morristown, N.J.

[29] Olley, R. H. and Bassett, D. C., "An Improved Permanganic Etchant for Polyolefines," *Polymer,* Vol. 23, 1982, pp. 1707-1710.

[30] Li, S., "Reference Ultra High Molecular Weight Polyethylene," Technical Report, Hospital for Special Surgery, New York, NY, 1996.

[31] Tsubakihara, S., Nakamura, A., and Yasuniwa, M., "Hexagonal Phase of Polyethylene Fibers under High Pressure," *Polymer Journal*, Vol. **23**, No. 11, 1991, pp. 1317-1324.

[32] Hsieh, Y-L. and Ju, J., "Melting Behavior of Ultra-high Modulus and Molecular Weight Polyethylene (UHMWPE) Fibers," *Journal of Applied Polymer Science*, Vol. 53, 1994, pp. 347-354.

Mohsen Mosleh[1]

AN UHMWPE HOMOCOMPOSITE FOR JOINT PROSTHESES

REFERENCE: Mohsen Mosleh, **"An UHMWPE Homocomposite for Joint Prostheses,"** *Alternative Bearing Surfaces in Total Joint Replacement, ASTM STP 1346*, J. J. Jacobs and T. L. Craig, Eds., American Society for Testing and Materials, 1998.

ABSTRACT: A homocomposite consisting of an ultra-high molecular weight polyethylene (UHMWPE) matrix and an ultra-high molecular weight polyethylene reinforcing phase is introduced. While the chemical compositions of the bulk and fibers are the same, the fibers have a higher strength and a higher melting temperature due to their high degree of molecular orientation. The homocomposite was manufactured by compression molding of randomly oriented fibers and UHMWPE resin in a mold. The molding temperature was chosen to be slightly higher than the melting temperature of the matrix but below that of the fibers. Mechanical properties of the homocomposite such as the elastic modulus, and tensile strength are improved when compared with the properties of ultra-high molecular weight polyethylene. The homocomposite also exhibits a lower friction coefficient and a significantly higher wear resistance in dry sliding which are desirable properties in bearing applications. Due to the biocompatibility of polyethylene, the homocomposite may be acceptable as a bearing material in joint prostheses pending exhibiting improved tribological behavior in lubricated and simulated wear testing.

KEYWORDS: homocomposite, UHMWPE, wear, joint prostheses

INTRODUCTION

Thermoplastic polymer-based composites consist of a polymeric matrix such as polyethylene and a reinforcement such as carbon or glass fibers. The high modulus and strength of the reinforcing component increase stiffness and strength of the composite, while the matrix provides increased toughness. The strength of the interfacial bond between the matrix and the reinforcing element is critical in determining the mechanical properties of the composite. Failure in establishing a strong interfacial bond will always prevent composites from achieving improved properties as predicted by the rule of mixture. The chemical incompatibility of the matrix and the fiber prevents bonding, and as a result debonding may occur when the composite experiences a large strain such as in frictional loading. The cyclic nature of frictional loading produces an incremental accumulation of plastic deformation in the surface and subsurface. In particular, poor fiber/matrix interfacial strength in composites subjected to frictional loading leads to the nucleation and propagation of cracks. The extension of cracks to the neighboring ones and subsequent shearing to the surface cause delamination wear [1].

Different approaches have been utilized to enhance matrix/fiber bonding, such as the use of coupling agents. A novel approach was that of Capiati, Mead, and Porter [2,3]

---

[1] Assistant Professor, Mechanical Engineering Department, Howard University, Washington, DC 20059.

to use different morphologies of the same polymer as both the matrix and the fiber in a "one polymer composite". The composite used the difference in the melting point between a high density polyethylene (HDPE) matrix and highly oriented HDPE fibers. The crystallinity of polyethylene fibers was increased due to their high orientation which resulted in a 5 to 9 $^{\circ}C$ increase in their melting point compared with that of the HDPE. Partial melting of the fibers at their outer sheath was observed when the fibers were embedded in the HDPE melts. This enhanced the interfacial bonding of the fibers to the matrix. A high interfacial shear strength of about 17 MPa was measured in pull-out tests which is greater than the bonding strength for glass fiber reinforced polyesters. Recently, Marais [4] described a manufacturing method for production of variety of PE/PE composites.

The fibers which had been used in the previous studies were produced using solid state fiber drawing, a method with a limited drawing ratio. More recent techniques such as gel/solution spinning and liquid crystal spinning can produce fibers with a much higher crystallinity [5]. For instance, UHMWPE fibers are manufactured by solution spinning with a crystallinity of about 60-85%. These fibers possess a tensile strength of 3 GPa which is comparable to aramid and S-glass fibers. UHMWPE fibers have been used with epoxy resin, but poor fiber/matrix bonding has been reported [6,7]. The poor adhesion of these fibers to different matrices have been a limiting factor in their use for composite material applications. Some modification techniques such as plasma treatment and chemical etching of ultra-high molecular weight polyethylene fibers for enhanced adhesion are reported in the literature [8,9].

The goal of this study is to produce and test composites made of UHMWPE fibers and matrix. It is hypothesized that by introducing high strength UHMWPE fibers in a UHMWPE matrix, the plastic deformation of the surface layer under cyclic frictional loading will be reduced. Also, the fibers can inhibit crack propagation in the subsurface and reduce delamination wear.

One potential application of an ultra-high molecular weight polyethylene composite is in joint prostheses as a bearing material. Currently UHMWPE is widely used in artificial hips and knees due to its good wear resistance and biocompatibility. However, although the wear rate of UHMWPE is small compared with other plastics, it is still large enough to produce many particles which elicit a biological response and ultimately cause implant failure [10]. The polyethylene homocomposite can satisfy the biocompatibility requirement and improve the mechanical and tribological properties of UHMWPE.

EXPERIMENTAL

Materials

The control material used in wear testing experiments was the extruded UHMWPE (GUR 415) whose physical properties (except for the melting point which was measured by DSC) are given by Hoechst Celanese Co. (Table 1). The control samples used in tensile and compression tests were manufactured by compression molding under 10.33 MPa pressure.

Table 1--Properties of Ram Extruded GUR 415 UHMWPE.

Property	Method	Value
Density (g/cm^3)	ASTM D1505	0.932
Melting Point (^{o}C)	DSC	138-143
Tensile Yield Strength (MPa)	ASTM D638	21
Tensile Ultimate Strength (MPa)	ASTM D638	45

The matrix that was used in the production of the homocomposite was ultra-high molecular weight polyethylene resin (GUR 415). The fibers (commercially called Spectra) are produced by solution spinning and their properties are given by Allied Signal Inc. (Table 2).

Table 2--Properties of Spectra 1000 fibers in comparison with other fibers

Property	**Fiber**		
	Spectra	Aramid (HM)	S-Glass
Density (g/cm^3)	0.97	1.44	2.49
Filament diameter (μm)	23	12	9
Tensile Modulus (GPa)	113	131	89.6
Tensile Ultimate Strength (GPa)	2.91	2.75	4.6
Elongation at Break (%)	2.9	2.5	5.4

The melting points of the fibers and the UHMWPE resin were measured by a differential scanning calorimeter (DSC). Figure 1 shows the melting temperature of fibers and the resin as a function of gamma irradiation dosage. Gamma irradiation (which is currently used in the sterilization of joint replacement materials) changes the crosslinking density of polymers and may alter their melting temperature. However, the melting temperature of fibers remained independent of the gamma irradiation dosage. The Spectra fibers showed two peaks in their DSC traces, one at a lower temperature and the other at a higher temperature.

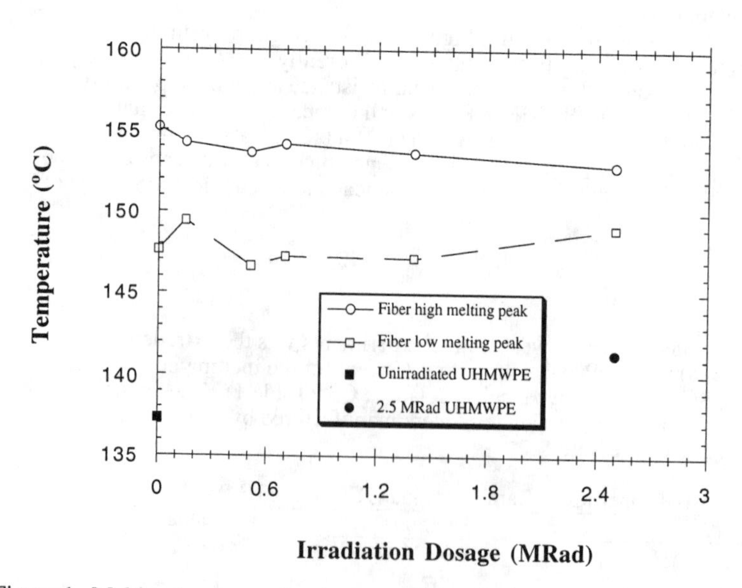

Figure 1--Melting temperatures of spectra fibers and GUR415 UHMWPE obtained by Differential Scanning Calorimetry (DSC).

Manufacturing

Spectra fibers were cut to a length of approximately 25 mm and then were mixed with the UHMWPE resin in a mixer. The mixer consisted of a container into which the resin and the fiber were placed and a high speed (10,000 rpm) propeller. In this process the filaments of each cut fiber tow are separated and mixed with the powder. The mixture was then compression molded. The compression molding cycle included heating the mixture under 10.33 MPa pressure, keeping the mixture at a steady state temperature and pressure for 30 minutes, and finally cooling down the mold and the composite under pressure. The steady state temperature was $152.5^{\circ}C$. The fiber weight fraction of the homocomposite was at values of 0.25, 0.50, and 0.75. The volume fraction of fibers in polyethylene homocomposites is approximately the same as their weight fraction due to similar densities for UHMWPE and spectra fibers (Tables 1, 2).

Testing

Mechanical and wear tests were performed with three to five samples of both homocomposites and UHMWPE. Tensile and compression tests were conducted according to ASTM standards D638 and D639, respectively. Friction and wear tests were also performed using a reciprocating tester shown in Figure 2. The testing direction for tension, compression and wear tests with respect to the compression molding direction is shown in Figure 3. In friction and wear tests, the applied normal load was 760 N and tests were run for 500,000 cycles at a sliding speed of 8 cm/s. Each cycle corresponds to 2.5 cm of sliding distance. The counterface was a cobalt chrome (CoCr) cylinder with a mean surface roughness of about 0.01 μm.

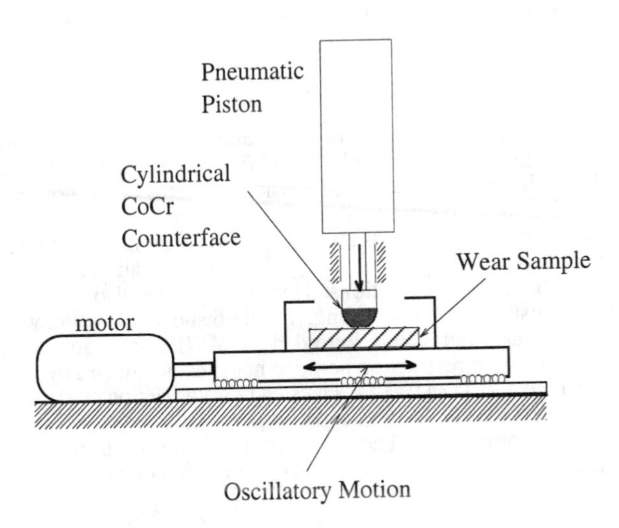

Figure 2--Schematic of friction and wear tester.

The mean surface roughness of the UHMWPE and homocomposite samples was about 0.4 μm. Since polymers may absorb lubricant during lubricated wear tests, the tests were run dry to obtain accurate weight measurements of the wear samples before and after testing.

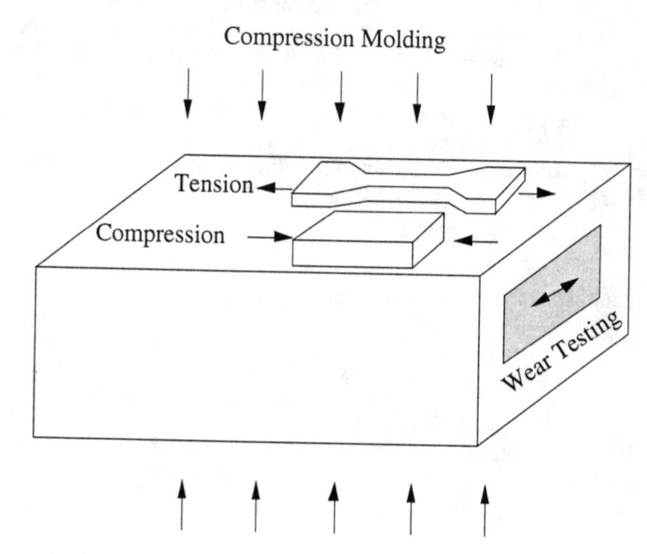

Figure 3--Compression molding and test directions in homocomposites

RESULTS

The tensile and compressive strengths of the fiber composites are increased compared with those of compression molded UHMWPE as shown in Figures 4 and 5. However, an increasing trend in tensile and compressive strengths of the homocomposite as the fiber volume fraction increases is not observed. For instance, the tensile strength dropped when the fiber volume fraction was above 0.5. This drop in tensile strength may be an indication of increased difficulty of achieving good mixing and bonding between fibers and resin at higher fiber volume fractions. Homocomposites also showed a significantly higher wear resistance in dry sliding. Figure 6 shows the mean wear and the standard deviation of the wear data for Ram Extruded UHMWPE and homocomposites. The mean wear of 0.75 fiber volume fraction homocomposites is reduced by 660% compared with the mean wear of UHMWPE. The steady state friction coefficient obtained with Ram Extruded UHMWPE was approximately 0.17. Figure 7 shows the friction coefficient of homocomposites. The lowest coefficient of friction was 0.1 and was obtained with the homocomposite having a fiber volume fraction of 0.75.

DISCUSSION

A difference of about $10^{\circ}C$ between the melting points of highly drawn UHMWPE fibers and an UHMWPE resin provides a processing range for the manufacture of polyethylene homocomposites by compression molding. The interaction of the matrix with the fibers is the primary factor affecting mechanical and physical

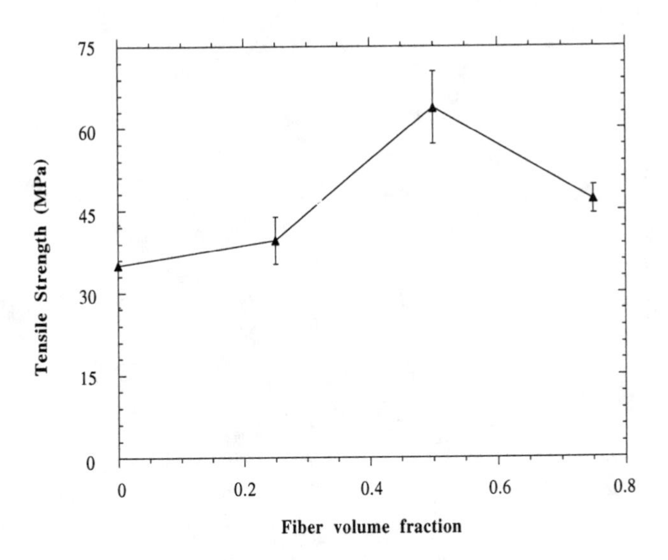

Figure 4--Tensile strength versus fiber volume fraction (V_f). Strain rate = 1.27 cm/min.

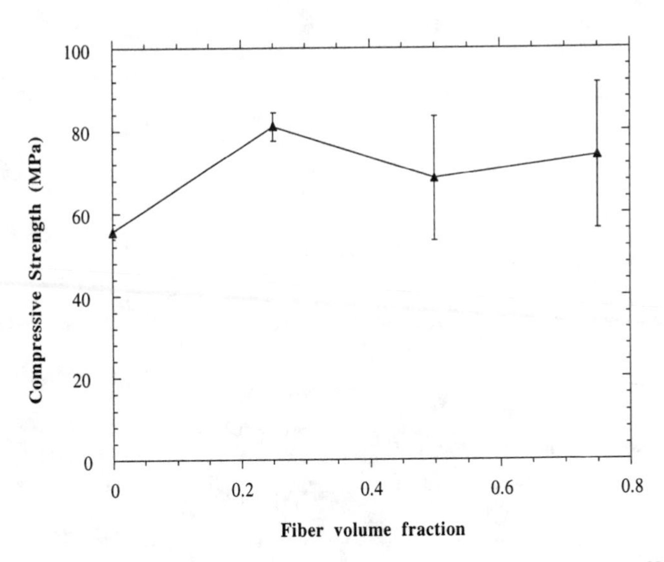

Figure 5--Compressive strength versus fiber volume fraction (V_f).
Strain rate = 0.127 cm/min.

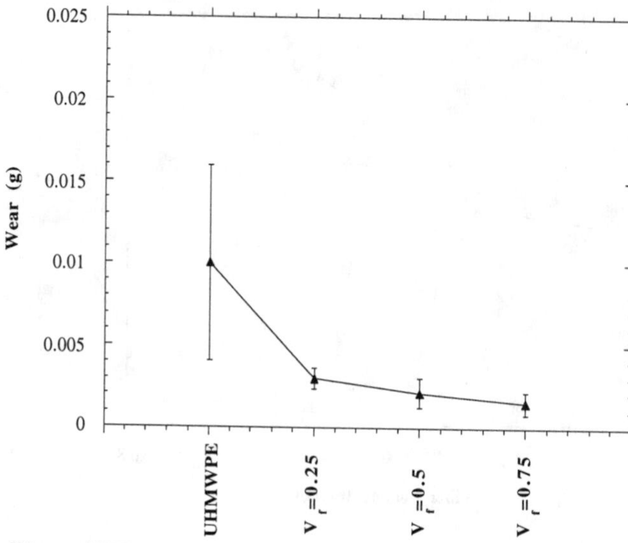

Figure 6--Wear of UHMWPE and fiber/resin composites after 500,000 cycles. Tests were run dry against a 3.175 *cm* diameter CoCr cylinder under a 760 *N* normal load.

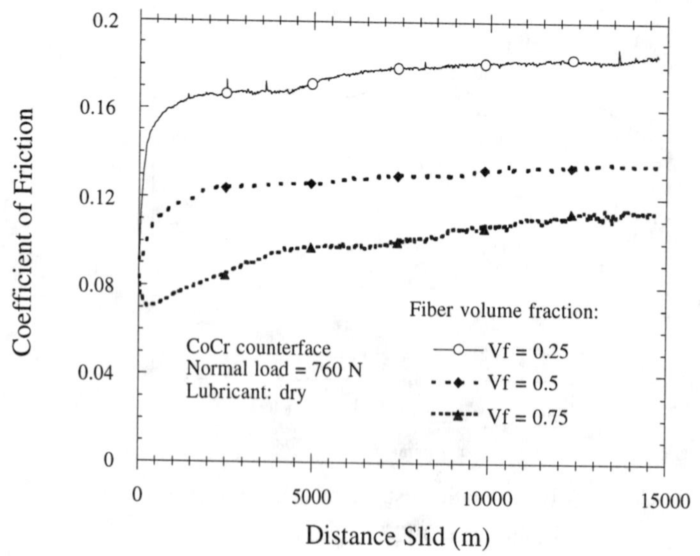

Figure 7--Friction coefficient of homocomposites. Tests were run dry against a 3.175 *cm* diameter CoCr cylinder under a 760 *N* normal load.

properties of the composite, and is a function of molding temperature and the physical and chemical states of the fiber surface. In addition to the above parameters, the uniformity of the mixing process and the uniformity of the temperature field in the compression molding material are issues associated with high volume production.

The ideal fiber/matrix interaction in homocomposites exists when the outer surface of the fibers is melted. This form of partial melting promotes improved interfacial adhesion with the matrix while the fiber core remains highly oriented. The mechanical properties of the homocomposite may be considered an indicator of the state of the fiber/matrix interaction. For example, the tensile strength of the homocomposites produced at a higher temperature (above 160 $^{\circ}C$) is the same as that of UHMWPE indicating that complete melting of fibers has occurred. On the other hand, homocomposites produced at a lower molding temperature (below 145 $^{\circ}C$) tend to have the same tensile strength as that of the fibers due to the negligible value of UHMWPE tensile strength compared with that of the fibers. The rule of mixtures can be used to find an approximate ideal value for the homocomposite properties. Assuming that fiber and matrix strains are equal in the fiber direction, the ideal ultimate tensile strength of the composite, σ_c may be calculated using:

$$\sigma_c = \sigma_f V_f + \sigma_m (1 - V_f) \tag{1}$$

where V_f is the fiber volume fraction, σ_f is the tensile stress of the fibers, and σ_m is the tensile stress of the matrix assuming that both the matrix and the fibers experience the same strain. In the case of fiber/resin composites, the fibers are randomly oriented and therefore the number of fibers in the tensile test direction is not known. The theoretical upper limits of the tensile strength of the fiber composites, assuming all fibers aligned in the pulling direction are 2258, 1517, and 776 MPa for 0.75, 0.50, and 0.25 fiber volume fractions, respectively. These values are significantly higher than those obtained in tensile tests of homocomposite samples. We can calculate the efficiency coefficient of the fibers (K) which is defined as:

$$K = \frac{P_c - (1 - V_f) P_m}{V_f P_f} \tag{2}$$

where the indices f, m, and c represent the fiber, the matrix, and the composite, and P is a property such as tensile strength. This coefficient is calculated for the fiber composites with respect to tensile strength as shown in Table 3. The efficiency coefficients are very low due to both the random orientation of the fibers and the partial or complete melting of some fibers during compression molding. In calculating K values, the tensile strengths of the matrix and fiber used were 45 MPa and 3000 MPa, respectively, and the mean tensile strength of the composites were taken from Figure 4. The efficiency coefficient cannot be calculated for wear or friction properties of the homocomposites because of the lack of information about such properties for the fibers.

Table 3--Efficiency coefficient of different homocomposites in tension

Fiber Volume Fraction (V_f)	Efficiency Coefficient
0.25	0.007
0.50	0.028
0.75	0.016

CONCLUSIONS

An ultra-high molecular weight polyethylene homocomposite was manufactured for meeting two distinct functional requirements: biocompatibility for possible use in joint replacements, and improved mechanical and wear properties for use as a bearing material. The homocomposite has shown significantly less wear in dry sliding than the currently used material in orthopaedic prostheses, i.e. UHMWPE, and improved mechanical properties. The promising tribological behavior observed from homocomposites needs to be further extended to lubricated sliding and simulated wear testing for a complete evaluation necessary for alternative bearing materials in joint prostheses. However, the UHMWPE homocomposite can be considered as an attractive bearing material for some current industrial applications.

REFERENCES

[1] Mosleh, M., and Suh, N. P., "Wear particles of polyethylene in biological systems", *Tribology Transactions*, Vol. 39, No. 4, pp. 843-848, 1996.

[2] Capiati, N.J., and Porter, R.S., "The concept of one polymer composites modeled with high density polyethylene", Journal of Materials Science, 1975, Vol. 10, pp. 1671-1677.

[3] Mead, W.T., and Porter, R.S., "The preparation and tensile properties of polyethylene composites", Journal of Applied Polymer Science, 1978, Vol. 22, pp. 3249-3265.

[4] Marais, C., and Feillard, P., "Manufacturing and mechanical characterization of unidirectional polyethylene-fiber/polyethylene-matrix composites", Composites Science and Technology, 1992, Vol. 45, pp. 247-255.

[5] Smith, P., and Lemstra, P.J., " Ultra-high strength polyethylene filaments by solution spinning/drawing", Journal of Materials Science, 1980, Vol. 15, pp. 505.

[6] Ward, I.M., and Ladizesky, N.J.H, "Ultra high modulus polyethylene composites", Pure and applied chemistry", 1985, Vol. 57, pp. 1641.

[7] Chang, H.W., Lin, L.C., and Bhatnagar, A., "Properties and applications of composites made of polyethylene fibers", 31st International SAMPE Symposium, SAMPE, 1986, pp. 859.

[8] Ward, I.M., and Ladizesky, N.J.H, "High modulus polyethylene fibers and their composites", Composites Interfaces, ed., H. Ishida, and J.L. Koenig, Elsevier Science Publishing Co., New York, 1986.

[9] Silverstein, M.S., Breuer, O., and Dodiuk, H., "Surface modification of UHMWPE fibers", Journal of Applied Polymer Science, 1994, Vol. 52, pp. 1785-1795.

[10] Mosleh, M., Arinez, J., and Suh, N.P., "Nanometer particles produced by the wear of polyethylene: Atomic force microscopy in the Tapping mode", Proceedings of the 41th Annual Meeting, Orthopaedic Research Society, Orlando, Florida, February 1995.

V. Krishna Polineni[1], Aiguo Wang[1], Aaron Essner[1], Ruey Lin[1], Ash Chopra[1], Cas Stark[1] and John H. Dumbleton[1]

CHARACTERIZATION OF CARBON FIBER-REINFORCED PEEK COMPOSITE FOR USE AS A BEARING MATERIAL IN TOTAL HIP REPLACEMENTS

REFERENCE: Polineni, V. K., Wang, A., Essner, A., Lin, R., Chopra, A., Stark, C., and Dumbleton, J. H., **"Characterization of Carbon Fiber-Reinforced PEEK Composite for Use as a Bearing Material in Total Hip Replacements,"** *Alternative Bearing Surfaces in Total Joint Replacement, ASTM STP 1346*, J. J. Jacobs and T. L. Craig, Eds., American Society for Testing and Materials, 1998.

ABSTRACT: A carbon fiber-reinforced polyetheretherketone (PEEK) composite acetabular cup was fabricated by injection molding. An extensive hip joint simulator test was conducted to evaluate the tribological performance of this CF-PEEK composite cup as a potential orthopaedic bearing surface. Hip joint simulator testing up to 10 million cycles showed that the wear of the composite cups is about 1% that of the UHMWPE cups. Hertzian contact stress analysis indicated that the CF-PEEK material had a lower maximum contact stress/yield strength ratio compared to air-irradiated UHMWPE acetabular cups. With prudent application of composite design principles, it is possible to engineer a composite insert that shows promise as an orthopaedic implant bearing surface in total hip replacements.

KEYWORDS: polyetheretherketone (PEEK), carbon fiber, composite, wear, hip

Nomenclature

a	radius of contact circle
ν	Poisson's ratio
σ_{max}	Maximum contact stress
σ_y	Yield strength
$\sigma_{contact}$	Normalized maximum contact stress, σ_{max}/σ_y
P	load applied
R	equivalent radius, $(1/R_{head} - 1/R_{cup})^{-1}$
E	equivalent elastic modulus, $((1-\nu_{head}^2)/E_{head} + (1-\nu_{cup}^2)/E_{cup})^{-1}$

[1] Research Engineer, Assistant Director, Senior Research Associate, Assistant Director (Retd.), Principal Research Engineer, Director and Vice-President, respectively, R&D, Howmedica, Inc., 309 Veterans Blvd., Rutherford, NJ 07055.

Introduction

Ultra-high molecular weight polyethylene (UHMWPE) has served as an excellent bearing material for orthopaedic applications for over three decades. Despite its success, UHMWPE wear debris generated *in vivo* has been identified as triggering a series of events that lead to the ultimate failure of the implant. The need for alternative bearing materials for total hip replacement such as ceramic-ceramic and metal-metal pairs exists. This study reports an alternative bearing material based on carbon-fiber reinforced polyetheretherketone (PEEK).

The addition of reinforcing agents, particularly in the form of fibers, significantly enhances the mechanical properties of polymers. This addition may also result in improved tribological properties. The use of fiber-reinforced polymeric composites as bearing materials has met with considerable success in high performance aerospace applications [1] and in industrial applications [2] where the bearings are expected to operate for extended periods under harsh environments including impact loading, dry sliding and abrasion. Several researchers have conducted studies into the mechanisms by which fibers reduce polymer wear [3, 4]. Studies have shown that fiber reinforcement in a tough, high temperature polymer matrix leads to improved wear resistance. In particular, Friedrich and co-workers [5, 6] demonstrated that carbon fiber reinforcement in a polyetheretherketone (PEEK) polymer matrix leads to superior wear resistance with reduced fiber-matrix delamination.

The previously mentioned studies involved the evaluation of tribological properties of composites under dry wear conditions. In the presence of a fluid lubricant, the wear performance of composites is not well researched, primarily because polymer composites were intended to be an alternative to traditional lubricated bearings. Earlier attempts at reinforcing UHMWPE with carbon fibers proved to be unsuccessful [7] for orthopedic bearing applications, especially as a tibial component in total knee replacement where fracture and delamination were the dominant wear mechanisms. In this study, an attempt is made to engineer a carbon fiber reinforced PEEK composite (CF-PEEK) that can perform successfully as a conforming bearing surface for acetabular cups. Extended duration hip joint wear simulator testing is conducted to validate the performance of the composite material.

Materials and Methods

Materials

(i) Acetabular Inserts: 28 mm System 12® design composite acetabular inserts injection molded from 70 wt.% polyetheretherketone(PEEK) (ICI, Grade 150G) and 30 wt.% pitch-based carbon-fiber (Amoco, Grade VMX-12) were used in the study. 28 mm UHMWPE acetabular inserts (System 12®, Size P3, Neutral, Howmedica, Inc.,) were also used to obtain a relative comparison of the wear behavior of the composite acetabular inserts. Both types of inserts were subjected to gamma-radiation sterilization at ~2.5 MRad (25 kGy) in air. The UHMWPE inserts were seated in acetabular shells made of Vitallium®

(Howmedica, Inc.). The composite inserts were seated in the same shells using a PEEK retaining ring. Three UHMWPE inserts and five composite inserts were used for testing.

(ii) Femoral heads: 28 mm zirconia heads (Zircone Prozyr®, Howmedica BG, France) were used for articulation against the acetabular inserts. Preliminary in-house tests had shown that zirconia heads were resistant to scratching by carbon fibers.

(iii) Lubricant: Bovine calf serum was used as lubricant in the wear tests. The serum was obtained from Hyclone Laboratories (Cat. #: SH30212.05) and contains carefully controlled levels of protein (41 grams/liter) and inorganic particulates. This controlled protein level helps in maintaining consistency of the lubricant during the test and also minimizes test variability. 20mM pH-balanced ethylenediaminetetraaceticacid (EDTA) solution was also added to the serum to eliminate any precipitate formation on the femoral head and to retard serum decomposition. The serum was then filtered before use through 0.2 μm capsule filters to eliminate any particles over 0.2 μm in size.

Test method

An eight-station MTS hip joint simulator [8] was used for testing the components. Each station consists of fixtures for accommodating the head and the insert which are aligned along the same vertical axis. An acrylic specimen chamber with a stainless steel baseplate is used. The spigot has an appropriate taper which accommodates the head. The specimen chamber fits onto a block inclined at 23°. The head and the insert are immersed in bovine calf serum and testing is conducted in the anatomical geometry: The insert is in the superior position and is stationary, the head articulates inside the insert. The inclined block rotates at a speed of 1 Hz and compressive loading is applied axially with a maximum load of 2450 N. The loading is cyclic in nature and follows the physiological profile determined by Paul [9]. Standard test protocols were used for cleaning, weighing and assessing the wear loss of the UHMWPE inserts [10].

Co-ordinate measuring machine (CMM) readings of the articular surface of the inserts were taken at 0, 1, 3, 5, 8 and 10 million cycles. The CMM machine has a resolution of 3 μm. The volume change of the inserts was monitored by calculating the volume of the mesh generated from the CMM readings. The linear penetration of the head into the insert was calculated from the CMM data. Gravimetric wear loss of the UHMWPE inserts was also determined at the same intervals. For the composite inserts, weight readings were taken only at 0 and 10 million cycles to reduce damage to the insert during removal from the shell. The weight loss values were converted to volume loss using the densities of the respective materials (UHMWPE = 0.935 g/cc, Composite = 1.5 g/cc). Soak controls were used for minimizing error due to moisture absorption.

Hertzian contact stress

Hertzian contact equations were used for estimating the maximum contact stress for UHMWPE/zirconia, CF-PEEK/zirconia couples. The maximum contact stress is given by

$$\sigma_{max} = (3P/2\pi a^2) \quad (1)$$

The relative maximum contact stress of each material is the ratio of its maximum contact stress to its yield strength and is given by

$$\sigma_{contact} = \sigma_{max} / \sigma_y \qquad (2)$$

Results

Wear was measured both by gravimetric analysis (weight loss) and by volume changes calculated from CMM readings. Table 1 shows the wear rates estimated by these methods. By the gravimetric method, the UHMWPE inserts show a total wear of 353.73 ± 54.36 mm^3 while the composite inserts show a total wear of only 3.91 ± 0.90 mm^3 after 10 million cycles (Figure 1). The wear of the composite inserts is only about 1% the wear of the conventional UHMWPE inserts.

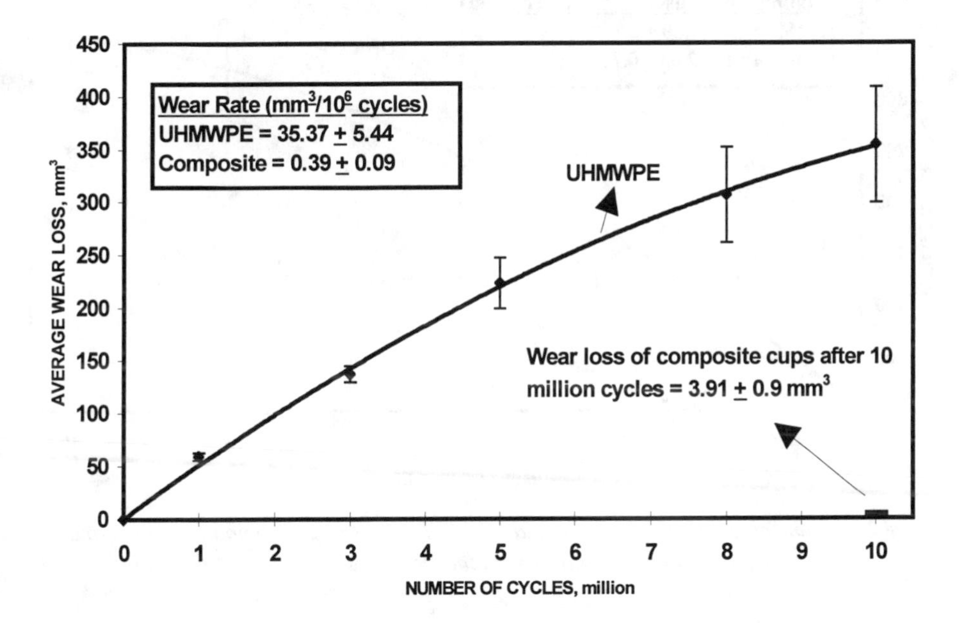

Figure 1: *Gravimetric wear loss of composite and UHMWPE acetabular components as tested on the MTS hip wear simulator. Testing conditions: Load: Paul profile with a peak load of 2450 N; Speed: 1 cycle/sec; Lubricant: 100% Hyclone bovine calf serum; Configuration: anatomical.*

The CMM method shows excellent agreement with the wear values observed for UHMWPE inserts through the gravimetric method. The wear of the CF-PEEK inserts is so low that the CMM readings give a negative volume change value indicating that the volume change of the composite inserts is beyond the resolution of the CMM machine (Figure 2).

It may be noticed that the values for UHMWPE from the CMM method are generally higher than obtained through the gravimetric method. This difference may be because the gravimetric method measures weight loss whereas the CMM method measures volume changes which include both wear and creep deformation. It may also be noticed that this difference occurs mostly during the first million cycles and does not drift higher with increasing number of cycles indicating that this is due to creep rather than any significant error in one of these methods. Further, it must be noted that the gravimetric method measures the wear of both the articular and back surfaces of the cup while the CMM method measures only the volume change on the articular surface.

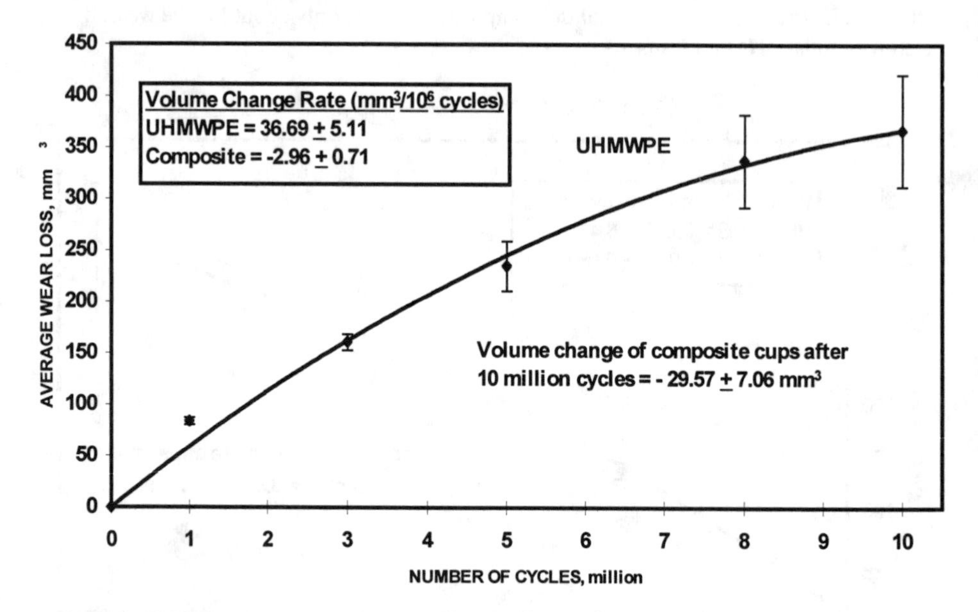

Figure 2: *Volume change of composite and UHMWPE acetabular components as tested on the MTS hip wear simulator with the CMM method. Testing conditions same as in Fig. 1.*

Table 1: *Wear rates of composite and UHMWPE acetabular inserts against zirconia femoral heads as evaluated on the hip joint wear simulator. Total number of cycles: 10 million.*

Cup Type	**Linear Penetration (μm/million cycles)**	**Wear Rate (mm^3/million cycles)**	
		Gravimetry	**CMM**
UHMWPE	66.41 ± 12.64	35.37 ± 5.44	36.69 ± 5.11
Composite	1.72 ± 1.36	0.39 ± 0.09	-2.96 ± 0.71

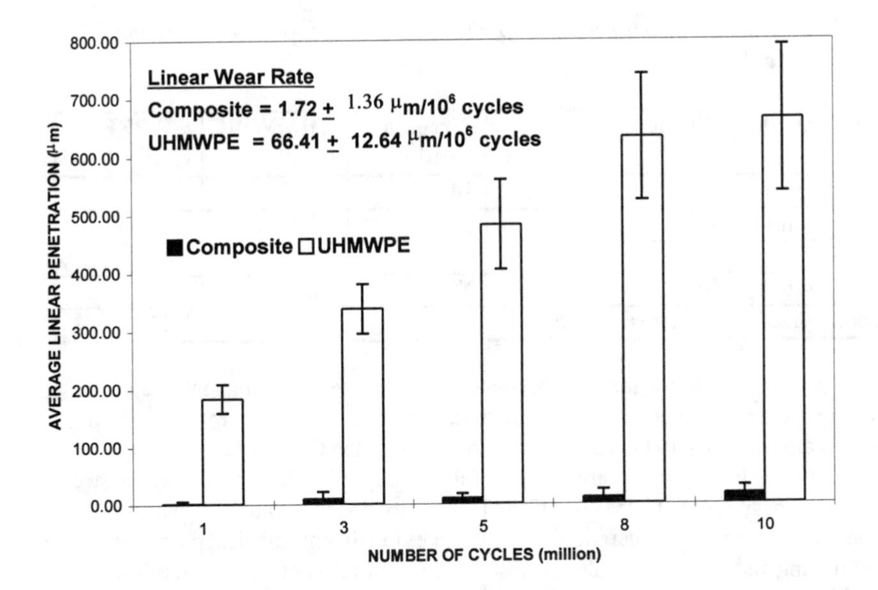

Figure 3: *Linear penetration of the femoral head into composite and UHMWPE acetabular components. Testing conditions same as in Fig. 1.*

Clinically, wear is measured in terms of linear penetration of the femoral head into the acetabular insert. The CMM method facilitates the estimation of this penetration at different stages of the test. Table 1 and Figure 3 show the linear penetration of the head into the composite and the UHMWPE acetabular inserts. The high standard deviation for the composite inserts indicates that the change is too small to be detected within the physical resolution of CMM. The UHMWPE inserts show an average linear penetration rate of 66.41 ± 12.64 μm per million cycles while the composite inserts show average penetration rates of 1.72 ± 1.36 μm per million cycles.

Discussion

The exceptionally low wear of the CF-PEEK composite acetabular cups may be due to a combination of factors. The PEEK resin during injection molding has a low viscosity which enables complete wetting of the carbon fibers. The wetting process enhances the fiber-matrix interfacial strength which allows for more effective load transfer behavior between the matrix and the fiber. The use of high strength/high modulus PEEK as the matrix, rather than UHMWPE, minimizes the elastic mismatch between the fiber and the matrix. This reduction helps to lessen the possibility of fiber/matrix debonding under load. Thus, the intrinsic wear resistance of the carbon fibers is properly utilized by using a PEEK matrix.

Table 2: *Material and geometric properties of the head and the cup used in Hertzian contact calculations.*

Geometric/Material Property	Zirconia Head	UHMWPE Cup	CF-PEEK Cup
Radius (mm)	14	14.25	14.25
Elastic Modulus (GPa)	210	0.80	15.2
Poisson's ratio	0.22	0.44	0.4
Yield Strength, σ_y (MPa)	N.A.	22.8	167.6
Max. normalized contact stress, σ_{max}/σ_y	N.A.	0.24	0.21

The proper selection of matrix/fiber materials to reduce elastic mismatch and possible improvement in fiber/matrix interfacial strength due to good fiber wet-out during fabrication is also reflected in the contact stress behavior of the CF-PEEK composite relative to UHMWPE. The results are given in Table 2. Earlier studies comparing the stress behavior of composites with UHMWPE [7, 11] tended to look at the absolute numbers of the contact stress without consideration for the changes in other mechanical properties. When comparing dissimilar materials, the absolute value of the contact stress has little meaning. Maximum contact stress normalized with respect to the yield strength of the respective materials is a better indicator in understanding the relative behavior of these materials. As shown in Table 2, the CF-PEEK composite material compares favorably with UHMWPE acetabular cups in terms of maximum normalized contact stress.

Further, the thermal conductivity of the CF-PEEK composite is 1.02 W/mK (as estimated by the rule of mixtures) while UHMWPE has a conductivity of 0.42 W/mK. The higher thermal conductivity of the composite may help to effectively transport frictional heat generated away from the articulating interface thus minimizing any detrimental thermal effects on the surface of the acetabular cups during motion.

Conclusions

A 10 million cycle hip joint wear simulator test comparing carbon fiber-reinforced PEEK composite acetabular inserts with conventional air-irradiated UHMWPE acetabular inserts has been conducted. Based on the study, the following conclusions may be drawn:

1. The composite acetabular inserts demonstrate superior wear resistance compared to the UHMWPE acetabular inserts; the wear rate was only about 1% of the UHMWPE acetabular inserts.
2. The CF-PEEK composite inserts show a reduced normalized contact stress compared to UHMWPE.

REFERENCES

[1] Lancaster, J. K., "Composites for aerospace dry bearing applications," in *Friction and Wear of Polymer Composites,* K. Friedrich (Ed.), Elsevier, Amsterdam, 1986, pp.363-396.

[2] Thorp, J. M., "Tribological properties of selected polymeric matrix composites against steel surfaces," in *Friction and Wear of Polymer Composites,* K. Friedrich (Ed.), Elsevier, Amsterdam, 1986, pp.89-136.

[3] Lancaster, J. K., "The effect of carbon fiber reinforcement on the friction and wear of polymers," *British Journal of Applied Physics*, 1, 5, 1968, 549.

[4] Tsukizoe, T. and Ohmae, N., "Friction and wear of unidirectionally oriented glass, carbon, aramid and stainless steel fiber-reinforced plastics," in K. Friedrich (Ed.), *Friction and Wear of Polymer Composites,* Elsevier, Amsterdam, 1986, pp.205-232.

[5] Friedrich, K., Lu, Z. and Hager, A. M., "Recent advances in polymer composites tribology," *Wear*, 190, 1995, pp.139-144.

[6] Friedrich, K., Lu, Z. and Hager, A. M., "Overview on polymer composites for friction and wear application," *Theoretical and Applied Fracture Mechanics*, 19, 1993, pp.-11.

[7] Wright, T. M., Fukubayashi, T. and Burstein, A. H., "The effect of carbon fiber reinforcement on contact area, contact pressure, and time-dependent deformation in polyethylene tibial components," *Journal of Biomedical Materials Research*, Vol. 15, 1981, pp. 719-730.

[8] Mejia, L. C. and Brierley, T. J., "A hip wear simulator for the evaluation of biomaterials in hip-arthroplasty components," *Biomedical Materials and Engineering,* 4, 1994, pp. 259-271.

[9] Paul, J., "Loading on normal hip and knee joints and on joint replacements," *Engineering in Medicine, Vol. 2, Advances in Artificial Hip and Knee Joint Technology,* M. Schaldach and D. Hohman (eds.), Springer-Verlag, New York, 1976.

[10] McKellop, H. and Clarke, I. C., "Evolution and evaluation of materials-screening machines and joint simulators in predicting *in vivo* wear phenomena," *Functional Behavior of Orthopaedic Biomaterials,* Vol. II, Applications, P. Ducheyne and G. Hastings (eds.), CRC Press, 1984.

[11] Bartel, D. L., Bicknell, V. L. and Wright, T. M., "The effect of conformity, thickness and material on stresses in ultra-high molecular weight components for total joint replacements," *Journal of Bone and Joint Surgery*, Vol. 68-A, 7, 1986, pp.1041-1051.

Author Index

Subject Index

L

M

N

O

P

R

S

T

V

Y

Z